Solid Organ Transplantation Imaging

Editors

AMIR A. BORHANI
ANIL K. DASYAM

RADIOLOGIC CLINICS
OF NORTH AMERICA

www.radiologic.theclinics.com

Consulting Editor
FRANK H. MILLER

September 2023 • Volume 61 • Number 5

ELSEVIER

1600 John F. Kennedy Boulevard • Suite 1800 • Philadelphia, Pennsylvania, 19103-2899

http://www.theclinics.com

RADIOLOGIC CLINICS OF NORTH AMERICA Volume 61, Number 5
September 2023 ISSN 0033-8389, ISBN 13: 978-0-443-18177-1

Editor: John Vassallo (j.vassallo@elsevier.com)
Developmental Editor: Isha Singh

Radiologic Clinics of North America (ISSN 0033-8389) is published bimonthly by Elsevier Inc., 360 Park Avenue South, New York, NY 10010-1710. Months of issue are January, March, May, July, September, and November. Periodicals postage paid at New York, NY and additional mailing offices. Subscription prices are USD 544 per year for US individuals, USD 1107 per year for US institutions, USD 100 per year for US students and residents, USD 643 per year for Canadian individuals, USD 1415 per year for Canadian institutions, USD 739 per year for international individuals, USD 1415 per year for international institutions, USD 100 per year for Canadian students/residents, and USD 315 per year for international students/residents. To receive student and resident rate, orders must be accompanied by name of affiliated institution, date of term and the signature of program/residency coordinatior on institution letterhead. Orders will be billed at individual rate until proof of status is received. Foreign air speed delivery is included in all *Clinics* subscription prices. All prices are subject to change without notice. **POSTMASTER:** Send address changes to *Radiologic Clinics of North America*, Elsevier Health Sciences Division, Subscription Customer Service, 3251 Riverport Lane, Maryland Heights, MO63043. **Customer Service: Telephone: 1-800-654-2452** (U.S. and Canada); **1-314-447-8871** (outside U.S. and Canada). **Fax: 1-314-447-8029. E-mail: journalscustomerservice-usa@elsevier.com (for print support); journalsonlinesupport-usa@elsevier.com (for online support).**

Reprints. For copies of 100 or more of articles in this publication, please contact the Commercial Reprints Department, Elsevier Inc., 360 Park Avenue South, New York, New York 10010-1710. Tel.: +1-212-633-3874; Fax: +1-212-633-3820; E-mail: reprints@elsevier.com.

Radiologic Clinics of North America also published in Greek Paschalidis Medical Publications, Athens, Greece.

Radiologic Clinics of North America is covered in *MEDLINE/PubMed (Index Medicus), EMBASE/Excerpta Medica, Current Contents/Life Sciences, Current Contents/Clinical Medicine, RSNA Index to Imaging Literature, BIOSIS, Science Citation Index,* and *ISI/BIOMED.*

Printed in the United States of America.

Contributors

CONSULTING EDITOR

FRANK H. MILLER, MD, FACR, FSAR, FSABI
Lee F. Rogers, MD, Professor of Medical
Education, Chief, Body Imaging Section,
Medical Director, MRI, Professor, Department
of Radiology, Northwestern Memorial Hospital,
Northwestern University Feinberg School of
Medicine, Chicago, Illinois, USA

EDITORS

AMIR A. BORHANI, MD
Associate Professor, Department of Radiology,
Northwestern University Feinberg School of
Medicine, Chicago, Illinois, USA

ANIL K. DASYAM, MD
Professor, Department of Radiology, University
of Pittsburgh School of Medicine; Department
of Surgery, Liver Transplantation, Thomas E.
Starzl Transplantation Institute, University of
Pittsburgh, Pittsburgh, Pennsylvania, USA

AUTHORS

RANISH DEEDAR ALI KHAWAJA, MD
Assistant Professor, Department of Radiology,
University of Colorado, Aurora, Colorado, USA

RYAN E. BAILEY, MD
Fellow, Department of Radiology, Section of
Body Imaging, Northwestern University
Feinberg School of Medicine, Chicago, Illinois,
USA

AMIR A. BORHANI, MD
Associate Professor, Department of Radiology,
Northwestern University Feinberg School of
Medicine, Chicago, Illinois, USA

DANIEL BORJA-CACHO, MD
Assistant Professor, Department of Surgery,
Northwestern University Feinberg School of
Medicine, Chicago, Illinois, USA

CONSTANTINE M. BURGAN, MD
Associate Professor, Department of Radiology,
University of Alabama–Birmingham,
Birmingham, Alabama, USA

CHRISTOPHER BUROS, MD
Assistant Professor, Department of Radiology,
University of Pittsburgh Medical Center,
Pittsburgh, Pennsylvania, USA

RUY J. CRUZ JR., MD, PhD
Associate Professor of Surgery, Director,
Intestinal Rehabilitation and Multivisceral
Transplant Program, Thomas E. Starzl
Transplantation Institute, University of
Pittsburgh, Pittsburgh, Pennsylvania, USA

ANIL K. DASYAM, MD
Professor, Department of Radiology, University
of Pittsburgh School of Medicine; Department
of Surgery, Liver Transplantation, Thomas E.
Starzl Transplantation Institute, University of
Pittsburgh, Pittsburgh, Pennsylvania, USA

NAVYA DASYAM, MD
Assistant Professor, Department of Radiology,
University of Pittsburgh Medical Center,
Pittsburgh, Pennsylvania, USA

ATMAN ASHWIN DAVE, MD
Abdominal Imaging Clinical Instructor,
Department of Radiology, University of
Pittsburgh Medical Center, Pittsburgh,
Pennsylvania, USA

SUBBA R. DIGUMARTHY, MD
Associate Professor, Division of Thoracic
Imaging and Intervention, Massachusetts

General Hospital; Harvard Medical School, Boston, Massachusetts, USA

GHANEH FANANAPAZIR, MD
Professor of Radiology, Department of Radiology, University of California, Davis, Health, Sacramento, California, USA

MYRA K. FELDMAN, MD
Associate Professor of Radiology, Cleveland Clinic Lerner College of Medicine, Case Western Reserve University, Section of Abdominal Imaging, Imaging Institute, Cleveland Clinic, Cleveland, Ohio, USA

ALESSANDRO FURLAN, MD
Associate Professor, Department of Radiology, University of Pittsburgh Medical Center, Pittsburgh, Pennsylvania, USA

REECE J. GOIFFON, MD, PhD
Department of Radiology, Division of Abdominal Imaging, Massachusetts General Hospital, Boston, Massachusetts, USA

CHRISTOPHER B. HUGHES, MD, FACS
Associate Professor of Surgery, University of Pittsburgh School of Medicine; Surgical Director of Liver Transplantation, Thomas E. Starzl Transplantation Institute; , University of Pittsburgh, Pittsburgh, Pennsylvania, USA

SARA A. HUNTER, MD
Assistant Professor of Radiology, Cleveland Clinic Lerner College of Medicine, Case Western Reserve University, Section of Abdominal Imaging, Imaging Institute, Cleveland Clinic, Cleveland, Ohio, USA

AVINASH R. KAMBADAKONE, MD, DNB, FRCR
Chief, Abdominal Radiology Division, Department of Radiology, Massachusetts General Hospital, Boston, Massachusetts, USA

JIYOON KANG, DO
Resident Physician, Division of Thoracic Imaging and Intervention, Massachusetts General Hospital; Harvard Medical School, Boston, Massachusetts, USA

VENKATA KATABATHINA, MD
Department of Radiology, University of Texas Health, San Antonio, Texas, USA

PATRICK YOON KIM, MD
Resident Physician, Department of Radiology, University of California, Davis, Health, Sacramento, California, USA

MARK E. LOCKHART, MD
Professor, Department of Radiology, University of Alabama-Birmingham, Birmingham, Alabama, USA

CHRISTINE O. MENIAS, MD
Chair, Division of Abdominal Imaging, Department of Radiology, Mayo Clinic at Scottsdale, Scottsdale, Arizona, USA

BENJAMIN M. MERVAK, MD
Associate Professor, Division of Abdominal Radiology, Department of Radiology, University of Michigan–Michigan Medicine, University Hospital, Ann Arbor, Michigan, USA

SRINIVASA R. PRASAD, MD
Professor, Department of Radiology, University of Texas MD Anderson Cancer Center, Houston, Texas, USA

ROSA ALBA PUGLIESI, MD
Fellow, Department of Radiology, Section of Body Imaging, Northwestern University Feinberg School of Medicine, Chicago, Illinois, USA

BALASUBRAMANYA RANGASWAMY, MD
Southwest Medical Imaging, Scottsdale, Arizona, USA

MOLLY E. ROSELAND, MD
Assistant Professor, Divisions of Abdominal Radiology and Nuclear Medicine, Department of Radiology, University of Michigan–Michigan Medicine, University Hospital, Ann Arbor, Michigan, USA

AZARIN SHOGHI, MS, MD
University of California, Davis, School of Medicine, Sacramento, California, USA

BIATTA SHOLOSH, MD
Southwest Medical Imaging, Scottsdale, Arizona, USA

DAVID SUMMERLIN, MD
Assistant Professor, Department of Radiology, University of Alabama–Birmingham, Birmingham, Alabama, USA

VARAHA SAI TAMMISETTI, MD
Associate Professor, Department of Radiology,
University of Texas Health, Houston, Texas,
USA

NIKHIL V. TIRUKKOVALUR, MBBS
Kamineni Academy of Medical Science and
Research Centre, LB Nagar, Hyderabad,
Telangana, India

DANIEL VARGAS, MD
Associate Professor, Department of Radiology,
University of Colorado, Aurora, Colorado, USA

ASHISH P. WASNIK, MD, FSAR, FSRU
Professor and Director, Division of Abdominal
Radiology, Department of Radiology,
University of Michigan–Michigan Medicine,
University Hospital, Ann Arbor, Michigan, USA

MARKUS Y. WU, MD
Associate Professor, Department of Radiology,
University of Colorado, Aurora, Colorado, USA

Contents

Deceased liver donor transplantation is increasing in prevalence resulting in larger volumes of posttransplant imaging studies. Radiologists should familiarize themselves with the spectrum of normal posttransplant anatomy. The key findings can be categorized into 4 systems reconstructed during surgery: hepatic venous, portal venous, hepatic arterial, and biliary ductal systems. Here we discuss the imaging findings seen with the most common surgical techniques, those that can be misidentified as complications, and some less common variations resulting from different surgical techniques.

Liver transplant is the definitive treatment of end-stage liver disease and early hepatocellular carcinoma. The number of liver transplant surgeries done is highly affected by the number and availability of deceased donor organs. Living donor liver transplantation has emerged as an alternative source of donors, increasing the availability of organs for transplant. Many factors must be considered when choosing living donor candidates to maintain a high level of donor safety and organ survival. To that end, potential donors undergo a rigorous pre-donation workup.

Other than rejection, hepatic artery and portal vein thrombosis are the most common complications in the immediate postoperative period with hepatic arterial thrombosis more common and more devastating. Hepatic artery stenosis is more common 1 month after transplantation, whereas portal and hepatic vein stenosis is more often seen as a late complication. Ultrasound is the first-line imaging examination to diagnose vascular complications with contrast-enhanced CT useful if ultrasound findings are equivocal. MR cholangiography is often most helpful in diagnosing bile leaks, biliary strictures, and biliary stones.

End-stage renal disease continues to grow worldwide, and renal transplantation remains the primary and most effective treatment to handle this burden. Living-donor transplantation is the ideal mechanism for transplant recipients to have a successful allograft but carries both medical and surgical risks. Cadaveric kidneys have their own risks and can have a high rate of success as well. Multimodality imaging is crucial and has improved greatly during the last 20 years. Finally, a robust understanding of current surgical techniques can facilitate better postoperative imaging when early complications are a consideration.

Kidney grafts are the most common transplanted solid organ. To optimize graft survival, radiologists should be familiar with the anatomy and potential complications unique to transplanted kidneys. In addition to being able to recognize the imaging characteristics to diagnose etiologies of kidney graft dysfunction, an understanding of the pathophysiology is a key to narrowing the differential diagnosis. This article provides a summary of the most common complications based on broad categories of type of complication and posttransplant timing.

Pancreatic transplantation is a complex surgical procedure performed for patients with chronic severe diabetes, often performed in combination with renal transplantation. Vascular and exocrine drainage anatomy varies depending on the surgical technique. Radiology plays a critical role in the diagnosis of postoperative complications, requiring an understanding of grayscale/Doppler ultrasound as well as computed tomography and MR imaging. In this review, we detail usual surgical methods and normal postoperative imaging appearances. We then review the most common complications following pancreatic transplants, emphasizing diagnostic features of vascular (arterial/venous), surgical, and diffuse parenchymal pathologic conditions on multiple imaging modalities.

Lung transplant is an established treatment for patients with end-stage lung disease. As a result, there is increased demand for transplants. Despite improvements in pretransplant evaluation, surgical techniques, and postsurgical care, the average posttransplant life expectancy is only around 6.5 years. Early recognition of complications on imaging and treatment can improve survival. Knowledge of surgical techniques and imaging findings of surgical and nonsurgical complications is essential. This review covers surgical techniques and imaging appearance of postsurgical and nonsurgical complications, including allograft dysfunction, infections, neoplasms, and recurrence of primary lung disease.

Heart transplantation has been increasingly performed for patients with end-stage heart failure most commonly related to ischemic and non-ischemic cardiomyopathies. The major complications are procedure-related complications, infection, acute rejection, cardiac allograft vasculopathy, and malignancy. Radiologists have an important role in the evaluation of transplant candidates and early detection of postoperative complications.

Intestinal transplantation and multivisceral transplantation are technically challenging and complex procedures mainly performed on patients with irreversible and non-medically manageable end-stage intestinal failure. Increasingly, other organs besides small intestines are included in the allograft for which the terms "composite intestinal transplantation" and "multivisceral transplantation" are used. Commonly, complex vascular reconstructions are used for these procedures. Knowledge of surgical anatomy hence is essential for accurate interpretation of postoperative imaging in these patients. This article reviews the indications and most common surgical techniques for intestinal and multivisceral transplantations.

Advancements in immunosuppression protocols, surgical techniques, and postoperative care in the last few decades have improved outcomes of intestinal transplant patients. Normal immediate postoperative imaging appearance can simulate pathology. Intestinal transplant recipients are prone for several postoperative complications due to the complex surgical technique, which involves multiple anastomoses, and immunogenic nature of the allograft intestine. Imaging plays a crucial role in detection of several major complications including infectious, immunologic, vascular, gastrointestinal, pancreaticobiliary, genitourinary, and neoplastic complications. The awareness of the posttransplant anatomy and normal imaging appearances helps radiologists anticipate and accurately detect posttransplant complications.

Uterus transplantation (UTx) is a novel procedure being studied as a treatment of absolute uterine factor infertility. Imaging plays an important role throughout the life cycle of a uterus transplant. In this review, we will first describe the surgical technique of UTx. The article will then focus on the importance of imaging in the evaluation of potential recipients and donors and during the immediate post-surgical time course as graft viability is established. Imaging as part of including in vitro fertilization, pregnancy, and complications will also be discussed.

Solid organ transplantation is the only long-term therapeutic option for patients with end-organ failure but cadaveric and living donor transplant pools are unable to meet the demand for organ transplantation. Newer techniques, innovative strategies and altruistic donors can help bridge this wide gap between the number of organ donors and recipients. Domino liver transplantation, paired organ donation, and ABO incompatible transplants are some of the ways to ensure increased transplant organ availability. Split liver transplantation and ex vivo liver resection and auto transplantation are considered surgically challenging but are being done at tertiary transplant centers.

The availability of effective immunosuppressive medication is primarily responsible for the dramatic improvement in long-term graft survival rates after solid organ transplantation. The commonly used drugs include monoclonal/polyclonal antibodies, corticosteroids, calcineurin inhibitors (cyclosporine and tacrolimus), antimetabolites, mammalian target of rapamycin, and many novel drugs. Prolonged immunosuppression is accompanied by several well-described potentially life-threatening complications. In addition to drug-related side effects, recipients of solid organs are unavoidably at a higher risk for infections and malignancies. Select infections and malignancies in solid organ transplant patients have distinctive imaging findings, and radiologists play a crucial role in the timely diagnosis and management of these conditions.

PROGRAM OBJECTIVE

The objective of the Radiologic Clinics of North America is to keep practicing radiologists and radiology residents up to date with current clinical practice in radiology by providing timely articles reviewing the state of the art in patient care.

TARGET AUDIENCE

Practicing radiologists, radiology residents, and other healthcare professionals who provide patient care utilizing radiologic findings.

LEARNING OBJECTIVES

Upon completion of this activity, participants will be able to:

1. Describe medical and surgical risks associated with living and deceased donors.
2. Discuss the imaging findings seen with the most common surgical techniques and those that can be misidentified as complications with transplantation.
3. Recognize the most common complications in the immediate postoperative period and the critical role Radiology plays in the diagnosis of postoperative complications.

ACCREDITATION

The Elsevier Office of Continuing Medical Education (EOCME) is accredited by the Accreditation Council for Continuing Medical Education (ACCME) to provide continuing medical education for physicians.

The EOCME designates this journal-based CME activity for a maximum of 13 *AMA PRA Category 1 Credit*(s)™. Physicians should claim only the credit commensurate with the extent of their participation in the activity.

All other healthcare professionals requesting continuing education credit for this enduring material will be issued a certificate of participation.

DISCLOSURE OF CONFLICTS OF INTEREST

The EOCME assesses conflict of interest with its instructors, faculty, planners, and other individuals who are in a position to control the content of CME activities. All relevant conflicts of interest that are identified are thoroughly vetted by EOCME for fair balance, scientific objectivity, and patient care recommendations. EOCME is committed to providing its learners with CME activities that promote improvements or quality in healthcare and not a specific proprietary business or a commercial interest.

The planning committee, staff, authors, and editors listed below have identified no financial relationships or relationships to products or devices they or their spouse/life partner have with commercial interest related to the content of this CME activity:

Ryan E. Bailey, MD; Amir A. Borhani, MD; Daniel Borja-Cacho, MD; Constantine M. Burgan, MD; Christopher Buros, MD; Ruy J. Cruz, Jr, MD, PhD; Anil K. Dasyam, MD; Navya Dasyam, MD; Atman Ashwin Dave, MD; Ghaneh Fananapazir, MD; Myra K. Feldman, MD; Alessandro Furlan, MD; Reece J. Goiffon, MD, PhD; Christopher B. Hughes, MD; Sara A. Hunter, MD; Avinash R. Kambadakone, MD, DNB, FRCR; Jiyoon Kang, DO; Venkata Katabathina, MD; Ranish Deedar Ali Khawaja, MD; Patrick Yoon Kim, MD; Kothainayaki Kulanthaivelu, BCA, MBA; Michelle Littlejohn; Mark E. Lockhart, MD; Christine O. Menias, MD; Benjamin M. Mervak, MD; Srinivasa R. Prasad, MD; Rosa Alba Pugliesi, MD; Balasubramanya Rangaswamy, MD; Molly Roseland, MD; Azarin Shoghi, MS; Biatta Sholosh, MD; David Summerlin, MD; Varaha Sai Tammisetti, MD; Nikhil Tirukkovalur, MBBS; Daniel Vargas, MD; Ashish P. Wasnik, MD, FSAR, FSRU; Markus Y. Wu, MD.

The planning committee, staff, authors, and editors listed below have identified financial relationships or relationships to products or devices they or their spouse/life partner have with commercial interest related to the content of this CME activity:

Subba R. Digumarthy, MD: Independent Contractor: Merck, Pfizer, Bristol-Myers Squibb, Novartis, Roche, Polaris, Cascadian, Abbvie, Gradalis, Bayer, Zai laboratories, Biengen, Resonance, Analise; Researcher: Lunit Inc, GE Healthcare, Qure AI, Vuno Inc.; Speaker/Advisor: Siemens

UNAPPROVED/OFF-LABEL USE DISCLOSURE

The EOCME requires CME faculty to disclose to the participants:

1. When products or procedures being discussed are off-label, unlabelled, experimental, and/or investigational (not US Food and Drug Administration (FDA) approved; and
2. Any limitations on the information presented, such as data that are preliminary or that represent ongoing research, interim analyses, and/or unsupported opinions. Faculty may discuss information about pharmaceutical agents that is outside of FDA-approved labelling. This information is intended solely for CME and is not intended to promote off-label use of these medications. If you have any questions, contact the medical affairs department of the manufacturer for the most recent prescribing information.

TO ENROLL

To enroll in the Radiologic Clinics of North America Continuing Medical Education program, call customer service at 1-800-654-2452 or sign up online at http://www.theclinics.com/home/cme. The CME program is available to subscribers for an additional annual fee of USD 340.00.

METHOD OF PARTICIPATION

In order to claim credit, participants must complete the following:

1. Complete enrolment as indicated above.
2. Read the activity.
3. Complete the CME Test and Evaluation. Participants must achieve a score of 70% on the test. All CME Tests and Evaluations must be completed online.

CME INQUIRIES/SPECIAL NEEDS

For all CME inquiries or special needs, please contact elsevierCME@elsevier.com.

RADIOLOGIC CLINICS OF NORTH AMERICA

SERIES OF RELATED INTEREST

Advances in Clinical Radiology
Available at: https://www.advancesinclinicalradiology.com/
Magnetic Resonance Imaging Clinics
Available at: https://www.mri.theclinics.com/
Neuroimaging Clinics
Available at: www.neuroimaging.theclinics.com
PET Clinics
Available at: www.pet.theclinics.com

Preface
Transplantation Imaging

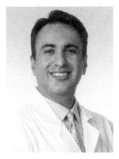   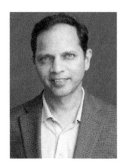

Amir A. Borhani, MD   Anil K. Dasyam, MD
Editors

Solid organ transplantation has become an established treatment option for end-stage organ failure, improving both the quality and the duration of life for many patients. Advances in surgical techniques, immunosuppression regimens, and postoperative care have led to significant improvements in outcomes following transplantation. However, despite these advances, successful transplantation remains a complex and challenging process that requires careful management and monitoring.

Imaging plays a crucial role in the evaluation and management of solid organ transplantation. It provides essential information about the preoperative evaluation of potential donors and recipients, as well as postoperative monitoring of organ function, complications, and rejection. The use of imaging modalities, such as ultrasound, computed tomography, MR imaging, and PET, has significantly improved the accuracy and reliability of the evaluation and management of solid organ transplantation.

This issue of *Radiologic Clinics of North America* provides an up-to-date and comprehensive review of solid organ transplantation imaging. Each article has been written by a leading expert in the respective field, providing a unique and authoritative perspective on the topic. The text is richly illustrated with high-quality images, providing readers with a clear understanding of the relevant imaging findings and their clinical implications. The articles cover all aspects of imaging in liver, lung, heart, pancreas, kidney, and intestinal transplantation,

including donor evaluation, pretransplant assessment of the recipient, intraoperative imaging, postoperative monitoring, and detecting complications and rejection. To ensure comprehensive coverage relevant to radiologists, the issue also includes articles on immunosuppression complications and special transplant scenarios, such as Domino transplantation and autotransplantation.

This issue is intended for practicing radiologists and radiology trainees, as well as other health care professionals involved in the care of transplant patients. It provides essential information for the effective evaluation and management of solid organ transplantation and will be a valuable resource for anyone involved in this complex and challenging field.

Amir A. Borhani, MD
Department of Radiology
Northwestern University
Feinberg School of Medicine
676 North St Clair Street, Suite 800
Chicago, IL 60611, USA

Anil K. Dasyam, MD
Department of Radiology
University of Pittsburgh School of Medicine
200 Lothrop Street
Pittsburgh, PA 15216, USA

E-mail addresses:
Amir.borhani@northwestern.edu (A.A. Borhani)
dasyamak@upmc.edu (A.K. Dasyam)

Radiol Clin N Am 61 (2023) xv
https://doi.org/10.1016/j.rcl.2023.05.001
0033-8389/23/© 2023 Published by Elsevier Inc.

radiologic.theclinics.com

Deceased Donor Liver Transplantation
Techniques and Surgical Anatomy

Reece J. Goiffon, MD, PhD*, Avinash R. Kambadakone, MD, DNB, FRCR

KEYWORDS

• Liver transplant • Surgical anatomy • Imaging techniques • Anatomic variants

KEY POINTS

- With liver transplant rates increasing globally, radiologists must be familiar with different posttransplant anatomies.
- Hepatic venous and inferior vena cava reconstruction is most commonly performed via either the "traditional" donor caval interposition or the "piggyback" technique in which the donor hepatic vein confluence/inferior vena cava is anastomosed to the recipient hepatic veins.
- Portal venous reconstruction is usually end-to-end but size mismatch and thrombectomy can cause the resulting portal vein to seem irregular.
- Hepatic arterial reconstruction is variable depending on donor and recipient anatomy but usually involves fish-mouth anastomoses that should not be confused for pseudoaneurysms.
- Biliary reconstruction is typically performed as end-to-end anastomoses between the native and recipient common bile ducts, unless a hepaticojejunostomy is required due to anatomic constraints or biliary disease.

INTRODUCTION

Deceased liver donor transplantation (DDLT) has evolved from an experimental technique resulting in perioperative death in the first 3 patients in 1963, a successful procedure by 1968, to a procedure today performed 20,000 to 30,000 times annually in more than 80 countries.[1–3] Although living donor transplantation has overtaken DDLT in Southeast Asia, DDLT remains the most frequent technique in Western Europe, the Eastern Pacific, and the Americas.[3] Notably, one-third of all global DDLTs are performed in the United States, driven there by the increase in alcoholic cirrhosis and hepatocellular carcinoma (HCC) outpacing the fall in hepatitis C-related cirrhosis. Other indications for DDLT include but are not limited to acute liver failure, biliary disease, venous hepatopathy, and inborn errors of metabolism.[4,5] Due to the shortage of deceased liver donors, other strategies have been developed including split-liver donation,

which is procedurally more similar to living donor transplantation.[6] Domino transplantation is another strategy to increase donor availability, in which a patient with end-stage liver disease receives a liver from a patient with a metabolic disease, who in turn receives a cadaveric donor liver.[7]

With the trend of increasing prevalence, it is more important than ever for radiologists to understand liver transplant anatomy and imaging appearance to identify abnormalities early and trigger interventions that can save or prolong the function of the graft. The complex surgical anatomy of a patient after DDLT can make interpretation difficult for radiologists, especially those unfamiliar with the techniques.

DECEASED LIVER DONOR TRANSPLANTATION STEPS

Even with modern advancements, DDLT is a complex, multistage procedure with some variation

Department of Radiology, Division of Abdominal Imaging, Massachusetts General Hospital, 55 Fruit Street, White 270 Boston, MA 02114, USA
* Corresponding author.
E-mail address: rgoiffon@mgh.harvard.edu

Radiol Clin N Am 61 (2023) 761–769
https://doi.org/10.1016/j.rcl.2023.04.001

between institutions. Donor hepatectomy is often performed at a different institution than the DDLT due to the geographic location of the donor's death. The donor liver is explanted and perfused with cooled preservation solution before being transported to the transplant institution, where further "back-table" preparation is carried out in the operating room as part of the DDLT procedure. If not already performed, the donor liver undergoes cholecystectomy. Any further necessary back-table reconstruction is then performed based on combined needs of the donor and recipient anatomy, notably of the hepatic arterial tree. The recipient hepatectomy is then performed and the donor liver is orthotopically placed in the recipient. Hepatic venous reconstruction follows, the donor hepatic venous outflow joined with the native inferior vena cava (IVC) by either end-to-end, piggyback, or side-to-side methods (described in detail later in this review).[8] If the IVC is interrupted during native liver explantation, venovenous bypass may be initiated during reconstruction. This was introduced to support venous return to the heart during the anhepatic phase, maintaining preload and thus cardiac output in order to prevent vital organ injury.[9] Since the 1980s, bypass has somewhat fallen out of favor and is only used by approximately half of transplant centers.[10] Next, the hepatic arterial and portal venous anastomoses are performed, the order per institutional preference, and the liver is reperfused.[11] Finally, the biliary tract is reconstructed.[12,13]

NORMAL ANATOMY AND IMAGING TECHNIQUE
Liver Anatomy and Pretransplant Imaging

The liver has 2 input systems, hepatic arterial and portal venous, and 2 output systems, biliary and hepatic venous. All 4 of these systems have variable anatomy that is important when evaluating a patient for living liver donation, covered separately in this issue. Deceased donors are not universally imaged with intravenous (IV) contrast preoperatively; instead, they are usually anatomically characterized during explantation. Donor imaging that is performed before DDLT is often to screen for malignancy or signs of hepatic steatosis or more severe organ dysfunction that would disqualify the donor, most often with ultrasound with or without a nonenhanced abdominal CT.[14,15]

The role of imaging in the recipient is to assess variant anatomy that may require additional planning and to ensure that there are no contraindications to transplantation, such as extensive HCC burden according to Milan or San Francisco

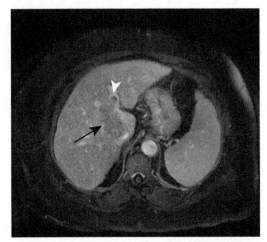

Fig. 1. T1-weighted transaxial MR with delayed-phase IV Gd contrast acquired as part of pretransplant imaging in a patient with steatocirrhosis showing a 6.3 cm mass (*arrow*) invading the proximal left portal vein (*arrowhead*). Both the size of the lesion and the vascular involvement were contraindications for DDLT for this patient. Pathology from a CT-guided biopsy performed 5 months later showed moderately differentiated HCC.

criteria.[16–18] The hepatic and portal veins must be assessed for extensive portal venous thrombus (**Fig. 1**). If portal or hepatic venous thrombus is identified, it is important to distinguish bland thrombus from vascular invasion of HCC that would disqualify the recipient. This is not to be confused with normal laminar flow artifact in the superior mesenteric and portal veins (**Fig. 2**). The radiologist's ability to distinguish these entities as well as characterize variant arterial anatomy depends on imaging technique used.

IMAGING TECHNIQUES

Liver transplant patients are imaged, both routinely and as further indicated by suspicion for complications, using ultrasound, computed tomography (CT), and magnetic resonance (MR).[19,20] Although ultrasound is useful in assessing for biliary, vascular, and perioperative complications, its limited field-of-view hinders assessment of posttransplant anatomy. Cross-sectional techniques such as CT and MR are preferred for pretransplant and posttransplant liver anatomy.

The superior intrinsic soft tissue contrast of MR shows most postoperative findings but depiction of transplant vasculature is improved with multiphase T1-weighted images with IV gadolinium (Gd) contrast. Acquiring arterial, portal venous,

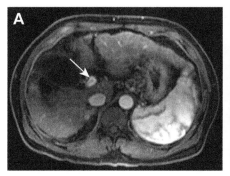 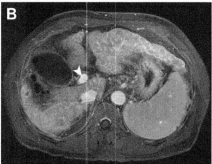

Fig. 2. T1-weighted transaxial MR images in (*A*) dynamic arterial and (*B*) delayed phase IV Gd contrast of a patient with hepatitis B cirrhosis and previously ablated HCC undergoing pretransplant evaluation. The superior mesenteric venous anatomy often causes peripheral enhanced blood to flow in a laminar fashion around central unenhanced blood, causing pseudothrombus in the portal vein (*arrow*), which resolves on delayed phase (*arrowhead*).

and delayed phases is also important to differentiate bland and tumor thrombus in the pretransplant patient with HCC. At our institution, these are acquired in transaxial plane with an additional coronal delayed image for colocalization. MR cholangiopancreatography (MRCP) or the use of a hepatobiliary contrast agent such as gadoxetic acid shows the biliary anatomy in greater detail.

Multiphase CT angiography acquired in pre-, arterial, and portal venous contrast phases is preferred for delineation of DDLT vascular anatomy. Reconstructions should be isometric with thin slices (<2 mm) to allow for multiplanar reconstruction. Technological advancements such as dual energy CT can allow improved characterization of the vasculature with low-iodinated contrast dose, assess parenchymal perfusion, and mitigate streak artifact from metallic surgical material in and around the transplant liver.

IMAGING FINDINGS
Hepatic Venous Reconstruction

There are 3 main techniques to return hepatic venous blood to IVC circulation.[8] The "classic" technique requires retrohepatic IVC resection from the recipient followed by donor caval interposition with end-to-end infrahepatic and suprahepatic IVC anastomoses (**Fig. 3**). As described above, this may be accompanied by venovenous bypass either by the surgeon's preference or in the case of insufficient cardiac preload in the absence of IVC return. With the second technique, termed "piggyback," the donor infrahepatic IVC is ligated and the suprahepatic IVC is anastomosed to the recipient hepatic veins in an end-to-end fashion, leaving the recipient IVC intact (**Fig. 4**). This eliminates the need for venovenous bypass,

and there is growing evidence that it may provide benefits such as lower transfusion requirements and shorter graft ischemic time.[21–23] The third technique involves creation of a side-to-side cavocavostomy without recipient retrocaval dissection. This technique is less common but shows promise in reducing operative time, hemorrhage, and hepatic venous insufficiency.[8,24,25]

Portal Venous Reconstruction

Compared with the other vascular anastomoses of DDLT, the portal venous reconstruction is usually more straightforward. The most common technique is an end-to-end anastomosis between the donor and recipient portal veins. To avoid redundancy, the donor vein is trimmed to the desired length so that the recipient vein is preserved in case a redo transplant is required. In order to allow for future expansion of the vein, a "growth factor" anastomosis is usually made, in which a running suture is knotted with 75% of the vein diameter remaining between the knot and the vein wall.[13,26,27] Because recipients often have chronic portal hypertension, there may be focal narrowing at the portal anastomosis that is not necessarily of clinical significance, usually most evident early in the postoperative window before the growth factor expands (**Fig. 5**).

Complications at the time of transplantation can lead to interventions identifiable on imaging. Patients with chronic, nonextensive portal venous thrombosis are still eligible for DDLT with improved outcomes after undergoing thrombectomy.[28] If successful, the patent portal vein will often seem irregular leading up to the anastomosis, at which point the donor vein will often be normal (**Fig. 6**). Although this appearance is

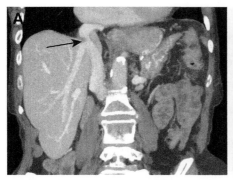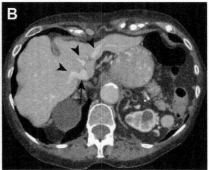

Fig. 3. Portal venous phase contrast CT of a DDLT with classic hepatic venous outflow technique using caval interposition performed approximately 30 years before imaging. (*A*) Oblique-coronal maximum intensity projection showing the right hepatic vein draining into a relatively normal IVC with only mild narrowing (*arrow*), made more pronounced by hypertrophy of the caudate lobe. In this case, the absence of metallic surgical clips renders the DDLT difficult to identify without also knowing the clinical history. (*B*) Transaxial slice of the same CT showing normal three-hepatic-vein configuration (*arrowheads*) converging on the interposed IVC (*arrow*).

not unexpected after thrombectomy, it should be scrutinized on subsequent imaging to exclude recurrent thrombus.

If the portal vein is surgically inadequate, alternative portal blood supplies can be used such as direct anastomosis from the superior mesenteric vein (SMV), splenic vein, or left renal vein in the presence of a large splenorenal shunt. Direct supply from the systemic circulation is not routinely used as animal model experiments in the 1970s suggest that trophic factors in splanchnic venous blood is required to support liver growth and function.[29] A synthetic or donor iliac vein jump graft from the SMV to the donor portal vein is sometimes used either as part of the primary DDLT procedure or as a rescue strategy after portal thrombectomy and/or stenting have failed (**Fig. 7**).[30]

Hepatic Arterial Reconstruction

The celiac and hepatic arterial tree is highly variable, as published by Nicholas Michels with his descriptions of 10 variants of celiac/hepatic arterial supply in the 1960s.[31] By his report, only around half of his 200 cadaveric dissections had "conventional" anatomy. In the context of DDLT, in which the liver is left whole and thus the intrahepatic arteries are not dissected, the variants of consequence are (1) conventional common hepatic artery from the celiac trunk, (2) replaced or accessory right hepatic artery from the superior mesenteric artery, (3) replaced or accessory left hepatic artery from the left gastric artery (LGA), (4) combined replaced or accessory left and right hepatic arteries, and (5) nonceliac origin of the common hepatic artery (**Fig. 8**). Larger studies have shown that conventional anatomy may be more prevalent than initially reported, with up to 75% showing a conventional branch pattern.[32,33]

Hepatic arterial anastomoses are typically made in a "fish mouth" fashion joining 2 branch patches, created by opening 2 arteries at a bifurcation into a wider, funnel-shaped end. Commonly in DDLT, a branch patch from the recipient common hepatic

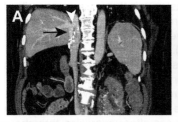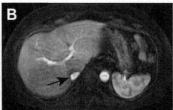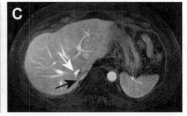

Fig. 4. DDLT with piggyback hepatic venous outflow configuration. (*A*) Portal venous phase contrast CT oblique-coronal MIP showing the blind-ending donor IVC (*arrow*) anastomosed end-to-end with the recipient hepatic veins (*arrowhead*). (*B*) Late arterial phase and (*C*) portal venous phase T1-weighted transaxial MR imaging of the same patient showing the typical appearance of 2 adjacent IVCs caudal to the anastomosis, the native IVC (*black arrow*) enhancing before the transplant IVC (*white arrow*).

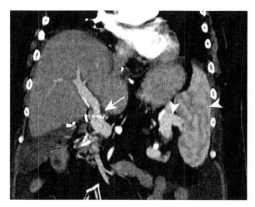

Fig. 5. Portal vein anastomotic diameter transition. Coronal CT with IV contrast shows the wider recipient proximal portal vein narrowing at the anastomotic level, demarcated with streak artifact from adjacent clips (*arrow*). Note the enlarged spleen and dilated splenic vein due to pretransplant portal hypertension (*arrowheads*).

bifurcation (into gastroduodenal and proper hepatic arteries) is sutured to either a branch patch from the celio-splenic bifurcation or an aortic patch created by cutting the aorta around the celiac ostium; the choice is often made due to surgeon preference and donor anatomy (**Fig. 9**).[19,34] The fish mouth anastomosis is less likely to develop stenosis compared with an end-to-end anastomosis and allows for different vessel diameters to be joined; this appearance should not be confused for a pseudoaneurysm (**Fig. 10**).

Jump grafts can be used as part of the initial transplantation to compensate for insufficient donor hepatic arterial supply or as a rescue method in the case of posttransplant hepatic artery thrombosis. Most grafts are constructed from an iliac artery harvested from the liver donor, although synthetic grafts are also an option.[35]

More rarely, a recipient vessel such as the external iliac artery can be used as a jump graft, or redundant branches of the superior mesenteric artery can be transposed to the common, right, and/or left hepatic arteries (**Fig. 11**).

Biliary Reconstruction

The biliary tree is reconstructed last, usually with a simple end-to-end anastomosis between the donor and recipient extrahepatic ducts. This is the more advantageous of the 2 biliary reconstruction strategies because it preserves choledochal sphincter function to prevent reflux of intestinal contents into the biliary tree. Typically, the length of remaining recipient bile duct remnant is maximized to provide tissue in case a second transplant is needed later, so the anastomosis is often near the liver hilum or cystic duct insertion. Although cholecystectomy is performed as part of the reconstruction, a cystic duct stump may seem prominent and be mistaken for a biloma (**Fig. 12**). In cases of low donor cystic duct insertion on the donor common bile duct, there may be 2 cystic duct stumps, one from the donor and one from the recipient.

There are multiple situations that preclude reapproximation of normal biliary anatomy, such as biliary disease (eg, sclerosing cholangitis), redo transplantation, or insufficient combined bile duct length. In these cases, a hepaticojejunostomy is instead used to drain bile into the enteric lumen. The biliary limb of divided jejunum is typically brought through the transverse mesocolon to the liver hilum, not to be confused for a fluid collection in the postoperative state. In some cases, the remnant native common bile duct may accumulate secretions from the epithelium, retained behind the functioning choledochal sphincter, giving the appearance of mild extrahepatic biliary dilatation,

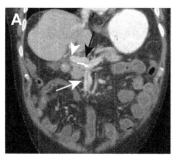
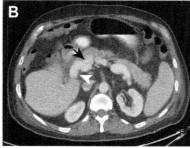
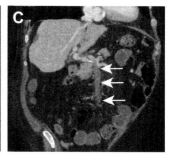

Fig. 6. DDLT after portal vein thrombectomy. (*A*) coronal oblique and (*B*) transaxial views showing irregularity of the proximal portal vein (*black arrows*) and SMV (*white arrow*) with normal postanastomotic appearance of the donor portal vein (*white arrowhead*). (*C*) Coronal oblique minimum intensity projection obtained 6 years later showing recurrent SMV thrombus (*white arrows*).

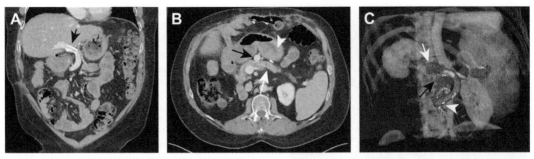

Fig. 7. Donor iliac vein jump graft between the SMV and portal vein. (*A*) Coronal CT showing the hilar configuration of the graft with a stent to maintain patency at the point of a prior portal thrombus (*arrow*). (*B*) Transaxial slice of the same CT showing the typical course of a jump graft (*black arrow*) through the transverse mesocolon, between the pancreas (*white arrow*) and stomach (*white arrowhead*). (*C*) 3D reconstruction showing the takeoff of the jump graft (*white arrowhead*), cutoff of the proximal native portal vein at the portosplenic confluence behind the graft (*black arrow*), and jump graft entrance into the liver hilum (*white arrow*).

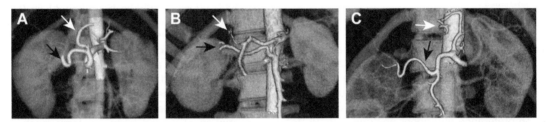

Fig. 8. Most common celiac-hepatic artery variants with different origins of the left (*white arrow*) and right (*black arrow*) hepatic arteries. (*A*) Traditional branching pattern in which the common hepatic artery bifurcates into the gastroduodenal artery and proper hepatic artery, the latter bifurcating into the left and right hepatic arteries. This anatomy is amenable to a branch patch anastomosis. (*B*) Replaced right hepatic artery from the superior mesenteric artery. The left hepatic artery originates from the bifurcation of the common hepatic artery. This donor configuration requires an additional anastomosis of the replaced right hepatic artery, for example, to the donor splenic or gastroduodenal arteries, to approximate "conventional" right hepatic artery perfusion from the celiac artery. (*C*) Replaced left hepatic artery from the LGA. This configuration can be managed with a donor aortic patch sewn to the recipient common hepatic artery, allowing for a single anastomosis to perfuse both the right and left hepatic arteries.

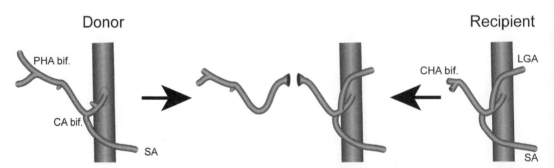

Fig. 9. Hepatic arterial reconstruction techniques. The donor arterial tree is prepared by either creating a branch patch by opening the celiac artery into the splenic artery (SA) at the celiac bifurcation (CA bif.) or by creating an aortic patch around the celiac ostium. The recipient branch patch is prepared by opening the common hepatic bifurcation (CHA bif.) into the gastroduodenal and proper hepatic arteries. Typically, the LGA and SA are preserved unless there is variant donor anatomy requiring additional arterial supply.

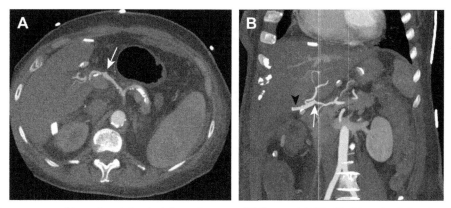

Fig. 10. Appearance of branch patch arterial anastomoses. (*A*) Transaxial CT with IV contrast showing a bulge at the hepatic arterial anastomosis consistent with the branch patch morphology (*arrow*). This should not be confused for a pseudoaneurysm. (*B*) Coronal oblique MIP shows irregularity at the hepatic arterial anastomosis (*arrow*) followed by diffuse relative enlargement of the donor artery (*arrowhead*), the result of a mismatch between donor and recipient artery diameters. Branch patch technique allows for arteries to be upsized or downsized to match donor to recipient.

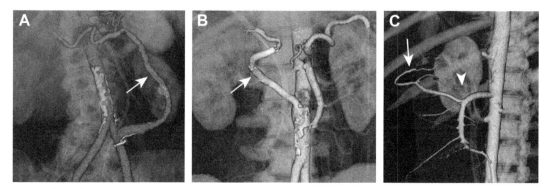

Fig. 11. Three-dimensional reconstructions of arterial jump graft techniques. (*A*) Cadaveric iliac artery from the liver donor used as a jump graft (*arrow*) from the left common iliac artery to the right and accessory left hepatic arteries. (*B*) Synthetic jump graft (*arrow*) from the aorta to the common hepatic artery. (*C*) Branches of the native superior mesenteric artery transposed to the right hepatic artery (*arrow*) and toward the small replaced left hepatic artery (*arrowhead*), the latter too small to render with this visualization technique.

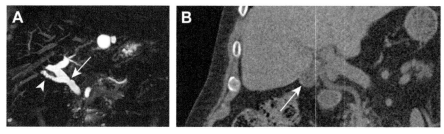

Fig. 12. End-to-end biliary anastomosis. (*A*) MRCP showing the anastomosis (*arrow*) immediately distal to the insertion of the donor cystic duct on the common hepatic duct, exaggerated by biliary dilatation in the setting of choledochal sphincter dysfunction. The cystic duct is also dilated, showing its typical corkscrew appearance (*arrowhead*). (*B*) Fluid-filled structure (*arrow*) adjacent to the otherwise normal posttransplant extrahepatic bile duct. This structure progressively enlarged over multiple routine CTs, identifiable as a remnant cystic duct mucocele.

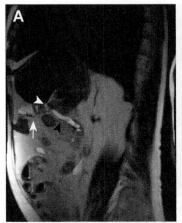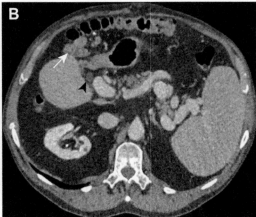

Fig. 13. DDLT with hepaticojejunostomy. (*A*) Sagittal T2-weighted MR imaging showing a loop of jejunum (*white arrow*) anastomosed to the common bile duct (*white arrowhead*). (*B*) Transaxial CT of the same patient showing jejunum (*white arrow*) passing posterior to the transverse colon and through the transverse mesocolon to the liver hilum. The tubular structure descending from the liver hilum in both images (*black arrowheads*) is the retained distal common bile duct; it can remain filled with secreted fluid due to the functioning choledochal sphincter.

usually of no consequence because this native duct no longer communicates with the intrahepatic biliary tree (**Fig. 13**).

SUMMARY

DDLT is an increasingly common procedure globally, and with increased patient survival and imaging utilization, it is ever more important that radiologists become familiar with the relevant preoperative anatomy and postoperative appearance. The highly variable nature of the surgery leads to a wide range of appearances on CT and MR. Understanding the scope of expected findings helps the radiologist guide management by better identifying abnormalities that require intervention and to prevent misidentification of normal anatomy as postoperative complications.

CLINICS CARE POINTS

- Donor imaging, when performed, is primarily used to confirm the absence of exclusion criteria such as severe hepatic steatosis or abdominal malignancy.
- All four systems requiring anastomoses in deceased donor liver transplantation (hepatic venous, portal venous, hepatic arterial, and biliary ductal) can have variable appearance depending on surgical technique. The documented surgical technique can guide the

radiologist in discerning expected appearances from complications.

- Recipient hepatic arterial supply may require pre-operative planning based on donor liver arterial anatomy and should be described in detail. The resulting hepatic arterial fish mouth anastomosis should not be confused for a pseudoaneurysm.
- The remnant common bile duct left *in situ* after hepaticojejunostomy may appear dilated and should not be interpreted as a post operative collection.

DISCLOSURE

RJG: Nothing to disclose. AKR: GE Healthcare - Research Grant (ongoing); PanCAN - Research Grant (ongoing); PanSU2C - Research Grant (ongoing); Philips Healthcare - Research Grant (ended); Bayer - Research Grant (ended); Bayer - Consultant Advisory Board (ended).

REFERENCES

1. Starzl TE, Marchioro TL, Vonkaulla KN, et al. Homotransplantation of the liver in humans. Surg Gynecol Obstet 1963;117:659–76.
2. Starzl TE, Groth CG, Brettschneider L, et al. Orthotopic homotransplantation of the human liver. Ann Surg 1968;168(3):392–415.
3. WHO-ONT collaboration. Global Observatory on Donation and Transplantation database. Published online

November 5, 2022. http://www.transplant-observatory.org/export-database/. Accessed November 5, 2022.

4. Kwong AJ, Ebel NH, Kim WR, et al. OPTN/SRTR 2020 Annual Data Report: Liver. Am J Transplant 2022;22(Suppl 2):204–309.

5. O'Leary JG, Lepe R, Davis GL. Indications for liver transplantation. Gastroenterology 2008;134(6):1764–76.

6. Azoulay D, Castaing D, Adam R, et al. Split-liver transplantation for two adult recipients: feasibility and long-term outcomes. Ann Surg 2001;233(4):565–74.

7. Celik N, Squires JE, Soltys K, et al. Domino liver transplantation for select metabolic disorders: Expanding the living donor pool. JIMD Rep 2019;48(1):83–9.

8. Chan T, DeGirolamo K, Chartier-Plante S, et al. Comparison of three caval reconstruction techniques in orthotopic liver transplantation: A retrospective review. Am J Surg 2017;213(5):943–9.

9. Shaw BW, Martin DJ, Marquez JM, et al. Venous bypass in clinical liver transplantation. Ann Surg 1984;200(4):524–34.

10. Schumann R, Mandell MS, Mercaldo N, et al. Anesthesia for liver transplantation in United States academic centers: intraoperative practice. J Clin Anesth 2013;25(7):542–50.

11. Czigany Z, Scherer MN, Pratschke J, et al. Technical Aspects of Orthotopic Liver Transplantation-a Survey-Based Study Within the Eurotransplant, Swisstransplant, Scandiatransplant, and British Transplantation Society Networks. J Gastrointest Surg 2019;23(3):529–37.

12. Pomposelli James J, Simpson Mary Ann, Simon Caroline J, et al. Liver transplantation. In: Forsythe JLR, editor. Transplantation. Fifth edition. Saunders/Elsevier; 2014.

13. Klintmalm GBG, Busuttil RW. Recipient Hepatectomy and Grafting. In: Transplantation of the liver. 3d edition. Elsevier Saunders; 2015. p. 600–10.

14. Chotkan KA, Mensink JW, Pol RA, et al. Radiological Screening Methods in Deceased Organ Donation: An Overview of Guidelines Worldwide. Transpl Int 2022;35:10289.

15. Mensink JW, Pol RA, Nijboer WN, et al. Whole Body CT Imaging in Deceased Donor Screening for Malignancies. Transplant Direct 2019;5(12):e509.

16. Varma V, Mehta N, Kumaran V, et al. Indications and Contraindications for Liver Transplantation. Bangladesh Liver J 2011;2011:1–9.

17. Mazzaferro V, Regalia E, Doci R, et al. Liver transplantation for the treatment of small hepatocellular carcinomas in patients with cirrhosis. N Engl J Med 1996;334(11):693–9.

18. Yao FY, Ferrell L, Bass NM, et al. Liver transplantation for hepatocellular carcinoma: expansion of the tumor size limits does not adversely impact survival. Hepatology 2001;33(6):1394–403.

19. Zhong J, Smith C, Walker P, et al. Imaging post liver transplantation part I: vascular complications. Clin Radiol 2020;75(11):845–53.

20. Allard R, Smith C, Zhong J, et al. Imaging post liver transplantation part II: biliary complications. Clin Radiol 2020;75(11):854–63.

21. Busque S, Esquivel CO, Concepcion W, et al. Experience with the piggyback technique without caval occlusion in adult orthotopic liver transplantation. Transplantation 1998;65(1):77–82.

22. Schmitz V, Schoening W, Jelkmann I, et al. Different cava reconstruction techniques in liver transplantation: piggyback versus cava resection. Hepatobiliary Pancreat Dis Int 2014;13(3):242–9.

23. Vieira de Melo PS, Miranda LEC, Batista LL, et al. Orthotopic liver transplantation without venovenous bypass using the conventional and piggyback techniques. Transplant Proc 2011;43(4):1327–33.

24. Navarro F, Le Moine MC, Fabre JM, et al. Specific vascular complications of orthotopic liver transplantation with preservation of the retrohepatic vena cava: review of 1361 cases. Transplantation 1999;68(5):646–50.

25. Lee TC, Dhar VK, Cortez AR, et al. Impact of side-to-side cavocavostomy versus traditional piggyback implantation in liver transplantation. Surgery 2020;168(6):1060–5.

26. Starzl TE, Iwatsuki S, Shaw BW. A growth factor in fine vascular anastomoses. Surg Gynecol Obstet 1984;159(2):164–5.

27. Kluger MD, Memeo R, Laurent A, et al. Survey of adult liver transplantation techniques (SALT): an international study of current practices in deceased donor liver transplantation. HPB 2011;13(10):692–8.

28. Seu P. Improved Results of Liver Transplantation in Patients With Portal Vein Thrombosis. Arch Surg 1996;131(8):840.

29. Starzl TE, Porter KA, Putnam CW. Intraportal insulin protects from the liver injury of portacaval shunt in dogs. Lancet 1975;2(7947):1241–2.

30. Chupetlovska KP, Borhani AA, Dasyam AK, et al. Post-operative imaging anatomy in liver transplantation. Abdom Radiol (NY) 2021;46(1):9–16.

31. Michels NA. Newer anatomy of the liver and its variant blood supply and collateral circulation. Am J Surg 1966;112(3):337–47.

32. Hiatt JR, Gabbay J, Busuttil RW. Surgical anatomy of the hepatic arteries in 1000 cases. Ann Surg 1994;220(1):50–2.

33. Noussios G, Dimitriou I, Chatzis I, et al. The Main Anatomic Variations of the Hepatic Artery and Their Importance in Surgical Practice: Review of the Literature. J Clin Med Res 2017;9(4):248–52.

34. Yilmaz S, Kutluturk K, Usta S, et al. Techniques of hepatic arterial reconstruction in liver transplantation. Langenbeck's Arch Surg 2022. https://doi.org/10.1007/s00423-022-02659-6.

35. Reese T, Raptis DA, Oberkofler CE, et al. A systematic review and meta-analysis of rescue revascularization with arterial conduits in liver transplantation. Am J Transplant 2019;19(2):551–63.

Imaging Evaluation of the Living Liver Donor: A Systems-Based Approach

Ryan E. Bailey, MD[a], Rosa Alba Pugliesi, MD[a], Daniel Borja—Cacho, MD[b], Amir A. Borhani, MD[c],*

KEYWORDS

- Living donor transplant • Liver transplant • Liver surgery • Hepatobiliary imaging
- Preoperative imaging

KEY POINTS

- Living donors have become an important supplemental source of liver allografts.
- Pre-donation imaging evaluation is important to discern anatomic variations and parenchymal factors which may increase risk to the donor or affect the transplantation outcome.
- The most common reason for donor exclusion is hepatic steatosis.
- Most of the biliary and vascular anatomic variations are not absolute contraindications to donation but may affect the decision on which lobe to harvest and may alter the surgical approach.

BACKGROUND

Liver transplant is the only definite therapy for end-stage liver disease and is one of the main curative treatment options for early hepatocellular carcinoma (HCC).[1] Unfortunately, demand for transplant organs far exceeds the supply. As of December 12, 2022, 10,847 patients in the United States remained on the liver transplant waiting list.[2] To increase the availability of donor organs, living donor liver transplant (LDLT) was developed as an alternative to the traditional deceased donor liver transplant (DDLT). First performed in the pediatric population in 1989[3] and in the adult population in 1998,[4] LDLT accounted for a record 569 of the 9236 adult liver transplants performed in the United States in 2021.[5] LDLT has become an important source of donor livers, and there is extensive evidence demonstrating its safety and efficacy.

Multiple studies have demonstrated improved survival benefit with LDLT versus DDLT.[6,7] LDLT has also demonstrated a unique survival benefit for patients with Model for End-Stage Liver Disease (MELD) scores less than 15, a finding not seen in prior studies of DDLT in these patients.[6] Immediate outcomes following LDLT are also improved relative to DDLT with decreased cost, length of hospital stay, and need for postoperative dialysis or blood transfusion.[7] Currently, the following major categories of patients are considered for LDLT in the United States: (1) patients with low MELD score who have major complications of cirrhosis or significantly decreased quality of life; (2) patients with low MELD who have cholestatic liver disease with recurrent cholangitis; (3) patients with large tumor burden HCC (outside of Milan criteria) with favorable tumor biology; (4) patients with low tumor burden HCC (within Milan criteria) who live in geographic regions with low deceased organ availability; and (5) patients with non-hepatocellular malignances not qualifying for DDLT.[8]

[a] Department of Radiology, Section of Body Imaging, Northwestern University, Feinberg School of Medicine, 676 North Street Clair Street, Ste 800, Chicago, IL 60611, USA; [b] Department of Surgery, Northwestern University Feinberg School of Medicine, Chicago, IL, USA; [c] Department of Radiology, Northwestern University Feinberg School of Medicine, 676 North Street Clair Street, Ste 800, Chicago, IL 60611, USA
* Corresponding author.
E-mail address: amir.borhani@northwestern.edu

Radiol Clin N Am 61 (2023) 771–784
https://doi.org/10.1016/j.rcl.2023.03.002
0033-8389/23/© 2023 Elsevier Inc. All rights reserved.

PREOPERATIVE ASSESSMENT OF LIVING LIVER DONOR CANDIDATES

One of the guiding principles of LDLT is minimization of donor risk. To that end, evaluation of living donor candidates is extensive and encompasses many facets of the potential donor's physical and mental health, as well as their social situation, support network, and additional psychosocial metrics. A comprehensive discussion of the clinical and social factors that contribute to living donor candidacy is beyond the scope of this article, and specific selection criteria, such as age, often vary by institution. Ultimately, most of the potential donors are rejected based on a combination of donor- and recipient-related factors. One study examining over 1000 potential living donors found that only 40% were accepted for donation. The most common reasons for rejection were comorbid medical conditions and incompatible anatomy with a lesser number rejected for steatosis or psychosocial factors.[9] Additional studies of donor evaluation have come to similar conclusions with roughly 30% to 40% of the evaluated donors meeting the necessary requirements to proceed to the operating room.[10,11]

Imaging assessment is performed to assess donor's eligibility and to provide information on vascular and biliary anatomy and to provide preoperative surgical roadmap. Comprehensive discussions of biliary and vascular hepatic anatomy have been previously published.[12] Here, the authors focus on the unique surgical and anatomic considerations inherent to LDLT and their impact on donor and recipient outcomes. Through this lens, the authors can better highlight the role of radiology in the donor selection process as well as several of the common and important anatomic variants of which the radiologist must be aware.

Donor Hepatectomy: Right Versus Left

To appropriately evaluate a potential living donor candidate, the radiologist must have a general understanding of the surgical techniques and relevant anatomic considerations for harvesting a donor graft. The graft in LDLT can be either a right or left lobe or, in the pediatric setting, a left lateral segment (**Fig. 1**). The resection plane for right lobe grafts parallels Cantlie's line (**Fig. 2**) running just lateral to the middle hepatic vein (MHV), thereby preserving the MHV in the donor.[7] The resection plane for left lobe grafts is variable and may include the MHV depending on the graft volume required.[13] In an ideal scenario, the graft will have a single outflow vein, a single arterial supply, and a single draining bile duct.

There are some data to suggest a lower rate of donor complications with left donor lobectomy.[14] In a matched case series of left versus right donations, overall complication rates were similar; however, donors who underwent right lobectomy had a higher incidence of Clavien grade 3 complications. A larger resection, or in other words a smaller liver remnant, correlated with a higher rate of postoperative complications and higher maximum international normalized ratio (INR) and bilirubin levels in the donor.[15] No significant difference in survival benefit has been shown based on the type of graft received.[16,17] Ultimately, the choice of left versus right lobectomy is related to several factors, most importantly safety of the donor. As a larger functional liver remnant supports this goal, when the volume is adequate for the recipient, left lobe grafts are often considered preferable. However, left lobe volume is often inadequate, and despite the slight advantages of left lobe donation reported by some authors, in recent years, there has been a trend toward a larger proportion of right lobe grafts in the setting of LDLT.[5]

Safety and Complications of Donor Hepatectomy

Although donor hepatectomy represents a major surgical procedure, it is relatively safe. In a study of noncirrhotic patients undergoing major hepatectomy, most commonly for metastasis resection, the overall complication rate was 43% and the incidence of death related to hepatic failure was 2.8%.[18] In the generally younger and carefully selected pool of potential living donors, complication and mortality rates are considerably lower. Reported overall complication and mortality rates are variable ranging from 19.5% to 40% and 0% to 0.4%, respectively.[7,10,19] National data from the Organ Procurement and Transplantation Network registry spanning 2016 to 2020 show that only a single medically related donor death out of 2128 LDLTs was reported within 1 year of donation.[5]

Complications following donor hepatectomy commonly involve postoperative infections, biliary complications, and incisional as well as diaphragmatic hernias (**Fig. 3**). Most of these tend to be mild and do not require intervention (Clavien grades 1 and 2). Approximately 1% of donors will experience residual disability.[10] There is also a minute risk of aborting the procedure, variably reported from 1% to 5% due to intraoperative findings in either the donor or recipient such as unexpected malignancy or unfavorable variant anatomy that was not seen on preoperative imaging.[10,19] In very rare cases, donors may experience complications severe enough to require liver transplant.[19]

Liver Transplantation: Anatomy Living Donor

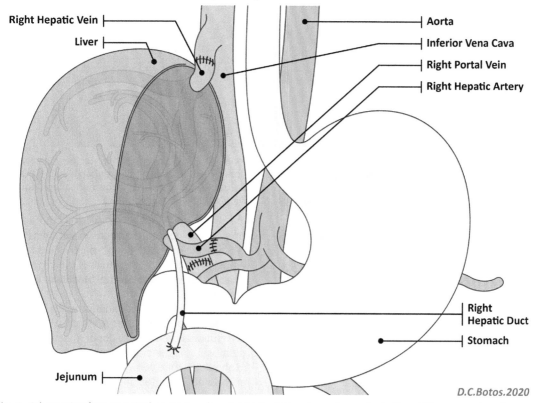

Fig. 1. Schematic of postsurgical anatomy after right lobe living donor transplantation. Biliary reconstruction can be done via duct-to-duct or biliary-enteric anastomosis (shown in this case). (*Courtesy of* D Botos, Chicago, IL.)

Graft Volume and Future Liver Remnant Volume

Although donors may be excluded from donation based on a number of imaging findings, insufficient graft volume is the most common cause. In a study of 159 potential donors, Hahn and colleagues found that of 61 potential donors excluded from imaging findings, 40 were excluded due to inadequate volume. Of the remaining 21 potential donors, 14 were excluded based on anatomic variation and 5 were excluded due to steatosis.[20] Similarly, Dirican and colleagues found inadequate volume to be the

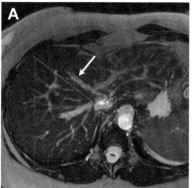
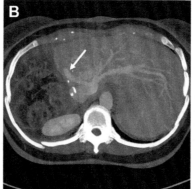
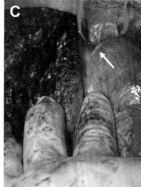

Fig. 2. (*A*) Axial maximum intensity projection (MIP) steady-state free precession image shows plane of hepatectomy in relation to the middle hepatic vein (*arrow*). (*B*) Axial MIP post-contrast CT in donor, obtained after hepatectomy, shows the remnant liver which contains the middle hepatic vein (*arrow*). (*C*) Intraoperative photograph shows the plane of resection lateral to the middle hepatic vein (*arrow*).

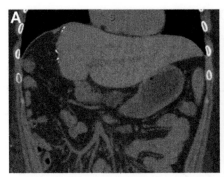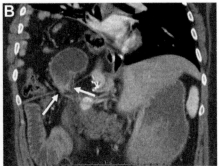

Fig. 3. (*A*) Coronal non-contrast CT obtained 3 months after donation shows post-right-hepatectomy anatomy in donor with appropriate compensatory hypertrophy of left lobe. (*B*) Coronal contrast-enhanced CT obtained 4 years later shows a defect through right hemidiaphragm (*arrows*) with associated large right diaphragmatic hernia containing bowel and mesenteric fat. (*Courtesy of* A Dasyam, MD, Pittsburgh, PA.)

most common imaging finding precluding donation, although a higher proportion of exclusion related to steatosis was noted in this study.[11]

It is no surprise that insufficient liver volume is the primary criteria for exclusion as inadequate graft volume has been clearly shown to correlate with poorer outcomes. The target graft size is greater than 0.8% of recipient body weight or greater than 40% recipient standard liver volume.[14] Early allograft dysfunction (defined as serum bilirubin $\geq$ 10 mg/dL on postoperative day 7, international normalized ratio (INR) $\geq$ 1.6 on postoperative day 7, or alanine transaminase (ALT) or aspartate transaminase (AST) >2000 IU/mL within the first 7 postoperative days) has been seen at a higher rate in patients who receive generally smaller left lobe grafts and correlates with a higher rate of graft loss.[21] A more severe consequence of inadequate graft volume is "small-for-size syndrome," a constellation of cholestasis, coagulopathy, and encephalopathy caused by inadequate metabolic capacity of the graft. Some centers have reported success with smaller grafts with the use of techniques such as portal inflow modulation and splenectomy. These techniques have allowed transplant using grafts as little as 0.5% of recipient body weight and are potentially opening the door to greater use of left lobe grafts and overall expansion of the donor pool.[17,22]

An important role of preoperative imaging is calculation of liver volumes. Liver volumetric measurements are most commonly performed on computed tomography (CT) due to its wider usage and inherent improved spatial resolution over magnetic resonanse (MR) imaging.[23] Although traditionally performed by slice-by-slice manual segmentation of liver contours, most centers now use semiautomatic methods (**Fig. 4**) for more time-efficient volumetry.[12] Both CT-based and MR imaging-based volumetric techniques tend to overestimate the true volume of the resected graft,

mainly due to inclusion of structures such as veins which do not reflect hepatic parenchyma, so a conversion factor of approximately 0.8 is generally applied to determine the actual functional graft tissue volume.[24]

Although there is some variation in the minimum accepted donor future liver remnant (FLR) based on institutional preference, donor age, and degree of steatosis, it is generally accepted that the donor FLR should, at minimum, be 30% of the donor total liver volume.[14,25] Residual liver volumes below 30% correlate with a higher rate of post-hepatectomy liver failure.[25] Hepatic parenchymal regeneration is robust in the donor population with remnant volumes usually reaching at least 79% and 88% of preoperative volume by 3 and 12 months post-donation, respectively.[26]

Back-Table Reconstruction

In cases of variant anatomy resulting in more than one hepatic venous outflow or draining bile ducts,

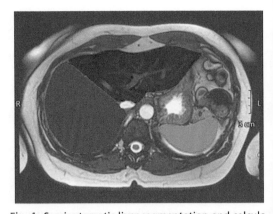

Fig. 4. Semiautomatic liver segmentation and calculation of allograft and remnant liver based on the plane of resection. Steady-state free precession MR imaging sequence was used for segmentation.

these structures are often reconstructed into a single channel on the back table, thereby facilitating a single anastomosis in the recipient and decreasing the risk of thrombosis/stricture.[22] The most common application of this principle is in reconstruction of the hepatic vein tributaries draining segments 5 and 8 (Fig. 5). This is performed on the back table before reimplantation and uses various graft materials and anastomotic techniques depending on availability and recipient anatomy.[27] In cases where large accessory veins are present but cannot be combined into a single anastomosis, additional anastomoses are required though smaller veins can be ligated.[28]

Assessment of Donor Liver Disease

The most common diffuse parenchymal abnormality resulting in donor exclusion is hepatic steatosis, which has an estimated prevalence as high as 34% in the United States.[29] The prevalence of steatosis in the living liver donor population is likely much lower (due to preselection of healthier individuals as donors) with a recent study of 143 donors finding steatosis in only 17%.[30] Detection of hepatic fat can be carried out with both CT and MR imaging. On unenhanced CT, hepatic attenuation less than 40 Hounsfield Units (HU) or hepatic attenuation of ≤ -10 HU relative to the spleen correlates with moderate steatosis on biopsy (ie, $\geq 33\%$ of hepatocytes containing fat on histopathological examination).[31] MR has largely replaced CT for detection of hepatic steatosis due to its greater sensitivity and ability to quantify steatosis with a high degree of accuracy.[32] More advanced MR imaging sequences, which are routinely used in clinical practice, allow for more accurate grading of hepatic steatosis by providing proton density fat fraction, a percentage value that correlates well with histopathologic analysis.[33]

The correlation of mild-to-moderate hepatic steatosis with donor outcomes is still being investigated. Donors with moderate steatosis are generally excluded from donation, as this degree of steatosis has previously been shown to correlate with a higher rate of graft loss.[34] One study examining donors with mild-to-moderate steatosis who successfully donated demonstrated encouraging results in this population. Donor remnant regeneration reached 82% of preoperative volume by approximately 100 days post-donation, and regeneration was similar regardless of steatosis severity. In addition, adverse outcomes in the recipients, including early allograft dysfunction, were not correlated with the degree of steatosis.[30]

Additional parenchymal abnormalities can result in donor exclusion but are less commonly encountered in the younger and healthier donor population. The most common diffuse parenchymal processes in this category other than steatosis are hepatic iron deposition or occult fibrosis. Some centers have included MR elastography in their preoperative workup, but its use is not universal.[23] Focal lesions such as large cysts, focal nodular hyperplasia, or hepatic adenoma are handled with a wide degree of variability, although it has been suggested that adenomas are a contraindication due to their potential for bleeding and malignant transformation.[35]

Variant Vascular and Biliary Anatomy

Although donor exclusion is less commonly due to anatomic variants, accurate delineation of the vascular and biliary anatomy is essential to facilitate preoperative planning. In the previously described study of 159 consecutive potential donors, of the 61 patients excluded based on imaging 14 were due to anatomic variation. Importantly, exclusion based on anatomic variation is often institution- and surgeon-dependent, and continually improving

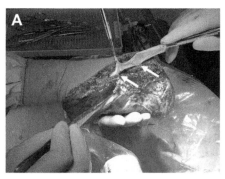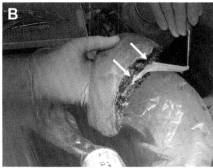

Fig. 5. (A, B) Back-table venous reconstruction for right lobe allograft. Cadaveric iliac vein was used to reconstitute drainage of segment 5 (V5) and segment 8 (V8) hepatic veins into recipient IVC. Orifices of V5 and V8 are annotated by arrows.

surgical techniques have resulted in many variants now being considered relative rather than absolute contraindications.[20,32]

Variant Arterial Anatomy

Conventional hepatic arterial anatomy refers to a common hepatic artery, which originates from the celiac artery and gives rise to the gastroduodenal and proper hepatic arteries. The proper hepatic artery then bifurcates into the left and right hepatic arteries (LHA and RHA). Variations in hepatic arterial anatomy are common and occur in up to 50% of the population. The most common variants are a replaced RHA arising from the superior mesenteric artery (SMA) and an accessory LHA arising from the left gastric.[12] The presence of arterial variation is not an absolute contraindication to donation, but it can increase case complexity. Some variants are favorable depending on the type of planned donation. For example, a replaced RHA arising from the SMA is beneficial in the setting of donor right hepatectomy due to its longer length (Fig. 6).[23]

Unlike in the case of DDLT, intrahepatic branching of hepatic arteries is important to be recognized and described in living donors. One specific arterial relationship vital to define preoperatively is that of the segment 4 arterial supply. At the population level, segment 4 supply is predominantly from the LHA in approximately 60% of people (Fig. 7).[23] The supply of segment 4 from the RHA is a relative contraindication to right lobe donation (Fig. 8), as hypertrophy of segment 4 of the liver remnant will be impaired following hepatectomy, although the procedure still may be

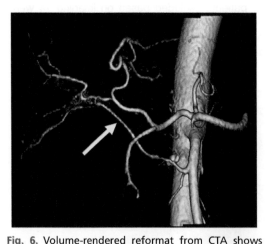

Fig. 6. Volume-rendered reformat from CTA shows variant arterial anatomy with a replaced right hepatic artery (*arrow*) originating from SMA. This is generally considered a favorable variant given the length of the replaced right hepatic artery.

performed provided the RHA can be ligated distal to the segment 4 branch takeoff (Fig. 9).[20] Alternatively, if a left lobe donation is planned, this necessitates arterial reconstruction and creation of two anastomoses to ensure adequate liver regeneration within the recipient. Hence, segment 4 arterial supply is one of the most critical pieces of radiologic information required for appropriate surgical planning.[14,23] An additional variant requiring particular attention is the arterial supply of segment 8 from the LHA. This is a relative contraindication to right lobe donation due to the need for two anastomoses and the associated increased risk of thrombosis.[20]

The two main noninvasive methods used for evaluation of arterial anatomy in potential living donors are CT angiography (CTA) and MR angiography (MRA). CTA has higher spatial resolution and is more widely available. Using MRA instead of CTA, however, allows for simultaneous assessment of vessels, biliary tree, and liver parenchyma, thereby simplifying the workup for potential donors. Performing high-quality MRA heavily relies on optimization of protocol and pulse sequences and might not be feasible on all MR imaging scanners. Multiple studies have evaluated MRA with both extracellular and hepatobiliary agents to determine its potential to serve as the sole imaging workup before donation. Using hepatobiliary agents has the added advantage of allowing simultaneous performance of T1-weighted MR cholangiography (Fig. 10).[32] MR imaging has been proven accurate for depiction of hepatic venous, portal venous, and biliary anatomy with accuracy rates of 94%, 100%, and 91%, respectively.[36] Studies using hepatobiliary agents have shown variable accuracy rates for depiction of arterial anatomy, in particular the segment 4 supply ranging from 73% to 100% and 55% to 85% for hepatic arterial anatomy and the segment 4 branch, respectively.[37–40] The reported rates of accurate depiction with extracellular agents are generally higher ranging from 92% to 100% for the hepatic arteries and up to 96% for the segment 4 supply.[41,42] To combine the added value of hepatobiliary agents for biliary imaging with the superior performance of extracellular agents for arterial imaging, few centers have proposed dual-agent MR imaging, where the MRA portion of the study is performed using extracellular agent followed by injection of hepatobiliary agent for purpose of delayed hepatobiliary phase imaging and contrast-enhanced T1-weighted cholangiography.

Despite the advantages of MRA, CTA remains the most common modality for arterial evaluation with a majority of centers reporting its use in their

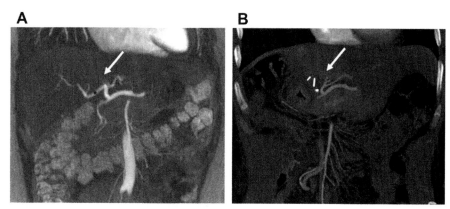

Fig. 7. (*A*) Coronal MIP MRA shows conventional anatomy with segment 4 artery (*arrow*) arising from the left hepatic artery. The right hepatic artery is annotated by an asterisk. (*B*) Coronal MIP CTA shows preserved segment 4 artery (*arrow*) in the donor remnant liver after hepatectomy.

donor evaluation protocol.[23] Although generally better to depict the hepatic arterial branches, CTA is not without limitations and, in certain patients, may be inferior to MR imaging.[39] In rare cases, complex anatomy may be difficult to delineate on cross-sectional imaging. Conventional angiography remains a viable option in those patients.[42] Given the advantages of MR imaging and its diagnostic accuracy in most patients, a prudent solution may be to use MRA/MR imaging as a first-line evaluation and reserve CT for troubleshooting.[39]

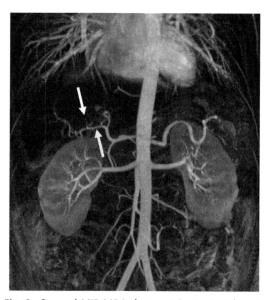

Fig. 8. Coronal MIP MRA shows variant arterial anatomy with segment 4 artery (*white arrow*) arising from right hepatic artery (*yellow arrow*). This is considered an unfavorable anatomic variant for living donor liver donation.

Variant portal venous anatomy

Conventional anatomy of the portal vein refers to a bifurcation of the main portal vein into right and left portal veins and the subsequent bifurcation of the right portal vein into anterior and posterior divisions. Variation in portal venous anatomy is less common than variation in hepatic venous or arterial anatomy. When present, it is often associated with biliary variation as these structures are intimately interrelated during embryological development. Portal vein variation occurs in 11% to 20% of the population.[43,44] The most common variants are portal vein trifurcation (7% incidence) and early branching of the right posterior portal vein from the main portal vein (5% incidence). Additional anatomic variants are rarer with an incidence of 3% or less but are nonetheless important to recognize as they can significantly increase case complexity and may prevent donation.[45] An example of these variants is origination of the right anterior portal vein from the left portal vein (**Fig. 11**). Right hepatectomy is relatively contraindicated in these patients because two anastomoses would be required in the recipient, and left hepatectomy is contraindicated as the left portal vein remnant within the graft is often too short to allow simple anastomosis in the recipient. Similar logic can be applied to origination of the left portal vein from the right anterior portal vein. Additional relative contraindications are present for right hepatectomy in patients with early branching of the right posterior division or segmental supply of segments 6 or 7 by an early branch as these variations require two anastomoses.[20,23,43]

Variant hepatic venous anatomy

Hepatic vein variation is similar in incidence to hepatic arterial variation, occurring in approximately 40% of the population. However, unlike portal,

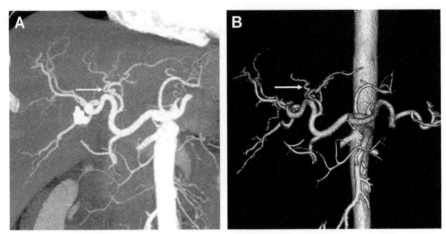

Fig. 9. Coronal MIP CTA (*A*) and volume-rendered reformat (*B*) show variant arterial anatomy with segment 4 artery (*arrows*) arising from right hepatic artery. Despite being an unfavorable anatomical variant, this candidate underwent right hepatectomy given the long length of right hepatic artery after segment 4 branch takeoff.

arterial, or biliary anatomy, no configuration of the hepatic veins represents a strong contraindication to transplant.[23] The primary need for describing hepatic venous anatomy in potential donors is to facilitate planning of the necessary reconstruction(s).

The most commonly encountered venous variant is the inferior right hepatic vein (**Fig. 12**). This vein and similar accessory veins draining directly into the inferior vena cava (IVC) must be described for two reasons: they can affect clamping techniques during the donor hepatectomy and also because they often necessitate back-table reconstruction or additional anastomoses during reimplantation in the recipient.[14] Techniques for hepatic vein reconstruction are variable including the use of synthetic, autologous, or cadaveric grafts. Anastomoses with the hepatic veins and IVC in the donor can be either direct or via an IVC patch.[27,28]

To ensure proper graft hypertrophy in the recipient, segmental veins draining segments 5 and 8, which are transected in the traditional MHV-sparing right donor hepatectomy, must be reconstructed to prevent venous congestion (**Fig. 13**). In general, hepatic vein tributaries measuring greater than 5 mm require reconstruction, whereas smaller tributaries can be safely ligated.[23,27] The radiologist should pay particular attention to larger tributaries of this type and report their location.

Variant biliary anatomy

Conventional biliary anatomy is similar to that of conventional portal anatomy with a right anterior

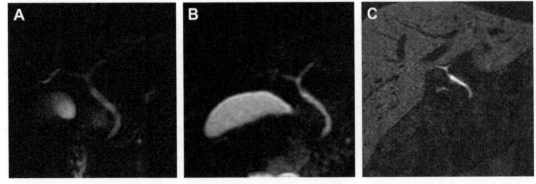

Fig. 10. Coronal 2D MR cholangiography (*A*) and coronal MIP 3D MR cholangiography (*B*) show conventional biliary anatomy in this candidate. Coronal contrast-enhanced MR cholangiography (*C*) further depicts the biliary anatomy. This additional sequence can increase accuracy and confidence of radiologist for assessment of biliary tree, especially when non-contrast T2-weighted MR cholangiography sequences are degraded by motion or when the bile ducts are not visualized due to their small size.

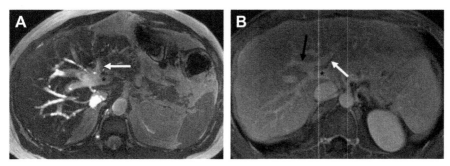

Fig. 11. (A) Axial MIP steady-state free precession MR imaging shows variant portal vein anatomy with "near-trifurcation" configuration and short length of right portal vein. The left portal vein is annotated by an arrow. (B) Axial contrast-enhanced T1-weighted MR imaging in a different candidate shows variant portal venous anatomy with right anterior portal vein branch (black arrow) arising from left portal vein (white arrow). Main portal veins are annotated by asterisks.

hepatic duct (RAHD) and right posterior hepatic duct (RPHD) joining to form a right hepatic duct (RHD). The RHD and left hepatic duct (LHD) then join to become the common hepatic duct (CHD) and following the junction of the cystic duct, the common bile duct (CBD). The accurate description of biliary anatomy is of the utmost importance in potential donor evaluation as biliary complications represent one of the most common etiologies of postoperative morbidity in the living donor population.[10] In addition, reported rates of biliary-related complications are higher when two2 or more biliary anastomoses are required.[46] Multiple anastomoses are required in many biliary tract variations such as trifurcation or drainage of RPHD to CHD.[23] Variations that result in drainage of the

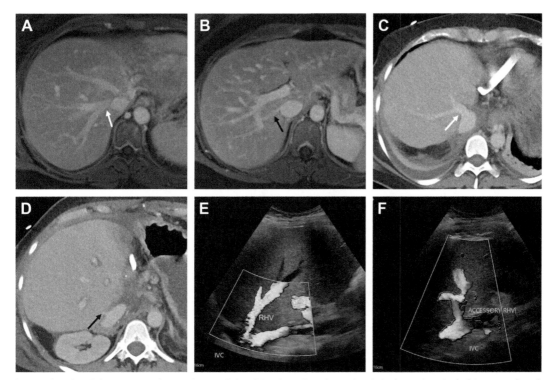

Fig. 12. (A, B) Axial contrast-enhanced T1-weighted MR imaging show the right hepatic vein (white arrow) and a large accessory right hepatic vein (black arrow). (C, D) Axial contrast-enhanced CT images in the recipient show separate anastomoses of right hepatic vein (white arrow) and accessory right hepatic vein (black arrow). (E, F) Color Doppler images in the recipient show patency of these two outflow veins. Radiologists should be aware of these venous reconstructions to fully evaluate the allograft.

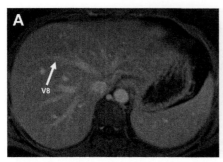
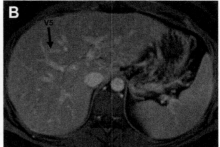

Fig. 13. (*A, B*) Axial contrast-enhanced T1-weighted MR imaging show large segment 8 (*white arrow*) and segment 5 (*black arrow*) hepatic veins draining into the middle hepatic vein. As these veins are transected during hepatectomy, venous reconstruction should be considered for adequate drainage of these segments to prevent hepatic congestion.

RAHD/RPHD into the LHD have particular importance (**Fig. 14**). In most instances, this is considered an absolute contraindication to left lobe donation as the donor would be subjected to complex biliary reconstruction. Right lobe donation is feasible in these individuals but will be more complex as two anastomoses are required in the recipient.[20] The opposite holds true for drainage of the main LHD or segmental LHDs into an RAHD/RPHD (**Fig.15**). This is an absolute contraindication to right lobe donation and increases the degree of complexity for left lobe donation.[43]

The widespread availability of MR imaging and utilization of hepatobiliary contrast agents (gadoxetate disodium being the most widely used) have contributed to making MR imaging the standard modality for assessment of biliary anatomy. MR imaging of bile ducts can be performed via two primary methods. The first utilizes heavily T2-weighted magnetic resonance cholangiography

sequences (MRC) without contrast. Conventional 2D MRC has an advantage in terms of image quality as these images are quick to acquire and can be obtained in a single breath. Three-dimensional (3D) MRCP is complimentary, allowing for better spatial resolution, though at the expense of increased acquisition time and requiring a respiratory trigger which can result in motion artifact.[47] Reported rates of concordance with intraoperative biliary anatomy are 85% to 90% when 2-dimentional (2D) and 3D techniques are used in combination (**Fig. 16**).[46,48] A potential drawback of the conventional T2-weighted MRC is nonvisualization (or suboptimal visualization) of small sectoral biliary branches which are often very small in these usually younger and healthy population. The second method, T1-weighted contrast-enhanced cholangiography, relies on delayed excretion of gadoxetate disodium into biliary system. T1-weighted images obtained after a roughly

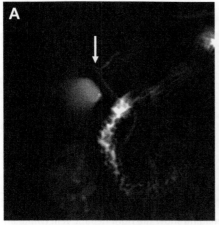
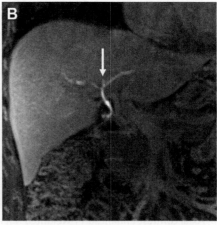

Fig. 14. (*A*) Coronal 3D MR cholangiography shows insertion of right posterior hepatic duct (*arrow*) into left hepatic duct. (*B*) Coronal contrast-enhanced MR cholangiography obtained 20 minutes after injection of gadoxetate disodium better shows this variant anatomy. This variant is unfavorable for right lobe transplant as it will require two separate biliary anastomoses.

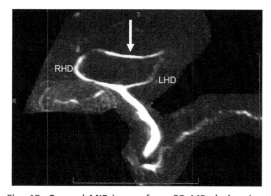

Fig. 15. Coronal MIP image from 3D MR cholangiography shows variant biliary anatomy with drainage of segment 4 duct (*arrow*) into the right hepatic duct. This is considered a contraindication for donor hepatectomy. (*Courtesy* of A Dasyam, MD, Pittsburgh, PA).

20-min delay during the hepatobiliary phase following gadoxetate acid (HBP) demonstrate excellent opacification of the biliary system (see **Fig. 10**). Utilization of a larger flip angle can improve detection of smaller branch ducts.[49] A secondary advantage of T1 MRC is the high contrast and spatial resolution of the liver seen on HBP provides excellent anatomic detail and an additional opportunity to measure the liver volume with precision.[12] Survey data suggests that the majority of living donor transplant programs utilize both T1-and T2-weighted MRC for donor evaluation.[23]

CLOSING REMARKS

Living liver donation is not without risk, both physical, as previously discussed, and psychological. Many donors face mental health challenges

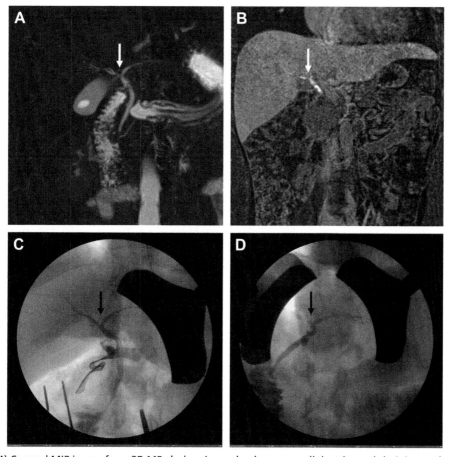

Fig. 16. (*A*) Coronal MIP image from 3D MR cholangiography shows a small duct (*arrow*) draining to the proximal right hepatic duct, believed to be duct of caudate lobe. (*B*) Coronal contrast-enhanced MR cholangiography, obtained 20 minutes after injection of gadoxetate disodium, further confirmed this finding. (*C*) Patient underwent intraoperative cholangiography for better delineation of this variant anatomy which again showed this small duct (*arrow*). (*D*) Post-hepatectomy cholangiogram shows transection of the right hepatic duct above the level of the small caudate duct (*arrow*). Recognition of these small ducts and communication to surgeons can improve surgical planning and prevent biliary complications in the donor and recipient.

following donation, including guilt if their recipient does not survive long-term. Despite these challenges, survey data suggests 95% of donors would donate again if given the same choice. This is encouraging, and further supports the idea that LDLT will be a consistent, if not increasing, source of liver donations in the future. For this reason, radiologists must understand the overall process of living donation and the donor outcomes as outlined here, so that they can best contribute to the future success of these transplant programs.

CLINICS CARE POINTS

- There is increasing number of living donor transplants performed. Familiarity with this technique is essential for correct interpretation of pre-operative imaging studies.
- Detailed assessment of liver parenchyma and vascular and biliary system, with special attention to anatomical variants, is the mainstay of pre-operative imaging.
- Radiology reports should be tailored to the type of transplant.

DISCLOSURES

None of the authors have relevant financial conflicts to disclose.

REFERENCES

1. Chu KK, Wong KH, Chok KS. Expanding Indications for Liver Transplant: Tumor and Patient Factors. Gut Liver 2021;15(1):19–30.
2. Organ Procurement and Transplantation Network - Data. Available at: https://optn.transplant.hrsa.gov/data/. Accessed December 12, 2022.
3. Strong RW, Lynch SV, Ong TH, et al. Successful liver transplantation from a living donor to her son. N Engl J Med 1990;322(21):1505–7.
4. Wachs ME, Bak TE, Karrer FM, et al. Adult living donor liver transplantation using a right hepatic lobe. Transplantation 1998;66(10):1313–6.
5. Kwong AJ, Ebel NH, Kim WR, et al. OPTN/SRTR 2020 Annual Data Report: Liver. Am J Transplant 2022;22(Suppl 2):204–309.
6. Abu-Gazala S, Olthoff KM. Status of Adult Living Donor Liver Transplantation in the United States: Results from the Adult-To-Adult Living Donor Liver Transplantation Cohort Study. Gastroenterol Clin North Am 2018;47(2):297–311.
7. Humar A, Ganesh S, Jorgensen D, et al. Adult Living Donor Versus Deceased Donor Liver Transplant (LDLT Versus DDLT) at a Single Center: Time to Change Our Paradigm for Liver Transplant. Ann Surg 2019;270(3):444–51.
8. Kim PT, Testa G. Living donor liver transplantation in the USA. Hepatobiliary Surg Nutr 2016;5(2):133–40.
9. Trotter JF, Wisniewski KA, Terrault NA, et al. Outcomes of donor evaluation in adult-to-adult living donor liver transplantation. Hepatology 2007;46(5):1476–84.
10. Abecassis MM, Fisher RA, Olthoff KM, et al. Complications of living donor hepatic lobectomy–a comprehensive report. Am J Transplant 2012;12(5):1208–17.
11. Dirican A, Baskiran A, Dogan M, et al. Evaluation of Potential Donors in Living Donor Liver Transplantation. Transplant Proc 2015;47(5):1315–8.
12. Borhani AA, Elsayes KM, Catania R, et al. Imaging Evaluation of Living Liver Donor Candidates: Techniques, Protocols, and Anatomy. Radiographics 2021;41(6):1572–91.
13. Samstein B, Cherqui D, Rotellar F, et al. Totally laparoscopic full left hepatectomy for living donor liver transplantation in adolescents and adults. Am J Transplant 2013;13(9):2462–6.
14. Cai L, Yeh BM, Westphalen AC, et al. Adult living donor liver imaging. Diagn Interv Radiol 2016;22(3):207–14.
15. Reichman TW, Sandroussi C, Azouz SM, et al. Living donor hepatectomy: the importance of the residual liver volume. Liver Transpl 2011;17(12):1404–11.
16. Olthoff KM, Smith AR, Abecassis M, et al. Defining long-term outcomes with living donor liver transplantation in North America. Ann Surg 2015;262(3):465–75 [discussion: 473-5].
17. Halazun KJ, Przybyszewski EM, Griesemer AD, et al. Leaning to the Left: Increasing the Donor Pool by Using the Left Lobe, Outcomes of the Largest Single-center North American Experience of Left Lobe Adult-to-adult Living Donor Liver Transplantation. Ann Surg 2016;264(3):448–56.
18. Mullen JT, Ribero D, Reddy SK, et al. Hepatic insufficiency and mortality in 1,059 noncirrhotic patients undergoing major hepatectomy. J Am Coll Surg 2007;204(5):854–62 [discussion: 862-4].
19. Cheah YL, Simpson MA, Pomposelli JJ, et al. Incidence of death and potentially life-threatening near-miss events in living donor hepatic lobectomy: a world-wide survey. Liver Transpl 2013;19(5):499–506.
20. Hahn LD, Emre SH, Israel GM. Radiographic features of potential donor livers that precluded donation. AJR Am J Roentgenol 2014;202(4):W343–8.
21. Pomposelli JJ, Goodrich NP, Emond JC, et al. Patterns of Early Allograft Dysfunction in Adult Live Donor Liver Transplantation: The A2ALL Experience. Transplantation 2016;100(7):1490–9.

22. Lee SG. A complete treatment of adult living donor liver transplantation: a review of surgical technique and current challenges to expand indication of patients. Am J Transplant 2015;15(1):17–38.

23. Hecht EM, Wang ZJ, Kambadakone A, et al. Living Donor Liver Transplantation: Preoperative Planning and Postoperative Complications. AJR Am J Roentgenol 2019;213(1):65–76.

24. Karlo C, Reiner CS, Stolzmann P, et al. CT- and MRI-based volumetry of resected liver specimen: comparison to intraoperative volume and weight measurements and calculation of conversion factors. Eur J Radiol 2010;75(1):e107–11.

25. Kim HJ, Kim CY, Hur YH, et al. Comparison of remnant to total functional liver volume ratio and remnant to standard liver volume ratio as a predictor of postoperative liver function after liver resection. Korean J Hepatobiliary Pancreat Surg 2013;17(4):143–51.

26. Emond JC, Fisher RA, Everson G, et al. Changes in liver and spleen volumes after living liver donation: a report from the Adult-to-Adult Living Donor Liver Transplantation Cohort Study (A2ALL). Liver Transpl 2015;21(2):151–61.

27. Hwang S, Lee SG, Ahn CS, et al. Cryopreserved iliac artery is indispensable interposition graft material for middle hepatic vein reconstruction of right liver grafts. Liver Transpl 2005;11(6):644–9.

28. Ito K, Akamatsu N, Tani K, et al. Reconstruction of hepatic venous tributary in right liver living donor liver transplantation: The importance of the inferior right hepatic vein. Liver Transpl 2016;22(4):410–9.

29. Kim D, Kim WR, Kim HJ, et al. Association between noninvasive fibrosis markers and mortality among adults with nonalcoholic fatty liver disease in the United States. Hepatology 2013;57(4):1357–65.

30. Qi Q, Weinstock AK, Chupetlovska K, et al. Magnetic resonance imaging-derived proton density fat fraction (MRI-PDFF) is a viable alternative to liver biopsy for steatosis quantification in living liver donor transplantation. Clin Transplant 2021;35(7):e14339.

31. Kodama Y, Ng CS, Wu TT, et al. Comparison of CT methods for determining the fat content of the liver. AJR Am J Roentgenol 2007;188(5):1307–12.

32. Kim B, Kim SY, Kim KW, et al. MRI in donor candidates for living donor liver transplant: Technical and practical considerations. J Magn Reson Imaging 2018;48(6):1453–67.

33. Tang A, Tan J, Sun M, et al. Nonalcoholic fatty liver disease: MR imaging of liver proton density fat fraction to assess hepatic steatosis. Radiology 2013;267(2):422–31.

34. Spitzer AL, Lao OB, Dick AA, et al. The biopsied donor liver: incorporating macrosteatosis into high-risk donor assessment. Liver Transpl 2010;16(7):874–84.

35. Gokcan H, Akdogan M, Kacar S, et al. Case of a successful liver transplantation from a living donor with focal nodular hyperplasia. Acta Gastroenterol Belg 2016;79(2):262–3.

36. Mu X, Wang H, Ma Q, et al. Contrast-enhanced magnetic resonance angiography for the preoperative evaluation of hepatic vascular anatomy in living liver donors: a meta-analysis. Acad Radiol 2014;21(6):743–9.

37. Lee MW, Lee JM, Lee JY, et al. Preoperative evaluation of hepatic arterial and portal venous anatomy using the time resolved echo-shared MR angiographic technique in living liver donors. Eur Radiol 2007;17(4):1074–80.

38. Xie S, Liu C, Yu Z, et al. One-stop-shop preoperative evaluation for living liver donors with gadoxetic acid disodium-enhanced magnetic resonance imaging: efficiency and additional benefit. Clin Transplant 2015;29(12):1164–72.

39. Jhaveri K, Guo L, Guimaraes L, et al. Mapping of hepatic vasculature in potential living liver donors: comparison of gadoxetic acid-enhanced MR imaging using CAIPIRINHA technique with CT angiography. Abdom Radiol (NY) 2018;43(7):1682–92.

40. Lee MS, Lee JY, Kim SH, et al. Gadoxetic acid disodium-enhanced magnetic resonance imaging for biliary and vascular evaluations in preoperative living liver donors: comparison with gadobenate dimeglumine-enhanced MRI. J Magn Reson Imaging 2011;33(1):149–59.

41. Streitparth F, Pech M, Figolska S, et al. Living related liver transplantation: preoperative magnetic resonance imaging for assessment of hepatic vasculature of donor candidates. Acta Radiol 2007;48(1):20–6.

42. Carr JC, Nemcek AA Jr, Abecassis M, et al. Preoperative evaluation of the entire hepatic vasculature in living liver donors with use of contrast-enhanced MR angiography and true fast imaging with steady-state precession. J Vasc Interv Radiol 2003;14(4):441–9.

43. Cahalane AM, Mojtahed A, Sahani DV, et al. Pre-hepatic and pre-pancreatic transplant donor evaluation. Cardiovasc Diagn Ther 2019;9(Suppl 1):S97–115.

44. Lee VS, Morgan GR, Lin JC, et al. Liver transplant donor candidates: associations between vascular and biliary anatomic variants. Liver Transpl 2004;10(8):1049–54.

45. Sureka B, Patidar Y, Bansal K, et al. Portal vein variations in 1000 patients: surgical and radiological importance. Br J Radiol 2015;88(1055):20150326.

46. Kashyap R, Bozorgzadeh A, Abt P, et al. Stratifying risk of biliary complications in adult living donor liver transplantation by magnetic resonance cholangiography. Transplantation 2008;85(11):1569–72.

47. Lim JS, Kim MJ, Myoung S, et al. MR cholangiography for evaluation of hilar branching anatomy in transplantation of the right hepatic lobe from a living donor. AJR Am J Roentgenol 2008;191(2):537–45.

48. Kim SY, Byun JH, Lee SS, et al. Biliary tract depiction in living potential liver donors: intraindividual comparison of MR cholangiography at 3.0 and 1.5 T. Radiology 2010;254(2):469–78.

49. Kim S, Mussi TC, Lee LJ, et al. Effect of flip angle for optimization of image quality of gadoxetate disodium-enhanced biliary imaging at 1.5 T. AJR Am J Roentgenol 2013;200(1):90–6.

Immediate and Late Complications After Liver Transplantation

Christopher Buros, MD, Atman Ashwin Dave, MD, Alessandro Furlan, MD*

KEYWORDS

- Liver transplantation complications • Hepatic artery thrombosis • Portal vein stenosis • Bile leak
- Biliary strictures • Biliary stones • Recurrent hepatocellular carcinoma
- Posttransplant lymphoproliferative disorder

KEY POINTS

- Hepatic artery thrombosis is the most worrisome complication in the immediate postoperative period following liver transplantation and has been associated with high mortality and graft failure rate.
- Vascular complications, which occur in both immediate and late postoperative periods, are the second most common cause of liver graft failure after rejection. Portal and hepatic venous complications are less common than hepatic arterial complications.
- Biliary complications, including bile leak, biliary strictures, and biliary stones, occur in up to a third of liver transplantation patients and most are diagnosed within 6 months of the transplant.
- Surveillance imaging is required to diagnose late complications such as recurrent malignancy, posttransplant lymphoproliferative disorder, or recurrence of primary liver diseases such as primary sclerosing cholangitis.

INTRODUCTION

It is estimated that more than 100 million people in the United States have some form of liver disease[1] with many people having undiagnosed fatty liver disease. Untreated, liver disease can lead to liver failure and cancer. In 2020, 51,642 adults in the United States died of liver disease (15.7 per 100,000 population)[2] with cirrhosis/chronic liver disease as the 12th leading cause of death. Liver transplantation is a lifesaving intervention and proven treatment in patients with end-stage liver disease. The liver transplant restores patient's health, lifestyle, and can extend lifespan by over 20 years.[3]

There were 9236 liver transplants performed in the United States in 2021—the largest number of liver transplants performed in a year to date.[4] Despite this increasing trend, there is still a shortage of liver donors with up to 2000 transplant candidates dying each year while on the waitlist.[5] Although living donor liver transplantation (LDLT) is one approach to increase organ availability, only 4% to 6% of liver transplants are from living donors and the rest are deceased donor liver transplantations (DDLTs).[4] The LDLT has a unique role in providing lifesaving transplantation for patients with less severe liver disease. Unfortunately, vascular and biliary complications have been shown to occur more often in LDLT than DDLT.[6–8] As more people receive liver transplantations, including LDLT, there is a greater need to recognize postoperative complications to initiate early treatment and prolong graft survival.

There is a general timeline for posttransplantation complications with some events more common in the immediate/early postoperative period and others occurring later (**Table 1**).[9] Knowledge

Department of Radiology, University of Pittsburgh Medical Center, Radiology Suite 200 East Wing, 200 Lothrop Street, Pittsburgh, PA 15213, USA
* Corresponding author.
E-mail address: furlana@upmc.edu

Radiol Clin N Am 61 (2023) 785–795
https://doi.org/10.1016/j.rcl.2023.04.002
0033-8389/23/© 2023 Elsevier Inc. All rights reserved.

Table 1
Liver transplant complications per expected time of occurrence after surgery (complication in bold indicates most likely time of occurrence)

	0–1 mo	1–12 mo	> 12 mo
Vascular complications	**Hepatic artery thrombosis (HAT)** **Portal vein thrombosis (PVT)**	**Hepatic artery stenosis (HAS)** HAT PVT PVS	**Hepatic vein stenosis** **Portal vein stenosis (PVS)** HAT PVT HAS
Biliary complications	**Bile leak**	**Biliary stricture** **Biliary sludge and casts**	**Biliary stones and casts** Biliary stricture
Parenchymal complications	**Post-op collection (hematoma, seroma)** **Acute rejection**	**PTLD** Recurrent HCC Rejection	**Recurrent HCC** **Recurrence of primary liver disease** **Chronic rejection** PTLD

of when complications are more likely to occur facilitates diagnosis and treatment. The imaging appearances and management of the most common complications following liver transplantation from deceased and living donors will be discussed.

VASCULAR COMPLICATIONS

Vascular complications are the most worrisome complication in the immediate postoperative period as they are associated with a high incidence of graft loss and mortality.[10,11] These events have been reported to occur in around 7% of DDLT and 13% of LDLT.[6] Overall, vascular complications are the second most frequent cause of graft failure, after rejection.

Postsurgical Anatomy and Imaging Approach

Hepatic artery, portal vein, and inferior vena cava (IVC) vascular anastomoses in the liver allograft are all potential sites of complications. The hepatic arterial anastomosis is the most variable and most frequently associated with complications. The donor common hepatic artery is most commonly attached to the recipient proper, right, or left hepatic artery depending on alignment and size match of the recipient and donor vessels. A "fish mouth" anastomosis (used in instances of caliber mismatch of the donor and recipient arteries) results in focal dilation of the vessel at the anastomosis and should not be confused with a pseudoaneurysm.[12] A donor iliac artery interposition graft is directly anastomosed to the recipient aorta to serve as a conduit for the donor hepatic artery in cases of severe atherosclerosis/narrowing of the recipient celiac or hepatic arteries.

End-to-end anastomosis between donor and recipient portal veins is commonly performed. The donor portal vein can also be anastomosed to the recipient superior mesenteric vein or preexisting portosystemic shunt using an interposition jump graft in cases of recipient chronic portal vein thrombus.[13] A piggyback technique for DDLT is commonly used for creating the IVC anastomosis where the donor IVC is anastomosed to the recipient hepatic vein confluence.[13] A less commonly used technique for IVC anastomosis involves resection of recipient retrohepatic IVC and anastomosis of donor IVC superiorly and inferiorly to recipient IVC. LDLT requires more complex venous reconstruction due to the need to preserve donor and recipient IVC. Autologous veins or synthetic grafts are often used to connect donor hepatic veins to the recipient IVC.

Doppler ultrasound is the initial imaging examination for evaluation of the liver transplant vasculature, as this examination can be performed at the bedside in the immediate postoperative period.[14] Abnormal spectral Doppler of the hepatic artery should prompt investigation of the more proximal artery to evaluate for vessel thrombosis or narrowing. Suspected vessel thrombus or stricture on gray scale ultrasound can be confirmed with Doppler examination or contrast-enhanced ultrasound.[15] Contrast-enhanced CT with both arterial and portal venous phases is useful in certain cases if the liver is not well visualized by ultrasound, vessel narrowing or thrombus is equivocal by ultrasound, and there is high clinical suspicion for vasculature complication.[16] Catheter angiography is useful in the treatment of vessel narrowing or thrombosis. MR angiography plays a limited role for acute assessment of vascular complications given the increased time it takes to perform the examination and the decreased spatial resolution limiting evaluation of smaller caliber arteries.

Hepatic Artery

Hepatic artery thrombosis (HAT) in the early postoperative setting is the most common vascular complication and carries high mortality and graft failure rate. Early recognition can allow for salvage of the graft with surgical revascularization (arterial reconstruction, thrombectomy, or re-transplantation). Ultrasound approaches nearly 100% sensitivity for detection of this condition, manifested as an absence of flow in the proper hepatic and intrahepatic arteries using color Doppler[17] (**Fig. 1**). Important pitfalls that can lead to false positive results include hepatic edema, hepatic artery stenosis (HAS), vasopressor use, or systemic hypotension. Elevated resistive indices (resistive index > 0.8) are nonspecific in the immediate postoperative period and should prompt follow-up in the context of otherwise normal flow. Correlation with clinical status, serum markers, and evaluation with dedicated CT or conventional angiography, or contrast-enhanced ultrasound can confirm the diagnosis in these cases. Late HAT leads to the development of collateral arterial vasculature manifesting as early as 2 weeks after surgery.[18] A more robust blood supply may fully supply the biliary tree and be asymptomatic, though arterial perfusion compromise may lead to some degree of biliary necrosis, causing cholangitis, abscesses, and bilomas. Imaging findings include non-visualization of the main hepatic artery, with Doppler demonstrating slow intrahepatic arterial flow and blunted systolic peaks, decreased resistive indices, and a mild parvus tardus Doppler waveform.[9]

Stenosis of the hepatic artery (**Fig. 2**) can be early or late in onset with clinical manifestations similar to late HAT. The combination of "*parvus tardus*" Doppler waveform, peak systolic velocity less than 48 cm/s in the hepatic artery distal to the stenosis, resistive index less than 0.4, and acceleration time longer than 0.12 s increases specificity and decreases false positive rate for diagnosis of HAS.[19,20] CT angiography is then helpful to localize the exact site of stenosis for treatment planning. Stenosis is most common at the hepatic arterial anastomosis. Management includes angioplasty with or without stent placement, surgical revision, or re-transplantation. Endovascular treatment is first line with a high technical success rate.[21] Although celiac artery stenosis may mimic HAS with findings of "*parvus tardus*" on spectral Doppler and decreased arterial resistive index, it can be distinguished from HAS by comparing hepatic artery waveform with splenic artery waveform. Both hepatic and splenic artery waveforms are abnormal with celiac artery stenosis, whereas only hepatic artery waveform is abnormal with HAS.[22] It is important to identify the presence of celiac artery stenosis in potential liver transplant recipients before transplantation as celiac artery stenosis compromises arterial blood flow to a transplanted liver more so than a native liver.[22] Unlike in a transplanted liver, collateral arterials develop to supply the native liver as celiac artery narrowing worsens.

Hepatic artery pseudoaneurysm after transplantation (**Fig. 3**) is an uncommon complication, typically asymptomatic and occurring at the site of the arterial anastomosis, usually mycotic in the setting of angioplasty.[12] Additional etiologies include hepaticojejunostomy with bile leak, primary sclerosing cholangitis (PSC), or biopsy. A ruptured pseudoaneurysm may present with hemorrhagic shock and intra-abdominal hemorrhage. Additional complication may involve fistulation with an adjacent biliary tree or bowel, presenting with upper gastrointestinal bleeding. At ultrasound, the diagnosis is made with identification of a cystic structure along

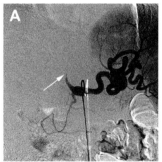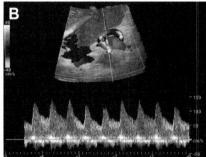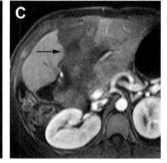

Fig. 1. Digital subtraction angiography shows completely occluded donor hepatic artery at the anastomosis (*arrow*, *A*). Hepatic artery is not visualized as a branch from the celiac artery on color Doppler ultrasound (*B*). Contrast-enhanced MR demonstrates occluded hepatic artery with development of large infarct/biloma (*arrow*, *C*).

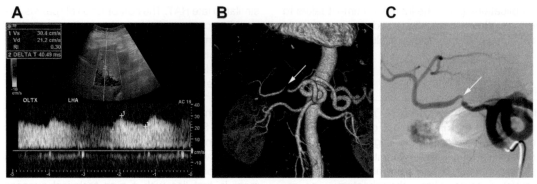

Fig. 2. Spectral Doppler ultrasound (*A*) downstream of hepatic artery stenosis shows "*parvus tardus*" waveform with decreased peak systolic velocity, low resistive index, and prolonged acceleration time. Coronal CT angiography 3D reconstruction (*B*) shows severe narrowing at the hepatic artery anastomosis (*arrow, B*), confirmed on Digital subtraction angiography (*arrow, C*).

the hepatic artery with internal turbulent swirling flow. CT and MR demonstrate an arterially enhancing, rounded lesion that follows the blood pool; distinction from a normal fish mouth arterial anastomosis is paramount. Management options include both surgical resection and endovascular embolization.

Portal Vein

Portal vein complications, including thrombosis and stenosis, are less common than arterial complications with an incidence of 1% to 3%.[23,24] Portal vein thrombosis (PVT) tends to occur in the first 4 weeks after transplant, whereas stenosis is most likely to present more than 12 months posttransplant.[9] Thrombosis of the portal vein typically affects the main extrahepatic segment. Ultrasound findings initially demonstrate an echogenic filling

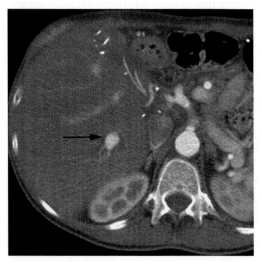

Fig. 3. Axial CT angiography shows focal dilation of right posterior hepatic artery (*arrow*) consistent with pseudoaneurysm post-right lobe liver transplantation.

defect with corresponding absent or partial flow on Doppler; thrombi eventually become anechoic. CT and MR can confirm the diagnosis. Treatment ranges from anticoagulation to direct intervention with stent placement, angioplasty, thrombolysis, or thrombectomy. On Doppler ultrasound, portal vein stenosis (PVS) (**Fig. 4**) demonstrates a peak anastomotic (AS) velocity greater than 125 cm/s, AS-to-pre-AS velocity ratio 3:1, and a velocity change of 60 cm/s across the anastomosis.[25,26] Potential pitfall when examining portal vein velocities can occur in the early postoperative period where portal vein velocities can be higher than in a native liver due to reduced portal venous resistance in the new organ. Mean portal vein velocity in a transplanted liver can be up to 58 cm/s, whereas normal native liver portal vein velocities are lower, ranging from 16 to 40 cm/s.[25] PVS can be treated with angioplasty and stent placement.

Hepatic Veins and Inferior Vena Cava

Complications involving the hepatic veins and IVC are uncommon. A higher incidence is appreciated in LDLT (up to 5%) due to the more complex venous reconstruction.[12] Patients with IVC/hepatic vein stenosis (HVS) and thrombosis can present with ascites and symptoms of acute Budd-Chiari due to the hepatic outflow obstruction. The piggyback AS technique preserves the recipient IVC by means of a blind-ending common stump. This technique has a slightly higher risk of acute hepatic outflow obstruction from kinking or graft torsion.[27,28] The blind-ending donor caval stump created during the piggyback technique often thromboses and this should not be mistaken for IVC thrombus. Abnormal monophasic venous waveform (normally triphasic waveform due to transmitted pressures from the right atrium) is sensitive for venous outflow obstruction, but not

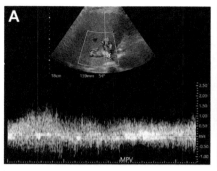
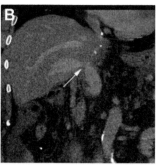
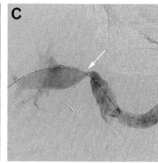

Fig. 4. Spectral Doppler ultrasound (*A*) demonstrates elevated velocity in the portal vein at the anastomosis. Contrast-enhanced CT (*B*) and DSA (*C*) demonstrate narrowing at the portal vein anastomosis consistent with severe stenosis (*arrow, B* and *C*).

specific for venous stenosis, as it can also be seen with extrinsic compression on the allograft from collections. A pulsatility index (quantifies phasicity of waveform), however, allows for more specificity as a value less than 0.45 has a 95% specificity for stenosis.[25] CT or MR venography in setting of HVS demonstrates the change in caliber of the vessel and usually heterogeneous hepatic enhancement due to venous congestion and sinusoidal dilatation (**Fig. 5**). Treatment includes venoplasty with or without stent placement and anticoagulation. Thrombosis of the IVC or hepatic vein can be visualized with ultrasound as an echogenic intraluminal filling defect and can be more readily assessed with a contrast-enhanced CT or MR.

BILIARY COMPLICATIONS

Biliary complications occur in up to a third of liver transplant patients. They are more frequent in LDLT than in DDLT, and most are diagnosed within 6 months of the transplant.

Postsurgical Anatomy and Imaging Approach

The liver transplant biliary reconstructions include a choledocholedochostomy (end-to-end or end-to-side duct-to-duct anastomosis) and a hepaticojejunostomy with creation of a Roux-en-Y loop. Although multiple factors drive the choice of the surgical approach, most DDLT are performed using a choledocholedochostomy, whereas a hepaticojejunostomy is commonly used in LDLT.[29] Hepaticojejunostomy is also preferred when there is a disparity between donor and recipient duct size or there is underlying biliary disease involving the recipient extrahepatic duct. Although ultrasound is the first-line imaging modality in liver transplant patients presenting with suspected biliary complications, most patients are evaluated with cross-sectional imaging including MR cholangiography (MRC) and contrast-enhanced CT.[30] In our institution, MRC is performed using axial and coronal T2-weighted single shot fast spin-echo imaging, 2-dimensional and 3-dimensional MRCP, axial T1-weighted gradient echo, and axial diffusion-weighted imaging.

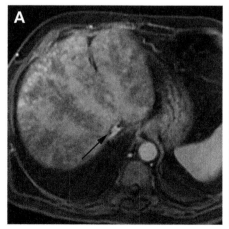
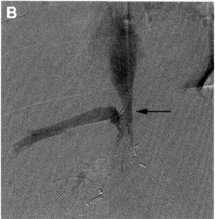

Fig. 5. Contrast-enhanced MR shows heterogeneous enhancement of the liver consistent with congestion/edema and tapering of the IVC near the cavocaval anastomosis (*arrow, A*). Right hepatic venogram confirms narrowing at the hepatic venous anastomosis (*arrow, B*). Liver biopsy demonstrated sinusoidal obstruction syndrome.

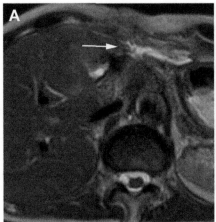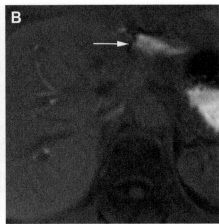

Fig. 6. Axial T2-weighted (*A*) and axial T1-weighted 30 minutes post-Gd-EOB-DTPA MR imaging show a perihepatic fluid collection (*arrow, A*) containing contrast on the hepatobiliary phase image (*arrow, B*) confirming the presence of a biloma. (Courtesy of R Girometti, MD, Udine, Italy.)

Pineapple juice or a solution containing diluted gadolinium can improve the MRC image quality decreasing the T2 signal of the fluid in stomach, duodenum, and proximal jejunum. A gadolinium-ethoxybenzyl-diethylenetriamine pentaacetic acid (Gd-EOB-DTPA) enhanced MRC may provide additional information in case of bile leak and AS strictures. When injecting Gd-EOB-DTPA, the T2-weighted MRCP images should be obtained before contrast administration, as the excretion of gadolinium into the bile ducts decreases their T2 signal and visualization.

Bile Leak

Bile leak is the most frequent biliary complication occurring in about 8% in DDLT and 10% in LDLT with the highest incidence in the first month after transplantation and usually due to ischemia or technical issues.[7] Common sites of leak include the entry site of the T-tube after tube removal, biliary anastomosis, and liver cut surface. CT and MRC are the preferred imaging methods for evaluation of a clinically suspected biliary leak. T2-hyperintense fluid collection is visible in the peri- and subhepatic space. Confirmation of a bile leak as the cause of the fluid collection can be achieved with a Gd-EOB-DTPA-enhanced MRC; the presence of contrast within the collection on the hepatobiliary phase (at least 20–30 minutes post-contrast administration) confirms the diagnosis of bile leak (**Fig. 6**).[31] Alternatively, a bile leak can also be confirmed using hepatobiliary

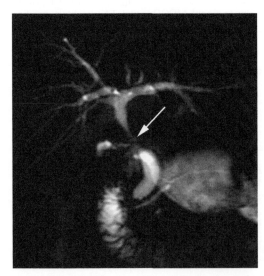

Fig. 7. MRC image shows severe narrowing (*arrow*) at the duct-to-duct anastomosis in a DDLT with mild intrahepatic biliary ductal dilatation.

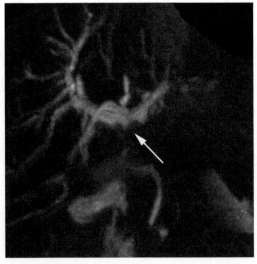

Fig. 8. MRC image shows biliary dilation upstream of hepaticojejunostomy (*arrow*) in a DDLT, consistent with anastomotic stricture.

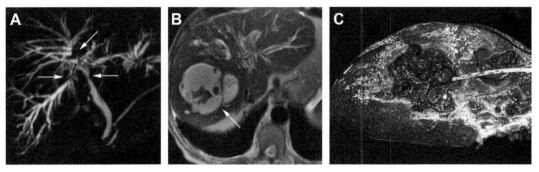

Fig. 9. MRC (A) showing multifocal ischemic-type biliary strictures (arrows). (B) Axial T2-weighted MR image obtained 1 year later shows new complex right hepatic fluid collection (arrow) most compatible with biloma, proven at explant (C).

iminodiacetic acid scintigraphy. Management options include the placement of a draining catheter using cross-sectional imaging guidance, surgery, endoscopic stent placement, or a percutaneous transhepatic cholangiogram (PTC) with internal–external drainage.[32]

Biliary Strictures

Biliary strictures can be classified as AS and non-AS (NAS) stricture. The AS stricture (Figs. 7 and 8) occurs in 5% to 15% of cases after DDLT and 28% to 32% of cases after LDLT[8] due to technical failure or late for ischemia or scarring. On MRC, it manifests as the absence of T2 signal in a short segment of bile duct at the anastomosis with or without ductal dilatation. A review of the thin-slice MRC images is recommended, as the maximum intensity projection may overestimate the degree of stenosis. The sensitivity of MRC for the diagnosis of AS is up to 92% in case of duct-to-duct anastomosis and up to 58% in case of a hepaticojejunostomy.[33]

Gd-EOB-DTPA-enhanced MRC may provide a functional assessment of the biliary stenosis and an improved visualization of the hepaticojejunostomy. The causes of non-AS biliary strictures include HAT (macroangiopathic damage), microangiopathic damage (patent hepatic artery; ischemic-type biliary lesions), infection, and recurrent biliary disease (eg, PSC). NAS ischemic-type biliary strictures are usually multifocal, located only in the biliary system of the donor, and are associated with variable degree of upstream biliary ductal dilatation. The most common site of ischemic injury is the hepatic confluence (Fig. 9). Treatment options include endoscopic stent placement and PTC with internal–external drainage. For ischemic cholangiopathy, the condition is not reversible, and definitive treatment may be retransplantation.[32]

Biliary Stones, Sludge, or Casts

Biliary stones and sludge may occur in association with biliary strictures due to the decreased flow of

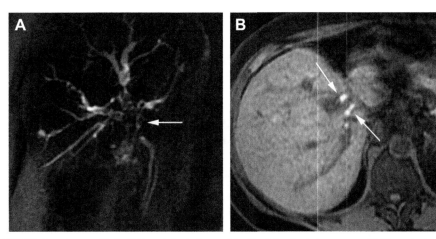

Fig. 10. MRC (A) showing multiple filling defects (arrow) in the bile ducts in a case of bilio-enteric anastomosis. (B) Axial T1-weighted unenhanced MR confirms shows corresponding high signal intensity in the bile ducts in keeping with stones (arrows).

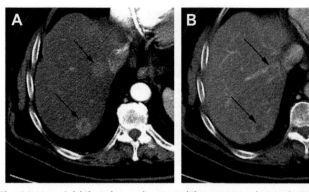
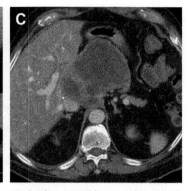

Fig. 11. Arterial (*A*) and portal venous (*B*) contrast-enhanced axial CT show multiple arterial hyperenhancing lesions with washout (*arrows* in *A* and *B*), consistent with multifocal recurrent hepatocellular carcinoma post-liver transplantation. Additional bulky periportal adenopathy reflecting extrahepatic disease (*C*).

bile. Biliary sludge is more problematic in the first-year posttransplantation, whereas stones are a more chronic complication.[34] Stones appear as round T1-hyperintense biliary filling defects (**Fig. 10**), whereas sludge appears as layering T1-hyperintense signal in the bile ducts. Biliary casts are from sloughed ischemic epithelium and appear as T1-hyperintense linear filling defects in the bile ducts.[34] Biliary stone, sludge, and casts can be differentiated from pneumobilia when in a dependent position in the dilated duct and when showing T1-hyperintense signal.

PARENCHYMAL COMPLICATIONS
Immediate Complications

The most common cause of graft failure is rejection with acute cellular rejection typically occurring within the first 90 days after transplantation.[35] Liver allograft heterogeneity on ultrasound may be the only imaging manifestation of rejection, but the finding is nonspecific.[36] Ultimately, the

diagnosis of rejection is achieved through histologic analysis of a liver biopsy with imaging used as an adjunct to rule out mechanical causes for allograft dysfunction.

Imaging plays a role in the diagnosis of immediate posttransplant fluid collections. Small volume perihepatic fluid is common in the immediate postoperative period and typically resolves within a few weeks without intervention. Larger perihepatic collections with mass effect on surrounding structures require drainage. Seroma and biloma are typically homogeneous collections that mimic water on imaging (anechoic on ultrasound, near-water attenuating on CT, and T1-hypointense/T2-hyperintense on MR imaging). Hematoma and abscess are heterogeneous collections with imaging appearance of hematoma changing over time. Acute hematomas are usually T1-hyperintense, attenuate around 45 to 70 HU on CT, and heterogeneous on ultrasound. Hematomas liquefy over time, developing complex internal septations on ultrasound to ultimately

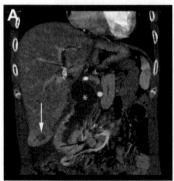
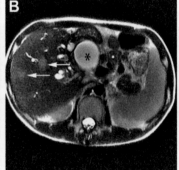
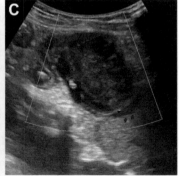

Fig. 12. Coronal contrast-enhanced CT (*A*) demonstrates circumferential jejunal mass involving hepatobiliary limb (*asterisk*), hypodense liver lesion (*white arrow*), and mesenteric adenopathy (*black arrow*). Axial T2-weighted MR (*B*) demonstrates multiple T2-hyperintense liver lesions (*arrows*) and upstream dilation of hepatobiliary limb from downstream mass (*asterisk*). Ultrasound-guided biopsy of jejunal mass (*C*) demonstrated PTLD.

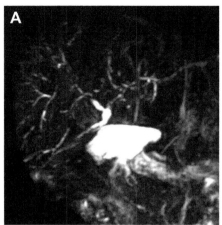 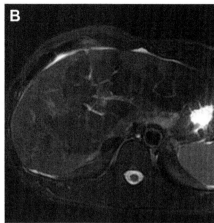

Fig. 13. MRC (*A*) demonstrates recurrent PSC in a DDLT with multiple short segment intrahepatic biliary strictures with normal caliber or slightly dilated intervening segment. Axial T2-weighted MR (*B*) demonstrates heterogeneous hepatic parenchymal signal with biopsy-proven recurrence of advanced fibrosis/cirrhosis.

become more homogeneous. Abscesses can have thick irregular rim enhancement and gas locules. Percutaneous aspiration with fluid analysis is the most reliable method to characterize post-transplant collections.

Late Complications

Chronic rejection occurs after 6 months in about 2% of patients.[37] Like acute rejection, diagnosis requires a liver biopsy with chronic rejection demonstrating ductopenia and cholestasis at histology.[38]

There is an increased risk for malignancy in the liver allograft due to long-term immunosuppression and risk factors that caused the end-stage liver disease such as viral hepatitis. Malignancies that develop in the transplanted liver include recurrent primary liver tumors, metastases when liver transplant is performed in patients with neuroendocrine tumor or colorectal primaries, tumors associated with immunosuppression such as Kaposi sarcoma, and posttransplant lymphoproliferative disorder (PTLD).[39] Most cases of recurrent hepatocellular carcinoma (HCC) occur within 2 years posttransplantation in up to 20% of cases.[40] Recurrent HCC in a transplanted liver is more likely to present with multiple lesions and extrahepatic disease due to immunosuppression[41] (**Fig. 11**). Recurrent cholangiocarcinoma post-liver transplant can manifest as a new malignant stricture at the biliary anastomosis or intrahepatic mass.[42] Older patients with higher preoperative cancer antigen 19-9 levels (>100 U/mL) and with larger tumors (>2 cm residual tumor in explant) are more likely to have cholangiocarcinoma recurrence in the transplant.[43] PTLD most commonly presents as new lymphadenopathy

mimicking lymphoma but can also manifest as a solid hypovascular tumor or multiple masses (**Fig. 12**). The tumors are known to affect the kidneys, adrenal glands, and bowel.[44]

The frequency of recurrent PSC significantly increases over time with 32% of liver transplant patients followed for greater than 15 years demonstrating recurrent disease.[45] PSC recurrence in liver transplant has similar imaging features to PSC in the native liver with the development of multiple short-segment strictures with normal caliber or slightly dilated (beading) of intervening segments (**Fig. 13**).

SUMMARY

As a growing number of liver transplantations are being performed, it is critical to promptly recognize and manage the postoperative complications so that the liver allograft is not lost. Imaging plays a central role in the diagnosis of vascular and biliary complications, perihepatic collections, and recurrent or new disease in the hepatic allograft. Knowledge of whether a complication is more common in the immediate or late postoperative period helps to direct the patient to the proper imaging study to narrow the differential diagnosis and tailor management.

CLINICS CARE POINTS

- Vascular and biliary complications have been shown to occur more frequently in living donor liver transplantation than deceased donor liver transplantation.

- Vascular complications, especially hepatic arterial thrombosis, are among the most worrisome liver transplantation complications in the immediate postoperative period. Doppler ultrasound serves as the initial imaging test of choice to evaluate for vascular complications.

- Most biliary complications occur within 6 months of liver transplantation. Although ultrasound is the first line imaging modality, most patients eventually undergo MR cholangiography. Common biliary complications include bile leak, biliary strictures, and biliary stones.

- Imaging plays an important role to diagnose late complications such as vessel stenosis, recurrent hepatocellular carcinoma, or recurrence of primary liver disease.

DISCLOSURE

A. Furlan provided consultation to Bracco Diagnostics for a topic unrelated to this article.

REFERENCES

1. American Liver Foundation. 2022. Available at: https://liverfoundation.org/about-your-liver/facts-about-liver-disease/how-many-people-have-liver-disease/. Accessed December 17, 2022.
2. Centers for Disease Control and Prevention. 2020. Available at: https://www.cdc.gov/nchs/fastats/liver-disease.htm . Accessed December 17, 2022.
3. Barber K, Blackwell J, Collett D, et al, UK Transplant Liver Advisory Group. Life expectancy of adult liver allograft recipients in the UK. Gut 2007;56(2):279–82.
4. Organ Procurement and Transplantation Network. 2022. Available at: https://optn.transplant.hrsa.gov/data/view-data-reports/national-data/# . Accessed December 17, 2022.
5. Thuluvath PJ, Guidinger MK, Fung JJ, et al. Liver transplantation in the United States, 1999-2008. Am J Transplant 2010;10(4 Pt 2):1003–19.
6. Khalaf H. Vascular complications after deceased and living donor liver transplantation: a single-center experience. Transplant Proc 2010;42(3):865–70.
7. Kochhar G, Parungao JM, Hanouneh IA, et al. Biliary complications following liver transplantation. World J Gastroenterol 2013;19(19):2841–6.
8. Lee HW, Shah NH, Lee SK. An Update on endoscopic management of post-liver transplant biliary complications. Clin Endosc 2017;50(5):451–63.
9. Craig EV, Heller MT. Complications of liver transplant. Abdom Radiol (NY) 2021;46(1):43–67.
10. Duffy JP, Hong JC, Farmer DG, et al. Vascular complications of orthotopic liver transplantation: experience in more than 4,200 patients. J Am Coll Surg 2009;208(5):896–905.
11. Piardi T, Lhuaire M, Bruno O, et al. Vascular complications following liver transplantation: A literature review of advances in 2015. World J Hepatol 2016;8(1):36–57.
12. Brookmeyer CE, Bhatt S, Fishman EK, et al. Multimodality Imaging after Liver Transplant: Top 10 Important Complications. Radiographics 2022;42(3):702–21.
13. Alhawsawi AM, del Rio MJ. Surgical techniques in liver transplantation. In: Wagener G, editor. Liver anesthesiology and critical care medicine. New York, NY: Springer; 2012. p. 83–95.
14. Crossin JD, Muradali D, Wilson SR. US of liver transplants: normal and abnormal. Radiographics 2003;23(5):1093–114.
15. Goh Y, Neo WT, Teo YM, et al. Role of contrast-enhanced ultrasound in the evaluation of post-liver transplant vasculature. Clin Radiol 2020;75(11):832–44.
16. Boraschi P, Della Pina MC, Donati F. Graft complications following orthotopic liver transplantation: Role of non-invasive cross-sectional imaging techniques. Eur J Radiol 2016;85(7):1271–83.
17. Horrow MM, Blumenthal BM, Reich DJ, et al. Sonographic diagnosis and outcome of hepatic artery thrombosis after orthotopic liver transplantation in adults. AJR Am J Roentgenol 2007;189(2):346–51.
18. García Bernardo CM, Argüelles García B, Redondo Buil P, et al. Collateral Development in Thrombosis of the Hepatic Artery After Transplantation. Transplant Proc 2016;48(9):3006–9.
19. Zheng BW, Tan YY, Fu BS, et al. Tardus parvus waveforms in Doppler ultrasonography for hepatic artery stenosis after liver transplantation: can a new cut-off value guide the next step? Abdom Radiol (NY) 2018;43(7):1634–41.
20. Park YS, Kim KW, Lee SJ, et al. Hepatic arterial stenosis assessed with doppler US after liver transplantation: frequent false-positive diagnoses with tardus parvus waveform and value of adding optimal peak systolic velocity cutoff. Radiology 2011;260(3):884–91.
21. Chen J, Weinstein J, Black S, et al. Surgical and endovascular treatment of hepatic arterial complications following liver transplant. Clin Transpl 2014;28(12):1305e12.
22. Horrow MM, Huynh ML, Callaghan MM, et al. Complications after liver transplant related to preexisting conditions: diagnosis, treatment, and prevention. Radiographics 2020;40(3):895–909.
23. Pérez-Saborido B, Pacheco-Sánchez D, Barrera-Rebollo A, et al. Incidence, management, and results of vascular complications after liver transplantation. Transplant Proc 2011;43(3):749–50.

24. Langnas AN, Marujo W, Stratta RJ, et al. Vascular complications after orthotopic liver transplantation. Am J Surg 1991;161(1):76–83.
25. Chong WK, Beland JC, Weeks SM. Sonographic evaluation of venous obstruction in liver transplants. AJR Am J Roentgenol 2007;188(6):W515–21.
26. Mullan CP, Siewert B, Kane RA, et al. Can Doppler sonography discern between hemodynamically significant and insignificant portal vein stenosis after adult liver transplantation? AJR Am J Roentgenol 2010;195(6):1438–43.
27. Parrilla P, Sánchez-Bueno F, Figueras J, et al. Analysis of the complications of the piggy-back technique in 1,112 liver transplants. Transplantation 1999;67(9):1214–7.
28. Settmacher U, Nüssler NC, Glanemann M, et al. Venous complications after orthotopic liver transplantation. Clin Transplant 2000;14(3):235–41.
29. Chupetlovska KP, Borhani AA, Dasyam AK, et al. Post-operative imaging anatomy in liver transplantation. Abdom Radiol 2021;46(1):9–16.
30. Girometti R, Como G, Bazzocchi M, et al. Post-operative imaging liver transplantation: state-of-the-art and future perspectives. World J Gastroenterol 2014;20(20):6180–200.
31. Boraschi P, Donati F. Postoperative biliary adverse events following orthotopic liver transplantation: assessment with magnetic resonance cholangiography. World J Gastroenterol 2014;20(32):11080–94.
32. Naidu SG, Alzubaidi SJ, Patel IJ, et al. Interventional radiology management of adult liver transplant complications. Radiographics 2022;42(6):1705–23.
33. Kinner S, Dechene A, Paul A, et al. Detection of biliary stenoses in patients after liver transplantation: Is there a different diagnostic accuracy of MRCP depending on the type of biliary anastomosis? Eur J Radiol 2011;80(2):e20–8.
34. Allard R, Smith C, Zhong J, et al. Imaging post liver transplantation part II: biliary complications. Clin Radiol 2020;75(11):854–63.
35. Neuberger J, Adams DH. What is the significance of acute liver allograft rejection? J Hepatol 1998;29(1):143–50.
36. Bhargava P, Vaidya S, Dick AAS, et al. Imaging of orthotopic liver transplantation: Review. Am J Roentgenol 2011;196:15–25.
37. NHS Blood and Transplant. Available at: https://www.nhsbt.nhs.uk/organ-transplantation/liver/benefits-and-risks-of-a-liver-transplant/risks-of-a-liver-transplant/rejection-of-a-transplanted-liver/. Accessed December 17, 2022.
38. Burton JR Jr, Rosen HR. Diagnosis and management of allograft failure. Clin Liver Dis 2006;10(2):407.
39. Chatrath H, Berman K, Vuppalanchi R, et al. De novo malignancy post-liver transplantation: a single center, population controlled study. Clin Transplant 2013;27(4):582–90.
40. Filgueira NA. Hepatocellular carcinoma recurrence after liver transplantation: Risk factors, screening and clinical presentation. World J Hepatol 2019;11(3):261–72.
41. Na GH, Hong TH, You YK, et al. Clinical analysis of patients with hepatocellular carcinoma recurrence after living-donor liver transplantation. World J Gastroenterol 2016;22:5790–9.
42. Herbener T, Zajko AB, Koneru B, et al. Recurrent cholangiocarcinoma in the biliary tree after liver transplantation. Radiology 1988;169(3):641–2.
43. Heimbach JK, Gores GJ, Haddock MG, et al. Predictors of disease recurrence following neoadjuvant chemoradiotherapy and liver transplantation for unresectable perihilar cholangiocarcinoma. Transplantation 2006;82(12):1703–7.
44. Baheti AD, Sanyal R, Heller MT, et al. Surgical Techniques and Imaging Complications of Liver Transplant. Radiol Clin North Am 2016;54:199–215.
45. Sagvand BT, McCullough A. Recurrent Primary Sclerosing Cholangitis in Transplanted Liver: A Longitudinal Cohort. Am J Gastroenterol 2018;113:S490–1.

Renal Transplantation
Pretransplant Workup, Surgical Techniques, and Surgical Anatomy

Constantine M. Burgan, MD[a],*, David Summerlin, MD[b],
Mark E. Lockhart, MD[c]

KEYWORDS

• Renal transplant • Pretransplant • Living donor • Deceased donor

KEY POINTS

- Renal transplantation remains the best treatment of end-stage renal disease.
- CT and MRI have become cornerstones in assessing donor kidneys and anatomy because they can assess kidney volumes, important incidental findings, and anatomic variants, thereby improving success and decreasing donor risks.
- Knowledge of current donor explant surgeries and techniques for implantation is helpful for radiologists assessing patients postoperatively.

INTRODUCTION, HISTORY, AND BACKGROUND

End-stage renal disease is a growing problem worldwide, driven in the United States largely by hypertension and diabetes mellitus. The preferred treatment that offers patients the best long-term outcome and quality of life is renal transplantation. Within the broader context of medical history, renal transplantation is a relatively recent development. Although the first renal transplant was performed in a dog in 1902, the first human-to-human renal transplant of a deceased donor did not occur until 1933. Although the recipient died shortly after transplantation, this prompted further interest and research into the field. A major advancement occurred in 1954 with the first successful renal transplantation involving a living renal donor. In spite of these surgical advances, long-term success of renal transplants was limited until the introduction of immunosuppressive medications in 1962. During the 1960s, 1-year graft survival rates increased from 67% to 92%. Through advancements in various imaging modalities including ultrasound in the 1950s and computed tomography (CT) in the 1970s, physicians were afforded better ways to evaluate patients both before and after renal transplantation.[1]

Although renal transplants may come from either deceased or living donors, living donor renal transplants demonstrate higher rates of graft survival. Advances in immunosuppressive medications and posttransplant management have contributed greatly to the success of transplantation programs; however, the expansion of living donor programs has driven much of the growth. More than 150,000 living donor renal transplants have been performed in the United States and more than 35,000 are performed annually across the globe.[2] Expansion of living donor programs can be attributed to both improvements to the process by which potential donors are identified as well as advances in surgical techniques. Traditionally, a donor nephrectomy was performed through an open approach, which presents significant challenges in the case of a living donor. However,

[a] Department of Radiology, University of Alabama-Birmingham, 625 19th Street South JT N316, Birmingham, AL 35233, USA; [b] Department of Radiology, University of Alabama-Birmingham, 625 19th Street South JT N370A, Birmingham, AL 35233, USA; [c] Department of Radiology, University of Alabama-Birmingham, 619 19th Street South JTN 344, Birmingham, AL 35233, USA
* Corresponding author.
E-mail address: cburgan@uabmc.edu

Radiol Clin N Am 61 (2023) 797–808
https://doi.org/10.1016/j.rcl.2023.04.003

through the development of laparoscopic donor nephrectomy in 1995, donors now experience less pain, shorter hospital stays, faster recovery times, and quicker return to work.[3]

Donor Risks of Renal Transplantation

Patient education and communication of risks and benefits are important elements in the early stages of the pretransplant donor evaluation. With respect to short-term risks of donor nephrectomy, the risk of minor complication such as nausea may be seen in up to 10% to 20% of patients. Risk of major complication (such as bleeding, infection, or death) is low, occurring in less than 3%, with even lower mortality risk (occurring in less than 0.03%). The long-term risk of donor nephrectomy has been a subject of debate with some recent studies identifying a small but not significantly increased risk of the donor developing end-stage renal disease when compared with healthy nondonors. As such, donor programs in the United States are required to inform potential donors of the small donor-attributable increased risk.[2]

Renal Donation Pretransplant Evaluation and Imaging Modalities

Pretransplant imaging of the potential donor is critical in identifying a suitable donor. In addition to dedicated imaging of the potential donor kidneys, a chest radiograph is recommended in order to screen for the presence of cardiopulmonary disease. There are numerous factors that would preclude a patient from donating a kidney including vascular pathologic condition, anomalies, or underlying renal pathologic condition such as malignancy, renal calculi beyond a certain threshold, or other underlying renal disease. Asymmetric renal size or function may also be a consideration. To assess the anatomy of potential donor kidneys, standard imaging protocols have been developed for the purposes of surgical planning and risk stratification. Contrast-enhanced computed tomography angiography (CTA) of the abdomen and pelvis is one such modality, which allows for detailed evaluation of both structural and vascular anatomy of the kidneys in a single study. Modern CTA renal donor protocols require a multiphase acquisition to evaluate anatomy of the arteries, veins, and renal collecting system, thereby resulting in higher patient radiation doses. Many institutions use a 4-phase protocol, which includes a noncontrast, series followed by additional series in the arterial, nephrographic, and excretory phases. Given radiation dose concerns associated with this technique, some institutions have used dual-energy technology in order to create a virtual

noncontrast series from iodine subtraction images, reducing the renal donor protocol to a 3-phase examination. Alternatively, as the primary utility of the noncontrast series relates to detection of renal collecting system calculi, some have argued that an appropriately timed arterial phase acquisition provides sufficient sensitivity for the detection of calculi given the absence of potentially confounding excreted contrast at this early phase of the examination. This strategy also effectively converts the examination to a 3-phase protocol, providing a significant dose reduction.[4]

The process of imaging donors may be considered a type of screening examination, and as such, the prospect of incidental findings is an important consideration when selecting the most appropriate study. In one study, incidental findings could be sufficiently characterized by multiphase CT in approximately 95% of cases with less than 5% requiring further imaging or workup.[4] Due to the sensitivity for stones and incidental lesions, the donor exclusion rate by imaging nearly doubled when CTA replaced the traditional workup. More than 50% of exclusions were due to the detection of stone disease not visible by radiographs.[5]

Contrast-enhanced magnetic resonance angiography (MRA) is another imaging modality that allows for detailed anatomic evaluation. Benefits of MRA technique include a lack of ionizing radiation as well as a lack of iodinated contrast, the latter representing a potentially significant benefit in specific patient populations, such as those with a severe contrast allergy. Although MRA has demonstrated a comparable level of accuracy to CTA in some studies, this has not been consistently demonstrated, particularly with respect to the evaluation of the venous anatomy or in detection of small accessory renal arteries.[3] Further, in comparison to CTA, MRA technique has been shown to be less sensitive in the detection of small urinary tract calculi or other calcifications—in which case, it may be coupled with noncontrast CT imaging. Additional potential limitations of MRA include artifact associated with patient motion as well as smaller coverage area, which could result in failure to identify accessory renal vessels originating from the distal aorta or iliac arteries.[4]

Imaging alternatives to CTA and MRA include Doppler ultrasound and digital subtraction angiography (DSA). Doppler ultrasound offers potentially useful information regarding both structural and vascular anatomy; however, there is a variety of inherent limitations with this technique including the potential for poor visualization. Although DSA provides excellent vascular assessment, this modality is invasive and provides limited information about renal structural anatomy. Given these limitations, these alternative imaging strategies are mostly utilized to evaluate specific concerns or to characterize abnormalities that are detected on CTA or MRA.

Postprocessing of images acquired by CTA or MRA has become a particularly useful part of the donor evaluation and a valuable tool for presurgical planning. Components of postprocessing include 3D reformatting for renal volume calculations as well as vascular anatomy. Maximal intensity projection (MIP) and multiplanar reformatting (MPR), including curved MPR, are also of particular value when performing measurements of the vascular anatomy and identifying accessory vessels. For example, small accessory renal arteries may seem less conspicuous on axial images than on reformatted MIP images. Although variance in renal vascular anatomy is not uncommon, the degree of complexity and type of variance is of primary importance when selecting an appropriate renal donor. Although the left kidney is often preferred for donor harvesting given the longer venous pedicle, the donor kidney with less complex vascular anatomy is often selected.[4]

Renal Donor Imaging Evaluation and Relevant Findings

Although a variety of factors contribute to a decision to select one imaging modality over another, CTA has remained the preferred modality in renal donor examinations given widespread availability, rapid acquisition, and high accuracy. Apart from evaluation of the relevant renal anatomy, CTA of the abdomen and pelvis also offers the potential to screen for malignancy outside the kidneys, which could preclude transplantation.[6] Regardless which method of renal donor imaging is selected, detailed evaluation of the renal parenchyma, vascular anatomy, and collecting system are crucial (**Fig. 1**).

STRUCTURED REPORT: CTA Abdomen Pelvis Renal Donor

RIGHT KIDNEY:
- RENAL ARTERY: [Single]
- RENAL VEIN: [Single]
- COLLECTING SYSTEM: [Single]
- RENAL CALCULI: [Absent]
- CYSTS/MASSES: [Absent]
- VOLUME: [ ] cm^3

LEFT KIDNEY:
- RENAL ARTERY: [Single]
- RENAL VEIN: [Single with conventional pre-aortic anatomy]
- COLLECTING SYSTEM: [Single]
- RENAL CALCULI: [Absent]
- CYSTS/MASSES: [Absent]
- VOLUME: [ ] cm^3

Fig. 1. Reporting template for renal donors at our institution. This includes the presence of renal lesions, stones, arterial/venous anomalies, and renal volumes.

As part of the renal parenchymal assessment, imaging is necessary to evaluate for the presence of an underlying cystic or solid lesion. The venous/nephrographic phase is most sensitive for small renal lesions but arterial phase can aid in the characterization. Small simple cysts and small benign neoplasms (<5 mm) are potentially eligible for renal donation. Even benign neoplasms larger than 5 mm may be eligible for renal donation as the neoplasm may be resected before transplantation. Because the kidney will be placed into an immunosuppressed recipient, any cancer risk is viewed with greater skepticism and may require surveillance or sampling before donation is allowed. Another important element of the parenchymal assessment includes measurements of renal length or volume, which have been shown to have prognostic value because it relates to function of a renal transplant during the first 36 months. In order to reduce the risk of renal insufficiency among living renal donors, estimation of renal function differences between kidneys plays an important role in donor kidney selection, particularly when there is a difference in renal length of more than 2 cm or when there is a renal parenchymal abnormality. Although split renal function has historically been calculated with radioisotope renal scintigraphy, this study is not available at all institutions. Subsequent studies have demonstrated renal volume to be an adequate surrogate to estimate relative function.[5] Given the ease with which volumetric data can be extracted from either CT or MR images, there is appeal in this method of estimating renal function.[7] One basic method of renal volume estimation involves entering multidimensional measurements into established formulas. Alternatively, volumetric data may be obtained either by manual tracing of the renal contour or, more recently, with automated segmentation techniques (**Fig. 2**). In the event that the function of one potential donor kidney is significantly less than the other, and in an effort to minimize risk to the donor, the kidney with lower function is generally chosen for transplantation in spite of complexity of vascular anatomy.[8] Criteria differ by institution but a 10% difference in volume is considered significant by our transplant surgeons, necessitating the smaller kidney be harvested. In these patients, the source image outlines are re-reviewed to ensure no measurement errors were present.

With respect to renal arterial anatomy, there are 2 principal categories, which include early or perihilar, branching and multiple or extrarenal arteries. Approximately 20% to 30% of kidneys will have multiple renal arteries historically, with a more recent series demonstrating 18% variance.[9]

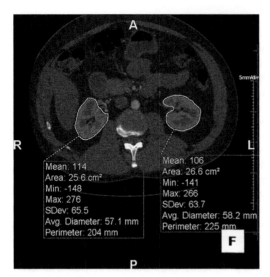

Fig. 2. Axial CT image with renal contour tracings, which are generated to calculate a 3-dimensional (3D) renal volume calculation. Studies have demonstrated 3D renal volume to be a useful tool for the estimation of relative renal function among potential renal donors.

Prevalence of early branching renal artery anatomy has been reported to be as high as 1 in 5 potential donors (**Figs. 3** and **4**). To classify as early branching, branching should be present within 20 mm of the origin, or in the case of the right renal artery, branching occurs either in a retrocaval location or within 10 mm of the right margin of the inferior vena cava (IVC). Extrarenal arteries constitute renal arteries that are of smaller caliber than the main renal artery and that have a separate origin. Extrarenal arteries include both accessory renal arteries, arteries which enter the kidney near the hilum, as well as aberrant renal arteries, which may course either through the renal parenchyma or along the renal capsule. Although the majority of extrarenal arteries originate via separate origin from the aorta, other sites have been reported including an iliac artery, superior mesenteric artery, inferior mesenteric artery, gonadal artery, and even an artery of the contralateral kidney. As it relates to donor selection, the presence of 2 or more extrarenal arteries or an extrarenal artery diameter of less than 3 mm results in higher risk of renal artery thrombosis. Furthermore, higher numbers of extrarenal arteries necessitates longer duration of the operation. Given the relatively small volume of renal parenchyma supplied, extrarenal arteries with a diameter of less than 2 mm could potentially be sacrificed. Importantly, however, even small extrarenal arteries of the lower pole must be preserved given higher rates of ureteral complications related to pyeloureteral necrosis that could result from sacrifice of a lower pole renal artery.[4] With respect to renal artery pathologic condition, fibromuscular dysplasia (FMD) and atherosclerotic disease are of particular importance. Although FMD has been traditionally considered a contraindication due to

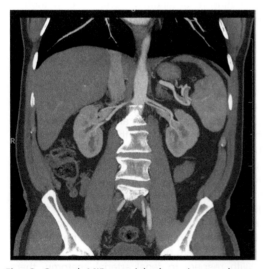

Fig. 3. Coronal MIP arterial phase image demonstrates early branching of involving the left renal artery. Identification of renal artery early branching is an important component of renal donor evaluation, both as it relates to donor kidney selection as well as surgical planning.

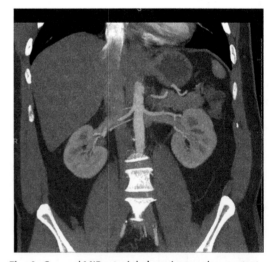

Fig. 4. Coronal MIP arterial phase image demonstrates early branching of the main right renal artery as well as a right extrarenal artery. Identification of renal artery anatomy including both early branching and extrarenal arteries are important components of renal donor evaluation, both as it relates to donor kidney selection as well as surgical planning.

presumed posttransplant hypertension risk, studies have shown that this may be performed safely, potentially with an arterial reconstruction.[10] Significant atherosclerotic disease is important to note given that endarterectomy may be necessary before renal donation.

Detailed evaluation of the venous anatomy is of particular importance in the donor presurgical evaluation. Variant renal venous anatomy is even more common than variant renal arterial anatomy, particularly on the left. Additionally, venous bleeding is the most common reason for the conversion from laparoscopic nephrectomy to open nephrectomy, further emphasizing the importance of careful characterization of venous anatomy. An accessory left renal vein is the most common anatomic variant of the renal veins, occurring in 15% to 30% of potential donors. Circumaortic (8%–11%) and retroaortic (3%) left renal veins are less common but not rare among potential renal donors. Potential tributaries to the left renal vein also require special attention, including gonadal, adrenal, lumbar and retroperitoneal veins. Duplicated or multiple renal veins are also common with the right kidney (**Fig. 5**). Given that renal vein thrombosis occurs with higher frequency in the setting of multiple renal veins, this may be a contraindication to renal donation. Although surgeons have often preferred to harvest the left kidney given the longer left renal vein, at least one study demonstrated shorter operating time with right donor nephrectomy and no significant difference in graft complication or survival.[4]

Anatomy of the donor renal collecting system is another key element of the pretransplant imaging evaluation. Congenital abnormalities of the renal collecting system including complete or partial ureteral duplication as well as ureteropelvic junction obstruction are not absolute contraindications to renal donation but should be characterized before renal donor selection. Criteria differ by institutional guidelines but donor kidneys containing a solitary small calculus (<5 mm) are typically eligible for transplantation. Even those with calculi larger than 5 mm or multiple calculi may be eligible, given the potential to extract larger stones from the donor kidney after nephrectomy but before transplantation. However, the presence of large or multiple calculi may prompt a more in-depth evaluation to evaluate for an underlying systemic or metabolic abnormality.[4] In our institution, patients with bilateral renal calculi are not considered for donation. A series of patients with "gifted stones" showed good clinical results with no significant morbidity or graft loss associated with obstructive nephrolithiasis at long-term follow-up.[11]

Transplant Recipient Imaging Evaluation and Relevant Findings

Given that one of the primary long-term risks of renal transplantation for the recipient relates to chronic immunosuppression, pretransplant imaging of the recipient is important to evaluate for a preexisting infection or malignancy, which could worsen with immunosuppression. In order to screen for any potential pulmonary infection or malignancy, a chest radiograph is recommended. A CT of the abdomen and pelvis is also recommended to evaluate for the presence of underlying malignancy or infection. In particular, given that many potential recipients have been on hemodialysis, there is an increased incidence of cystic renal disease and associated renal malignancy. Further, a CT of the abdomen and pelvis allows for optimal evaluation of the vascular anatomy, particularly because it relates to the extent and degree of atherosclerotic calcifications. Although arterial wall calcifications can be detected adequately without contrast, intravenous contrast enhancement allows for the evaluation of noncalcific atherosclerotic plaque and, therefore, is better to evaluate potential inflow abnormalities to the renal transplant. The iliac fossa is often chosen as the site for renal transplant placement, and as such evaluation of the common, external and internal iliac artery calcifications is a critical element of presurgical planning given the potential for calcific plaque to significantly complicate creation of the transplant arterial anastomosis (**Fig. 6**).[12] Donated kidneys have been lost due to inability to anastomose into the recipient before the routine use of

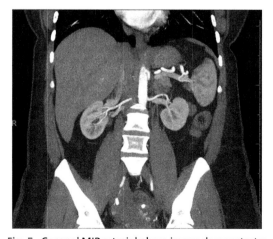

Fig. 5. Coronal MIP arterial phase image demonstrates 2 right renal veins. Identification of renal vein anatomy an important component of renal donor evaluation, both as it relates to donor kidney selection as well as surgical planning.

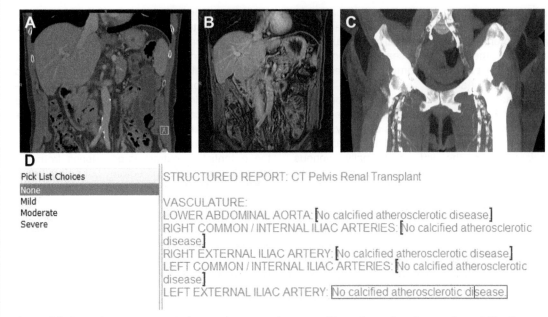

Fig. 6. (A) Coronal postcontrast CT image demonstrating aorto-iliac atherosclerotic vascular calcifications, an important aspect of surgical planning for renal transplant recipients. (B) Coronal postcontrast magnetic resonance (MR) image of the same patient demonstrating inconspicuous nature of atherosclerotic vascular calcifications on MR relative to CT. (C) Maximum intensity projection (MIP) images from a routine pretransplant noncontrast pelvic CT demonstrates heavy calcification without an appropriate calcific free interval (2 cm at our institution)—a relative contraindication for transplantation. (D) Sample reporting template for transplant candidates at our institution denoting the presence or absence as well as severity of calcifications in the caudal abdominal aorta, common iliac, and external iliac arteries.

iliac artery imaging of the recipient. Our transplant surgeons require 2 cm of artery essentially free of calcific plaque for anastomosis, and will generally use the less-involved side. All else equal, the right iliac artery is chosen among other reasons to remove any potential unmasking of May-Thurner syndrome due to increased flow through the left common iliac vein from the allograft.

Evaluation with CT also provides an opportunity to evaluate anatomy of the urinary bladder and any other adjacent structures in the lower abdomen and pelvis, particularly if there have been earlier failed transplants. Ultrasound or noncontrast MR are imaging alternatives that may also be considered as part of this evaluation; however, these modalities are suboptimal for evaluation of atherosclerotic calcifications. Potential recipients who have autosomal dominant polycystic kidney disease should also be screened for intracranial aneurysms with CTA or MRA given the higher incidence of aneurysms within this patient population.[6]

SURGICAL ANATOMY AND TECHNIQUES
Donor Retrieval (Deceased vs Living Donor)

Living donor renal transplants are a strategy to combat renal transplant shortages as the need

outpaces availability. In 2019, living donor renal transplants reached their highest level after many years of lack of growth, followed by the lowest level since 1999 due to the COVID-19 pandemic.[13] The year 2021 marked a return to average levels. It has been previously reported that living donor transplants confer a higher graft survival rate compared with deceased-donor transplants; however, donor nephrectomy is not without risk.

In addition to the aforementioned risks, donor nephrectomy confers numerous surgical risks, namely bleeding, infection, poor wound healing, inadvertent damage to structures in the area, adynamic ileus, and death, which are mandated to be discussed in the informed consent process by the Organ Procurement and Transplantation Network.[14] Complications have been reported to occur in 16.8% of patient undergoing donor nephrectomy, with major complications only affecting 2.5%.[15] Black donors had a significantly higher risk than white donors, including up to 56% increase in major complications. Patients with bleeding disorders, obese patients, and those with psychiatric conditions conferred higher risks while larger hospital volumes conferred lower risks. Postprocedurally, there have also been reported increased risks of hypertension and potentially of gestational hypertension and preeclampsia.[16]

The majority of patients undergoing donor nephrectomy in the United States undergo laparoscopic donor nephrectomy (**Fig. 7**). These patients have less morbidity, shorter hospital stays and return to work faster than those undergoing open surgery.[17] A 2015 meta-analysis comparing technique modifications[18] demonstrated that a retroperitoneoscopic approach resulted in less complications and warm ischemic times were reduced with hand-assistance. Additionally, surgeons with less experience had potential increases in safety. Studies have demonstrated mortality rates are low with both techniques.[19]

Greater than 75% of all donor nephrectomies performed as of 2016 were with a laparoscopic (or hand-assisted) approach. The remainder performed included retroperitoneoscopic, laparoendoscopic single site (LESS), robot-assisted and mini-open procedures, although the mini-open procedures are less studied and data are less defined (**Fig. 8**).[20] LESS is a single umbilical site nephrectomy that seems to have similar outcomes and complications.[21] These may have cosmetic advantages and potentially less postoperative pain and port site complications including hernias. Robotic procedures have been performed increasingly during the last 20 years. Data demonstrating benefits have been mixed, although at least 1 review[22] demonstrated lower rates of surgical site infections, most pronounced in obese recipients.

If an open donor nephrectomy is required, the most common approach involves the patient in the operating room on their side with angulation to open the space between the iliac crest and ribs. A flank incision extends from the level of the umbilicus to under the ribs is performed. The ureter is typically dissected first, followed by the kidney from Gerota's fascia. Once free, the artery and vein are dissected freely, and the ureter to the level of iliac bifurcation is then freed. The distal ureter is clamped and resected. This position is held until the recipient is prepared, at which point the artery and vein are clamped, divided and removed. A "back-table" preparation is then performed, where the kidney is flushed with a cold, heparinized solution (**Fig. 9**). More preparation and reconstruction are required for a laparoscopic nephrectomy since much of the preparation in the open nephrectomy can occur before removal. Before closing, the surgeons oversew/ligate the vascular stumps.[23,24] Laparoscopic surgeries are similar but use an intraperitoneal approach. Alternative open techniques have been described, including mininephrectomy and muscle splitting

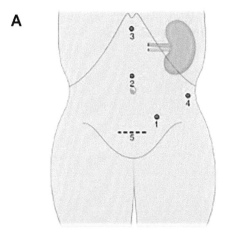

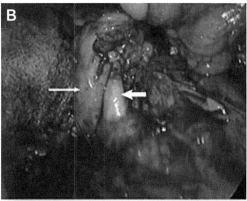

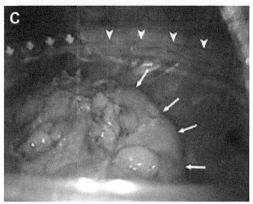

Fig. 7. Technique for laparoscopic donor nephrectomy. (*A*) Positions for 4 laparoscopic ports (1–4) and Pfannenstiel incision (5) through which the kidney is removed. (*B*) Intraoperative view showing left renal artery (*short arrow*) and vein (*long arrow*) prepared for control and division. (*C*) Intraoperative view showing the kidney (*arrows* mark lateral margin) placed in the endoscopic retrieval bag (*arrowheads* mark the edge of the bag). (*From* Barlow AD, Nicholson ML. Bacterial diseases. In: Johnson R, Feehally J, Floege J, Tonelli M, editors. Comprehensive Clinical Nephrology. USA: Elsevier; 2018. p. 103.)

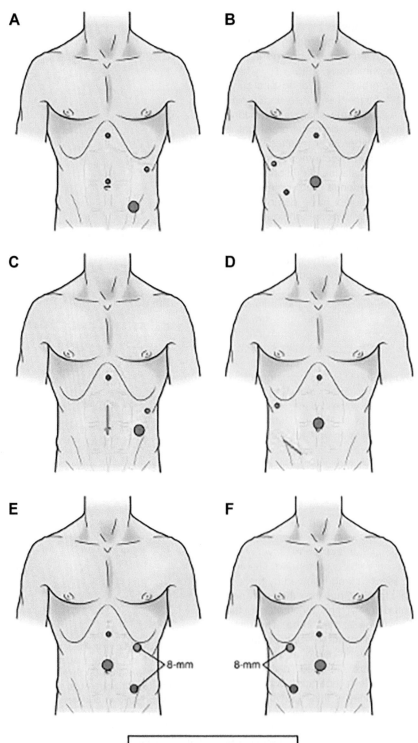

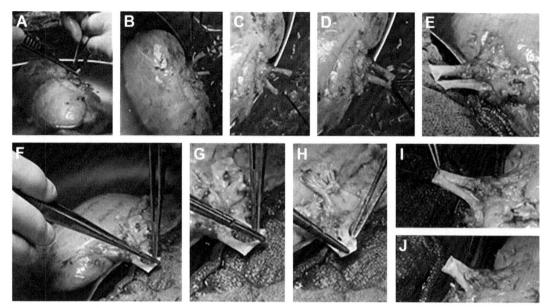

Fig. 9. Intraoperative images showing consecutive phases of extracorporeal (ex vivo) bench vascular reconstruction before robot-assisted kidney transplantation in case of a graft with 2 separate renal arteries of approximately the same caliber from a living donor. (*A–E*) After careful preparation of the 2 renal arteries, vascular reconstruction was carried out using a conjoined (side-to-side) arterial anastomosis in pantaloon fashion to create (*F–J*) a common arterial ostium for subsequent single arterial anastomosis to the external iliac artery. (*From* Siena G, Campi R, Decaestecker K, et al. Robot-assisted Kidney Transplantation with Regional Hypothermia Using Grafts with Multiple Vessels After Extracorporeal Vascular Reconstruction: Results from the European Association of Urology Robotic Urology Section Working Group. Eur Urol Focus. 2018;4(2):175 to 184.)

open donor nephrectomies more recently using smaller incisions, and compared with laparoscopy in limited fashion. These techniques could improve warm ischemia and operative time but other factors were mixed and patient populations have been small.[25]

When a deceased donor surgery is performed, there are differences in the dissection and what is removed from the donor because there is not a need to preserve major vascular structures. The kidneys are often the last organ to be harvested, as the upper abdominal organs must be removed and the bowel mobilized to expose the kidneys in the retroperitoneum. An aortic catheter is used in the meantime to flush a cold solution to preserve the kidneys in situ. The renal arteries and veins are typically procured with a cuff from the donor aorta and IVC—and in some cases, the entire donor IVC or iliac vein in the case of right

kidney procurement if the renal vein is short. This cuff of aorta, or "Carrel patch," is used to prevent anastomotic stenosis. More tissue around the kidneys and ureters are also typically taken in comparison to living donor retrievals. Most kidneys are removed "en bloc," as a whole with both kidneys and the transected aorta/IVC (**Fig. 10**). Following this, the kidneys are separated, although pediatric kidneys (typically less than 2 years old) may be transplanted entirely in an "en bloc" fashion. A "back-table" preparation is also performed, which can become challenging should there be multiple renal arteries or inadvertently ligated arteries because there is no collateral arterial flow to the transplant.[26,27]

Implantation

When a transplant kidney is implanted, many factors come into play to determine its location. Most

Fig. 8. Trocar placement for conventional laparoscopic donor nephrectomy (left and right), and hand-assisted laparoscopic donor nephrectomy (left and right). (*A*) Conventional laparoscopic left donor nephrectomy. (*B*) Conventional laparoscopic right donor nephrectomy. (*C*) Hand-assisted laparoscopic left donor nephrectomy. (*D*) Hand-assisted laparoscopic right donor nephrectomy. (*E*) Robot-assisted laparoscopic left donor nephrectomy. (*F*) Robot-assisted laparoscopic right donor nephrectomy. (*From* Glickman L, Munver R. Laparoscopic Live Donor Nephrectomy. In: Smith J, Howards S, Preminger G, Roger D, editors. Hinman's Atlas of Urologic Surgery Fourth Edition. USA: Elsevier; 2019. p. 189 to 196.)

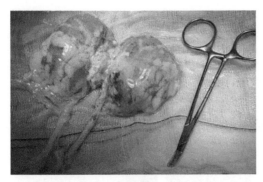

Fig. 10. En bloc kidneys. Pediatric en bloc kidneys on the operating room table ready for pretransplant bench surgery. Note the scarce perirenal fat and the size compared with a mosquito clamp. (*From* López-González JA, Beamud-Cortés M, Bermell-Marco L, et al. A 20-year experience in cadaveric pediatric en bloc kidney transplantation in adult recipients. Actas Urol Esp (Engl Ed). 2022;46(2):85 to 91.)

commonly, it is placed in a heterotopic position, typically in the iliac fossa to avoid entering the abdominal cavity.[28] In the case of a large graft or smaller (including pediatric) patient, an intraperitoneal transplant can be performed to avoid compartment syndrome/compression on the allograft. Bilateral failed transplants may necessitate a transperitoneal approach.[29] Short ureters may require a retrovesicular position, although uncommon. Although the right lower quadrant is the most common location due to the longer and more horizontal right external iliac vessels (in addition to May-Thurner unmasking concerns described earlier), the left may also be used in the case of prior right lower quadrant transplant or heavy atherosclerotic calcifications asymmetrically seen on the right.

A lower quadrant incision creates a potential space in the retroperitoneum and the inferior epigastric vessels and lymphatics are ligated and divided. The round ligament is also divided in women before peritoneal mobilization to access the external iliac vessels. An end-to-side anastomosis of the donor vein with the recipient external iliac vein is created first, followed by a similar anastomosis of the renal artery and external iliac artery. Anomalous anatomy creates challenges for the surgeon. Small, 1-mm branch arteries may be ligated if they perfuse less than 10% of the cortex. Larger branch arteries may be anastomosed to the external iliac or inferior epigastric arteries. This is considered to be more important in the lower pole because the ureteral vessels typically originate in this location. Multiple main renal arteries can be anastomosed side-to-side together or separately to the iliac vessels.[29]

After flow is restored, the ureter is then implanted with a ureteroneocystostomy, typically in an extravesicular fashion (typically the anterolateral aspect of the bladder) (**Fig. 11**); in some institutions (ours included), a stent is placed across the anastomosis. This stent may be removed cystoscopically in a delayed fashion or removed at discharge. If the graft ureter is small or ischemic, the native ureter may be used with a utereroureterostomy, pyeloureterostomy, or pyeloneocystostomy; alternatively, a pyelovesicostomy can be performed if both are unusable.

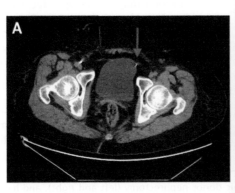
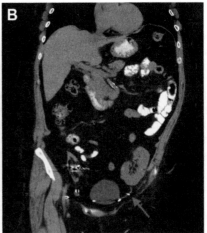

Fig. 11. (*A*) Axial pelvic CT images from a demonstrate bilateral ureteral anastomoses, one of which was from a failed transplant (*blue arrow*). The functioning allograft is anastomosed to the left (*red arrow*). These are placed in the anterolateral bladder. (*B*) Coronal CT images on this same patient better delineate the course of the ureter and anastomosis (*red arrow*).

Considerations for Children

Pediatric end-stage renal disease differs as most cases develop from congenital anomalies, cystic disease, congenital nephrotic syndrome, and dysplasia/aplasia. As such, typical anastomoses may be challenging or not suitable—for example, in cases of neurogenic bladder or chronic obstruction. Bladder augmentation or potentially a urinary diversion may be required in this setting. Children may require native nephrectomies in massive proteinuria, polyuria, refractory hypertension, urinary tract infection (UTI) and dilated tracts, or malignancy. These may be performed in a staged fashion or at the time of transplant. Pediatric kidney implantations are performed similarly, with the exception that with small children the iliac vessels may be too small to anastomose with the kidney, potentially requiring aortic/IVC anastomoses. Adult-sized kidneys may have a risk of kinking or twisting of the pedicle in children given the asymmetry of the vascular size relative to a smaller child.[30]

Considerations for Failed Transplant Candidates

In the setting of a failed or failing transplant kidney, the 2014 British Society Guidelines recommend preemptive evaluation for repeat transplant if graft survival is estimated less than 1 year unless the initial graft failed within 1 year. Dialysis on a short-term basis is suggested in this setting because data have shown patients have significantly higher graft failure risks without dialysis.[31] Prolonged waiting times increase the risks of rejection, graft failure, and mortality every year that a patient is delayed in the retransplant process. Should an early graft failure occur, these patients may undergo transplant nephrectomy, whereas if failure is on a more long-term basis, this is typically reserved for patients with a complication related to rejection or necrosis. If left in situ, the imaging appearance is typically that of progressive atrophy/decrease in size followed by calcification of the allograft (**Fig. 12**).

SUMMARY

End-stage renal disease continues to grow worldwide and renal transplantation remains the primary and most effective treatment to address this burden. It is important to recognize the risks of living-donor transplantation, both medical and surgical because this is the ideal mechanism for transplant recipients to achieve success. Knowledge of the factors that are important pretransplant for both donor and recipient success can allow for the radiologist to contribute greatly to the continued progress of renal transplantation programs at their institutions. Multimodality imaging is crucial and has evolved over the years. Finally, a robust understanding of current surgical techniques can facilitate better postoperative imaging when early complications are a consideration.

CLINICS CARE POINTS

- CT/CTA is the best choice for pretransplant donor and recipient imaging.
- Donor imaging is crucial to the success of transplantation programs for incidental findings and anatomical variants.
- Surgical approaches are varied in terms of living-donor nephrectomies as well as implantation approaches based on the clinical scenario.

DISCLOSURES

Dr M.E. Lockhart discloses book royalties from Elsevier and JayPee Brothers Medical Publishers, and Deputy Editor salary from Journal of Ultrasound in Medicine. Nonmonetary leadership/fiduciary role disclosures include Executive Board of Society of Radiologists in Ultrasound, Chair of ACR Appropriateness Criteria Committee, Chair of AIUM Future Fund Research Committee, and Chair of ABR Ultrasound Certifying Committee.

REFERENCES

1. Benjamens S, Moers C, Slart RHJA, et al. Kidney Transplantation and Diagnostic Imaging: The Early Days and Future Advancements of Transplant Surgery. Diagnostics 2020;11(1):47.

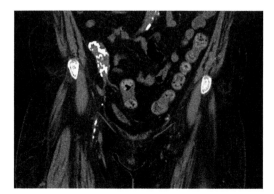

Fig. 12. Coronal pelvic CT images demonstrate a calcified soft tissue mass-like structure in the right lower quadrant. This patient had a renal allograft that failed year prior and has become heavily calcified and atrophic.

2. Lentine KL, Lam NN, Segev DL. Risks of Living Kidney Donation: Current State of Knowledge on Outcomes Important to Donors. Clin J Am Soc Nephrol 2019;14(4):597–608.

3. Ghonge NP, Gadanayak S, Rajakumari V. MDCT evaluation of potential living renal donor, prior to laparoscopic donor nephrectomy: What the transplant surgeon wants to know? Indian J Radiol Imaging 2014;24(4):367–78.

4. Aghayev A, Gupta S, Dabiri BE, et al. Vascular imaging in renal donors. Cardiovasc Diagn Ther 2019; 9(Suppl 1):S116–30.

5. Summerlin AL, Lockhart ME, Strang AM, et al. Determination of split renal function by 3D reconstruction of CT angiograms: a comparison with gamma camera renography. AJR Am J Roentgenol 2008;191(5):1552–8.

6. Harmath CB, Wood CG 3rd, Berggruen SM, et al. Renal Pretransplantation Work-up, Donor, Recipient, Surgical Techniques. Radiol Clin North Am 2016;54(2):217–34.

7. Habbous S, Garcia-Ochoa C, Brahm G, et al. Can Split Renal Volume Assessment by Computed Tomography Replace Nuclear Split Renal Function in Living Kidney Donor Evaluations? A Systematic Review and Meta-Analysis. Can J Kidney Health Dis 2019;6. 2054358119875459.

8. Vernuccio F, Gondalia R, Churchill S, et al. CT evaluation of the renal donor and recipient. Abdom Radiol (NY) 2018;43(10):2574–88.

9. Pradhay G, Gopidas GS, Karumathil Pullara S, et al. Prevalence and Relevance of Multiple Renal Arteries: A Radioanatomical Perspective. Cureus 2021;13(10): e18957.

10. Kolettis PN, Bugg CE, Lockhart ME, et al. Outcomes for live donor renal transplantation using kidneys with medial fibroplasia. Urology 2004;63(4):656–9.

11. Strang AM, Lockhart ME, Amling CL, et al. Living renal donor allograft lithiasis: a review of stone related morbidity in donors and recipients. J Urol 2008;179(3):832–6.

12. Benjamens S, Rijkse E, Te Velde-Keyzer CA, et al. Aorto-Iliac Artery Calcification Prior to Kidney Transplantation. J Clin Med 2020;9(9):2893.

13. OPTN (Organ Procurement and Transplantation Network) National Data. Available at: https://optn. transplant.hrsa.gov/data/view-data-reports/national-data/. Accessed November 1, 2022.

14. OPTN (Organ Procurement and Transplantation Network)/UNOS (United Network for Organ Sharing). OPTN Policies, Policy 14: Living Donation. Available at: https://optn.transplant.hrsa.gov/media/eavh5bf3/optn_policies.pdf. Accessed November 1, 2022.

15. Lentine KL, Lam NN, Axelrod D, et al. Perioperative Complications After Living Kidney Donation: A National Study. Am J Transplant 2016;16(6):1848–57.

16. Ibrahim HN, Akkina SK, Leister E, et al. Pregnancy outcomes after kidney donation. Am J Transplant 2009;9(4):825–34.

17. Nanidis TG, Antcliffe D, Kokkinos C, et al. Laparoscopic versus open live donor nephrectomy in renal transplantation: a meta-analysis. Ann Surg 2008; 247(1):58–70.

18. Özdemir-van Brunschot DM, Koning GG, van Laarhoven KC, et al. A comparison of technique modifications in laparoscopic donor nephrectomy: a systematic review and meta-analysis. PLoS One 2015;10(3):e0121131.

19. Segev DL, Muzaale AD, Caffo BS, et al. Perioperative mortality and long-term survival following live kidney donation. JAMA 2010;303:959.

20. Kortram K, Ijzermans JN, Dor FJ. Perioperative Events and Complications in Minimally Invasive Live Donor Nephrectomy: A Systematic Review and Meta-Analysis. Transplantation 2016;100:2264.

21. Aull MJ, Afaneh C, Charlton M, et al. A randomized, prospective, parallel group study of laparoscopic versus laparoendoscopic single site donor nephrectomy for kidney donation. Am J Transplant 2014;14: 1630.

22. Tzvetanov I, Bejarano-Pineda L, Giulianotti PC, et al. State of the art of robotic surgery in organ transplantation. World J Surg 2013;37(12):2791–9.

23. Scantlebury V. Cadaveric and living donation. In: Shapiro R, Simmons R, Starzl TE, editors. Renal transplantation. Appleton & Lange; 1997.

24. Yanaga K, Podesta LG, Broznick B, et al. Multiple organ recovery for transplantation. In: Starzl TE, Shapiro R, Simmons RL, editors. Atlas of organ transplantation. New York: Gower Medical Publishing; 1992.

25. Kok NF, Alwayn IP, Lind MY, et al. Donor nephrectomy: mini-incision muscle-splitting open approach versus laparoscopy. Transplantation 2006;81(6):881–7.

26. Shapiro R. The transplant procedure. In: Shapiro R, Simmons RL, Starzl TE, editors. Renal transplantation. Stamford, CT: Appleton & Lange; 1998.

27. Ellis D, Gilboa N, Bellinger M, et al. Renal transplantation in infants and children. In: Shapiro R, Simmons RL, Starzl TE, editors. Renal transplantation. Stamford, CT: Appleton & Lange; 1998.

28. Kakaei F, Nikeghbalian S, Malekhosseini SA. Kidney Transplantation Techniques. In: Current issues and future direction in kidney transplantation. IntechOpen; 2013. https://doi.org/10.5772/54829.

29. Hossain MA, Chadha R, Bagul A, et al. Kidney Transplantation. In: Díaz-Nieto R, editor. Procurement and transplantation of abdominal organs in clinical practice. Cham, Switzerland: Springer; 2019. p. 69–117.

30. Gunawardena T, Sharma H, Sharma AK, et al. Surgical considerations in paediatric kidney transplantation: an update. Ren Replace Ther 2021;7:54.

31. Andrews PA, Standards Committee of the British Transplantation Society. Summary of the British Transplantation Society Guidelines for Management of the Failing Kidney Transplant. Transplantation 2014;98(11):1130–3.

Renal Transplantation
Immediate and Late Complications

Patrick Yoon Kim, MD[a], Azarin Shoghi, MS, MD[b], Ghaneh Fananapazir, MD[a],*

KEYWORDS

- Transplant kidney • Renal transplant complications • Immediate and late
- Imaging of renal allografts

KEY POINTS

- Perinephric fluid collections are common after kidney transplantation; the four main types are hematoma, urinoma, abscess, and lymphocele.
- Vascular complications can be found in the immediate to late postoperative period. Timing to diagnosis is critical for early intervention and prognosis of the allograft when perfusion is jeopardized.
- Mild degree of hydronephrosis may be a normal finding in kidney grafts owing to denervation of the ureters and vesicoureteral reflux from the ureteroneocystostomy. It is important to correlate with clinical signs of allograft dysfunction when evaluating for ureteral obstruction.
- Malignancy is the third most common cause of death in renal transplant patients with an increased risk of malignancy in this population due to chronic immunosuppression and unregulated oncogenic viruses. These can be a new malignancy, recurrent malignancy in the recipient, or donor-related.
- Renal allografts undergoing acute rejection often appear normal on ultrasound. Urothelial thickening can be a sensitive finding but ultimately is a histopathological diagnosis.

INTRODUCTION

Since 1954, when the first kidney transplant was performed, much has improved regarding surgical technique, organ preservation, and immunosuppressive medications, which has led to longer graft survival. The recognition of complications based on imaging to optimize graft survival plays an important role. To narrow the differential diagnosis or identify a complication, it is important to understand the pathophysiologies that affect kidney grafts as well as the timelines in which such processes are to be expected. Complications can be grouped based on broad categories, such as perinephric fluid collections, vascular issues, diseases that affect the parenchyma, those that affect the ureter, and malignancies, but also based on expected timeline, such as immediate postoperative (first 2 weeks after transplantation), early (within the first year), and late (Fig. 1).

Imaging is still the primary modality in surveillance and evaluation of the renal graft. Duplex ultrasound plays the dominant role in the initial assessment as a fast, noninvasive diagnostic study. Color and pulsed Doppler allows for the evaluation of the hilar vasculature and parenchymal perfusion of the allograft. CT (computed tomography) and MR (magnetic resonance) imaging are useful adjunct imaging modalities with contrast given sparingly due to the risk of acute kidney injury. Nuclear medicine studies and invasive angiography also play important roles elucidating the etiology of renal graft dysfunction; however, for purposes of this review article, the focus will be primarily on ultrasound, CT, and MR imaging.

Perinephric Fluid Collections

The four main types of peritransplant fluid collections are hematomas, urinomas, lymphoceles,

a Department of Radiology, University of California Davis Health, Sacramento, CA 95817, USA; b University of California, Davis School of Medicine, Sacramento, CA 95817, USA
* Corresponding author.
E-mail address: fananapazir@ucdavis.edu

Radiol Clin N Am 61 (2023) 809–820
https://doi.org/10.1016/j.rcl.2023.04.004

Timeline of Renal Transplant Non-Infectious Complications

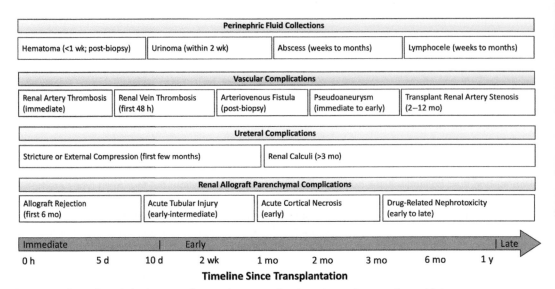

Fig. 1. Timeline of noninfectious renal transplant complications: immediate, early, and late.

and abscesses. Imaging features among the fluid collections can have overlap regardless of imaging modalities, and most will require fluid sampling in order to be definitive about the diagnosis.[1,2]

Hematomas

Hematomas are collections of blood products with the age of the blood determining the appearance on imaging. Hematomas are very common in the immediate postoperative setting but can also occur in the setting of iatrogenic injury (usually from biopsy or percutaneous nephrostomy tube placement).[2] Although most small hematomas have little consequence on the function of the kidney graft, larger hematomas may have a higher propensity to become infected and potentially exert mass effect on the kidney graft and may need to be evacuated.[3]

On ultrasound, hematomas have a variable appearance, often based on the acuity of the hematoma. Hyperacute hematomas may appear anechoic, whereas acute hematomas may appear more echogenic and heterogenous.[2] As hematomas become more chronic, they may become more anechoic, usually with a lace-like appearance from the fibrinous septations (Fig. 2). On CT, the acute hematoma may appear hyperdense (>28 HU) and the more chronic hematomas appear more hypodense[4] (see Fig. 2). On MR imaging, T1 and T2 appearances also vary depending on chronicity of the blood products. Acutely, will tend to have low T1 (deoxyhemoglobin) and low T2 signal, when subacute will demonstrate high T1 signal

(methemoglobin) and high T2 signal (fluid/edema). Chronic hematomas exhibit low T1 signal with varying appearances on T2-weighted images. Hematomas will generally not enhance unless they become infected, at which point they will appear as abscesses (rim-enhancing fluid collections).

In addition to the size of the hematoma, the location is important and can direct management.[5] Incisional hematomas are usually remote from the graft and are usually self-limiting. Hematomas lateral to the graft are usually caused by venous oozing. Most are self-limiting, though very large lateral hematomas may need to be evacuated. Subcapsular hematomas cause compression of the renal parenchyma.[3] Color Doppler or contrast-enhanced ultrasound in assessing perfusion to the cortex of the graft is useful to be able to identify these hematomas as they can sometimes be difficult to visualize, especially when the echogenicity of the hematoma is similar that of the parenchyma. On pulsed Doppler, the resistive index is usually elevated and can often demonstrate diastolic reversal of flow.[6] The mass effect on the kidney graft can lead to kidney dysfunction and hypertension, and these usually must be surgically evacuated. Finally, medial hematomas can be the most concerning location of a hematoma as these can sometimes indicate an anastomotic breakdown.[5] Either exquisite visualization of the anastomotic region by ultrasound with Doppler to assess for this complication or a contrast-

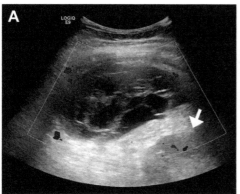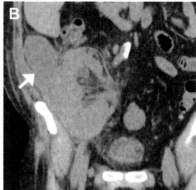

Fig. 2. A 57-year-old male status post deceased donor kidney transplant 2 months prior presents with right flank pain and hemoglobinemia. (*A*) Color Doppler US image shows a complex avascular fluid collection superficial and lateral to the right iliac fossa renal allograft (*arrow*). (*B*) Coronal non-enhanced CT image shows correlating hyperattenuating lateral perinephric hematoma (*arrow*) in the right iliac fossa.

enhanced CT is important when encountering medial hematomas.

Urinomas

Urinomas are collections of urine resulting from a disruption in the urothelium, which can occur at the level of the kidney to the bladder. They can result from an incisional injury, anastomotic leak along the ureteroneocystostomy, or urothelial necrosis owing to ischemia or rupture. These collections usually present within the first few weeks in cases of iatrogenic injury and in the first few months in cases of ureteral necrosis.[7]

Urinomas often appear as simple fluid collections around the graft, usually in the vicinity of the renal hilum or the bladder. On ultrasound, they appear anechoic. Similarly on CT and MR imaging, they appear as simple, non-enhancing fluid collections on non-delayed imaging, with correlating T2 hyperintensity on MR. On suspicion of a urine leak, a CT or MR during the urinary excretory phase can be obtained, with excretion of contrast into the collection being diagnostic of a urinary leak. In addition, radionuclide scintigraphy can also evaluate for the leak of urine into a fluid collection.

Image-guided aspiration, usually by ultrasound, may be used to collect and analyze the fluid for a creatinine level greater than that of serum. A simultaneous serum creatinine level should be obtained as these patients may have elevated baseline levels owing to renal dysfunction.

Lymphoceles

Lymphoceles are common perinephric fluid collections that contain lymphatic fluid and occur anywhere from the early to late postoperative period.[7] Histologically, these lack a true epithelial lining and occur along the lymphatic channels in the postoperative space. While benign in composition and often asymptomatic, when large enough, they can cause locoregional mass effect along the transplanted kidney, renal hilum, or the urinary collection system. It is the most common perinephric collection resulting in allograft hydronephrosis.

On ultrasound, they appear as distinct, anechoic collections of fluid with occasional internal thin septations. With more advanced imaging, they tend to follow characteristics of simple fluid organized within a barely perceptible, non-enhancing, thin wall (Fig. 3). On CT, the internal fluid is the density of water and hence appears T2 hyperintense on MR imaging.

Definitive diagnosis is made with analysis of the aspirated fluid. Lymphoceles are characterized by concentrations of creatinine and potassium equal to that of serum. Although most are benign, lymphoceles are often drained percutaneously when they cause mass effect. However, they are known to re-accumulate even when drains are left in place,[7] which can be further treated with sclerotherapy or surgery.

Abscesses

Abscesses are organized collections of infected purulent fluid. Patients may present with a clinical picture of infection, though this may be diminished owing to immunosuppressive medications. Abscesses typically develop within a few weeks to months posttransplantation[3] and manifest as a superinfection of an existing perioperative fluid collection or occur from spread from pyelonephritis.

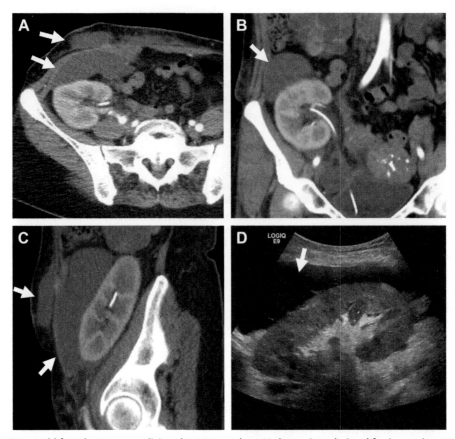

Fig. 3. A 45-year-old female status post living donor transplant 14 days prior admitted for increasing serum creatinine and large perinephric fluid collection. (*A*) Axial, (*B*) coronal, and (*C*) sagittal contrast-enhanced CT demonstrate a large, perinephric fluid collection as well as a superficial fluid collection (*arrows*) overlying the right iliac fossa renal allograft. Attenuation of the fluid measures that of simple fluid. (*D*) Gray scale US in the same patient shows a large, relatively simple-appearing anechoic fluid collection (*arrow*). Fluid analysis confirmed that this represented a lymphocele.

On imaging, abscesses appear as complex fluid collections with thick walls and possible loculations. They generally appear anechoic or hypoechoic by ultrasound with echogenic internal debris and increased wall vascularity on color Doppler. On CT and MR, they appear as rim-enhancing collections of simple to complex fluid (**Fig. 4**). On MR, the fluid will appear T2 hyperintense and restrict diffusion.

Given most transplant patients are on immunosuppressants, prompt treatment with antibiotics is required, often with percutaneous drainage or surgical evacuation. Ultimately, the maturity and size of the fluid collection will drive the management.

VASCULAR COMPLICATIONS

Vascular complications occur in 3% to 15% of kidney graft recipients.[8] The five main vascular complications are renal artery and vein thrombosis, transplant renal artery stenosis (TRAS), arterial-venous fistulas, and pseudoaneurysms. As these

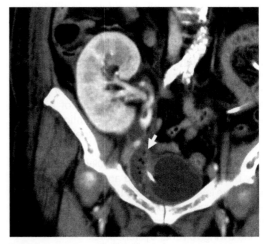

Fig. 4. A 53-year-old female status post renal transplantation 2 weeks prior presents with right lower quadrant abdominal pain. Coronal contrast-enhanced CT shows a rim-enhancing fluid collection with multiple foci of gas inferior to the right iliac fossa allograft (*arrow*).

complications affect the perfusion of the renal graft, early diagnosis is important. Ultrasound is again the dominant initial imaging modality in evaluation with the utility of CT and MR imaging as adjunctive modalities.

Renal Artery Thrombosis

Renal artery thrombosis is a rare complication with an incidence of 0.4%, typically occurring within the early postoperative period.[9] Arterial blood flow to the renal graft is occluded, often resulting from anastomotic occlusion, kinking of the transplant renal artery, or arterial dissection. Other factors such as external compression, embolism, or even vasculitis can thrombose the transplant renal artery. Clinically, most patients present in the early postoperative period with abrupt anuria and hypertension in the setting of acute renal failure. Graft pain is also a common symptom resulting from local inflammation and swelling which irritates the adjacent peritoneum.[4,7]

The imaging features vary depending on the site of occlusion, resulting in global or segmental infarction. On ultrasound, the graft may appear normal in size and appearance acutely. Infarcted renal tissue will become more hypoechoic and thinner with increasing chronicity. On color Doppler, involved areas will lack perfusion. The transplanted renal artery may demonstrate a lack of flow on Doppler and rarely show visible echogenic intraluminal thrombus. On contrast-enhanced ultrasound, CT, and MR imaging, areas of lack of enhancement will correlate to areas of infarct. CT or MR angiography and/or invasive digital subtraction angiography may further demonstrate an abrupt obstruction of the renal artery with lack of contrast perfusion to the kidney. Renal scintigraphy is also a modality to evaluate for perfusion with a reduced or lack of perfusion on the time activity curve.

In the setting of global infarct with total vascular occlusion, an accurate early diagnosis is critical for immediate intervention. Prognosis is generally poor with outcomes determined by the time to intervention with surgical or endovascular thrombectomy and graft reperfusion.

Renal Vein Thrombosis

Renal vein thrombosis is occlusion of the venous outflow of the graft kidney, resulting in reduced blood flow of the graft and ultimately jeopardizing perfusion. The incidence ranges from 0.3% to 4.2% but can account for up to 8% of graft failures[4,7,9] and typically have poor outcomes with a high likelihood of graft failure. Renal vein thrombosis usually occurs in the early postoperative period with peak incidence within the first

48 hours.[7] Clinically, patients present with acute renal failure, hypertension, and graft pain.

Venous outflow obstruction leads the kidney graft to become edematous and engorged. On ultrasound (US), there may be a loss of corticomedullary differentiation with perinephric fluid, which usually represents hematomas resulting from venous hypertension. On color Doppler, there is decreased global perfusion with elevated arterial resistive indices (**Fig. 5**), often demonstrating reversal of diastolic flow. However, the reversal of flow can be seen with other processes, such as acute tubular injury.[6] The absence of demonstrable venous outflow in the setting of elevated resistive indices requires careful consideration of renal vein thrombosis as the etiology for graft dysfunction. Rarely, the echogenic thrombus can be visualized within the renal vein. CT and MR may show perinephric stranding with possible adjacent hematomas. On contrast-enhanced imaging (CT, MR, or US), there is delayed or absent normal parenchymal enhancement and a filling defect within the transplant renal vein and possible thrombus propagation to the ipsilateral iliac vein can be seen.

Transplant Renal Artery Stenosis

TRAS is luminal narrowing of the graft renal artery with subsequent decreased vascular flow to the graft kidney, thus jeopardizing graft perfusion and graft function. This is the most common vascular complication, occurring in 5% to 10% of patients and typically manifests 2 to 12 months posttransplantation.[10] Patients can present with a variable clinical picture including refractory hypertension, fluid retention, and acute kidney injury. The etiology of the stenosis is likely multifactorial, including prolonged cold ischemic time and surgical revisions.[9] Stenosis of the renal artery usually occurs distal to the anastomosis, though it can occur proximal to or at the anastomosis.

When there is concern for TRAS, the initial evaluation usually involves ultrasound. There are three major parameters that have proven useful to evaluate the risk of TRAS: (1) peak main renal artery velocity greater than 300 cm/s, (2) spectral broadening in the distal segment artery, and (3) delayed upstroke of the intraparenchymal arteries on spectral Doppler of greater than 0.1 s[7,9,11] (**Fig. 6**). Depending on how many of the three criteria are present, the risk for TRAS is higher.[11] Confirmation can be obtained with contrast-enhanced CT or MR angiogram. Invasive angiography serves as a diagnostic and therapeutic study with the ability to take pressure measurements across the stenosis and treat endovascularly with angioplasty and/or stenting.

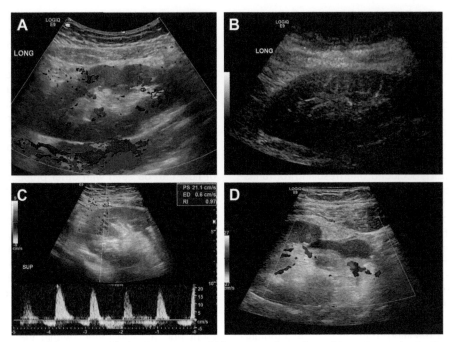

Fig. 5. A 34-year-old woman with day 0 status post kidney transplantation with acute renal vein thrombosis in the immediate postoperative period. Ultrasound (*A*) color and (*B*) B-flow demonstrate global hypoperfusion of the right iliac fossa renal allograft. (*C*) Spectral Doppler shows elevated parenchymal resistance with reversal of diastolic flow. (*D*) Color Doppler ultrasound of the renal hilum fails to show venous outflow. Layering echogenic debris, compatible with hematomas from venous hypertension.

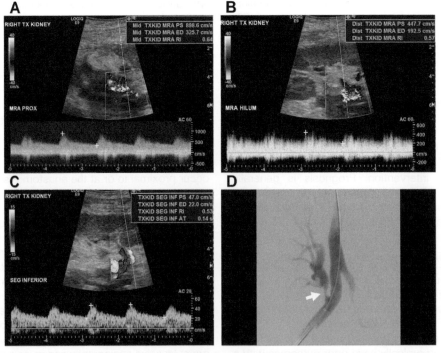

Fig. 6. A 43-year-old male status post renal transplantation 5 months prior presents with refractory hypertension. Ultrasound images show (*A*) elevated velocity at the proximal graft artery, (*B*) spectral broadening more distally in the renal artery indicative of turbulence, and (*C*) delayed systolic upstroke in the segmental arteries. (*D*) Digital subtraction angiography confirms juxta-anastomotic high-grade stenosis of the transplanted renal artery (*arrow*).

Arteriovenous Fistulas

Arteriovenous fistulas are almost always acquired communications between an artery and vein within the renal parenchyma. The most common etiology is iatrogenic where a point-to-point connection is created as a complication during percutaneous biopsies of the transplanted kidney. These are often discovered at the time of biopsy using ultrasound. Small fistulas may remain asymptomatic and close spontaneously, often treated with compression at the time of biopsy. However, some may enlarge overtime necessitating treatment.

Given the use of ultrasound guidance in most biopsies, arteriovenous fistulas are predominantly discovered using pulsed or color Doppler and typically not visualized on gray scale. The intraparenchymal artery will demonstrate high-velocity and low-resistance waveforms with the fistulized vein showing arterialized waveform on spectral Doppler. On color Doppler, a flash of color (color bruit artifact) caused by the vibration of adjacent tissues from the turbulence of the fistula will often point to its presence and location.

On other modalities, such as CT, MR, or angiography, the best diagnostic clue is simultaneous enhancement of the transplant renal artery and vein during the arterial phase. These can be treated using invasive angiography should there be a clinical need.

Pseudoaneurysms

Pseudoaneurysms are contained vascular injuries of the transplanted renal graft. The vascular injury involves all three layers of the vessel with blood contained by the surrounding tissues. These can be categorized as intraparenchymal or extrarenal, and like arteriovenous fistulas, pseudoaneurysms are usually post-biopsy complications, though they can be infectious in origin.[9,12]

Similar to arteriovenous fistulas, the soft tissue reverberation from pseudoaneurysms can lead to the color bruit artifact sign on color Doppler imaging. The neck of the pseudoaneurysm connecting the vessel with the contained rupture will show intermittent forward and reverse flow depending on the cardiac cycle. Within the pseudoaneurysmal sac, the blood flow circulates within it creating a "yin-yang" sign (Fig. 7), which indicates swirling of blood toward and away from the probe. With any contrast-enhanced imaging, a rounded region of enhancement matching arterial blood pool density/intensity will indicate the presence of a pseudoaneurysm.[12]

The management of pseudoaneurysms will vary depending on the size, location, and etiology. Small pseudoaneurysms, less than 2 cm in diameter, are often managed conservatively.[9,12] However, over time, these can grow and potentially rupture or cause mass effect within the graft parenchyma or adjacent hilar structures, if extrarenal. Larger pseudoaneurysms can be treated percutaneously with direct puncture and injection of thrombin, or they can be treated endovascularly with coiling or stenting.[9,12] When concerned for anastomotic pseudoaneurysms surgical repair may be necessary.

URETERAL COMPLICATIONS

Ureteral obstruction of the transplanted ureter is most commonly caused by a stricture, stone, or external compression. Strictures most commonly occur in the few months after transplantation.[7] Early occurrence is relatively uncommon and can be due to perioperative complications such as ureteral kinking, compression, or problems with the bladder anastomosis.

When a ureteral obstruction is suspected, the severity must be considered along with clinical factors to drive the management. Those with acute

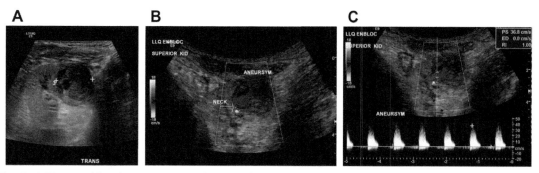

Fig. 7. A 50-year-old male status post pediatric en bloc renal transplant with a recent history of percutaneous transplant kidney biopsy presented for worsening hematuria for 10 days. Ultrasound demonstrates (A) 2.6 cm heterogenous, hypoechoic superior pole lesion in the kidney transplant (B) with Color and (C) pulsed Doppler showing feeding arterial flow consistent with a pseudoaneurysm.

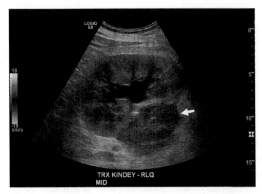

Fig. 8. A 59-year-old male status post renal transplantation 15 days prior presents with inability to urinate after nephroureteral stent removal. Gray scale US demonstrates moderate hydronephrosis of the renal allograft secondary to compression and obstruction from medial hilar hematoma (*arrow*).

allograft dysfunction with hydronephrosis require a more urgent investigation. If severe enough, urinomas can develop from elevated intraluminal pressures.

On imaging, kidney grafts with ureteral obstruction will show dilation of the calyces, renal pelvis, and ureters. A mild degree of hydronephrosis may be a normal finding in kidney grafts owing to denervation of the ureters and vesicoureteral reflux from the ureteroneocystostomy.[7] Moderate or increasing dilation of the renal pelvis and calyces with cortical thinning (**Figs. 8** and **9**) may suggest a more clinically relevant process. Following the ureter to the level of obstruction by CT, MR, or ultrasound can help determine the etiology of the obstruction (stone, stricture, or external compression). Delayed nephrograms on CT, MR, and renal scintigraphy may be useful in assessing the degree of obstruction.

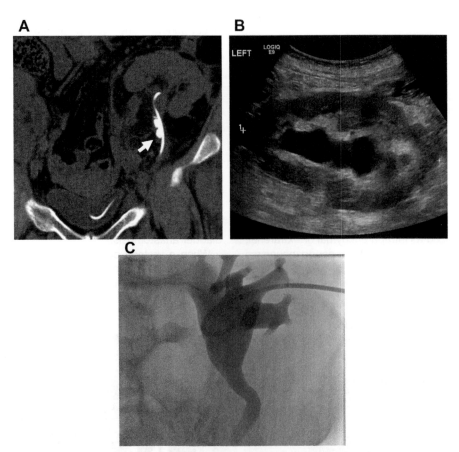

Fig. 9. A 53-year-old woman with left iliac fossa renal graft transplantation 1 week prior presents with sepsis from urinary tract infection. (*A*) Unenhanced coronal CT shows obstructive renal calculi adjacent to the intraoperatively placed ureteral stent (*arrow*). There is mild ureteral wall thickening with adjacent fat stranding and hydronephrosis of the kidney upstream from the obstruction. (*B*) Gray scale ultrasound shows moderate hydronephrosis. (*C*) Fluoroscopic nephrogram with newly placed percutaneous nephrostomy tube shows moderate dilation of the renal collecting system with distal obstruction.

Treatment options include percutaneous nephrostomy with ureteral stent placement and sometimes ureteroplasty. Surgical revision may also be necessary.

RENAL ALLOGRAFT PARENCHYMAL COMPLICATIONS

The transplanted graft can also be subject to complications intrinsic to the graft parenchyma. These include allograft rejection, acute tubular injury, acute cortical necrosis, and drug-related nephrotoxic effects.[7] Although acute cortical necrosis can be diagnosed confidently by imaging, the other parenchymal complications are diagnosed primarily by biopsy. The role of imaging in parenchymal disease is mostly to assess for alternative vascular or ureteral etiologies of graft dysfunction.

Rejection

With advances in immunology and transplant nephrology, clinicians and pathologists have a better grasp of allograft rejection. The traditional classification divided rejection into a temporal relationship to graft implantation (hyperacute, acute, and chronic rejection). However, since 1991, the Banff classification has standardized the way for histopathological diagnosis and management.[13,14]

Rejection is now categorized into antibody-mediated and T-cell mediated subtypes. Rejection can occur any time after transplantation but most commonly occurs within the first 6 months.[7,14] The recipient's immune system is activated by recognition of foreign donor antigens via antibodies or T cells, resulting in damage to the allograft.

On ultrasound, grafts undergoing acute rejection are often normal, though urothelial thickening has been shown to be a sensitive finding[15,16] (Fig. 10). Traditionally held ultrasound parameters of increased size of the graft, loss of corticomedullary differentiation, increased resistive indices, and decreased perfusion have not shown to be useful in identifying rejection.[7,15] Ultimately, diagnosis of rejection is assessed via biopsy of the renal graft.

Acute Tubular Injury

Acute tubular injury is typically an early cause of renal allograft dysfunction.[7] Damage occurs at the level of the tubules, typically from hypoperfusion from prolonged cold ischemic times.[17] Diagnosis can be suggested based on imaging but ultimately is reliant on biopsy.

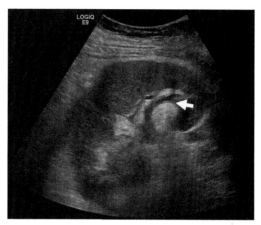

Fig. 10. A 43-year-old female status post renal transplantation. Gray scale US demonstrates nonspecific findings of urothelial thickening (*arrow*) with otherwise normal appearing renal allograft. This nonspecific finding overlaps with many other parenchymal processes, however, at times may be the only indicator of rejection.

On ultrasound, the graft may appear normal to mildly enlarged with subtle changes in parenchymal echogenicity. Doppler often shows decreased cortical perfusion with elevated intraparenchymal arterial resistive indices (>0.8). In severe cases, there may even be reversal of diastolic flow.

Acute Cortical Necrosis

Acute cortical necrosis is a rare entity which is of uncertain etiology, though often seen in the setting of hypotension. Reperfusion injury may provide a mechanism for acute cortical necrosis in the renal graft, particularly in the recent postoperative period.[17] Acute cortical necrosis is irreversible and, depending on the amount of graft involved, can lead to varying levels of permanent renal dysfunction.

On ultrasound, absent perfusion on Doppler ultrasound in the peripheral cortical portion of the kidney should raise concern, though decreased perfusion can be seen in other parenchymal etiologies of dysfunction such as acute tubular injury.[17,18] In distinction to acute tubular injury, intraparenchymal arterial resistive indices in patients with acute cortical necrosis can be normal, owing to shunting of blood away from the cortex through the Trueta phenomenon.[19] The use of contrast-enhanced ultrasound can confidently discriminate between these two entities. More chronically, the infarcted cortex will appear more hypoechoic on gray scale images, known as the hypoechoic rim sign.

Drug-Related Toxicity

Calcineurin inhibitors can produce nephrotoxic effects which can be difficult to discriminate from imaging findings of acute tubular injury. Diagnosis is usually made using a combination of biopsy and laboratory findings.

INFECTIOUS COMPLICATIONS

Owing to immunosuppressive medications, transplant recipients are at an increased risk of infection. Although there are large variations in the types of infections, there are predictable patterns of many infectious complications based on the length of time since transplantation.[20] In the first month after transplantation, infectious complications are mostly surgical wound infections, urinary tract infections, or pneumonia.[7] Donor-related infections are rare and caused by viral pathogens. In the late period, the graft is susceptible to opportunistic infections and routine community-acquired infections in the setting of prolonged immunosuppression.[7] Given that the transplanted ureter and the native bladder may lack a sphincter, pathogens may ascend from the urethra to the bladder, increasing risks of allograft pyelonephritis.[21] Occasionally, transplant pyelonephritis can occur as a result of bloodstream or surgical site infections.

Although the infectious appearance of many pathogens is nonspecific, patients generally present with classic signs of fever, graft pain, and positive urine cultures, although the clinical picture can be muted owing to immunosuppression. Imaging can show a thickened urothelium and wedge-shaped abnormalities on ultrasound, CT, and MR imaging. Adjacent fat may show inflammatory changes. With contrast-enhanced imaging, there may be a discrete rim-enhancing fluid collection to suggest an abscess. On Doppler ultrasound, affected portions may show decreased perfusion. On contrast-enhanced imaging, striated nephrograms can be seen (**Fig. 11**).

Pyonephrosis, which is hydronephrosis with superimposed infection, often has urothelial thickening and layering debris in a dilated collecting system and is a surgical emergency. Rarely, necrotizing infections of the parenchyma by gram-negative bacteria such as *Escherichia coli* can rapidly progress to emphysematous pyelonephritis, where the treatment is often emergent allograft nephrectomy.

As a measure of preventing opportunistic infections, inactivated vaccinations are administered 3 to 6 months following transplantation. In addition,

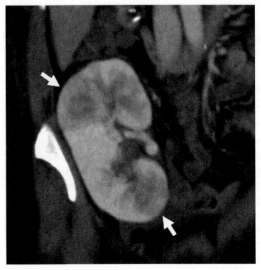

Fig. 11. A 47-year-old woman with pyelonephritis of the right iliac fossa with sepsis. Coronal contrast-enhanced CT image shows wedge-shaped areas of hypoattenuation (*arrows*) compatible with acute pyelonephritis.

antimicrobial and antiviral prophylaxis are given 6 months to 1-year posttransplant.

MALIGNANCY

Malignancy is the third most common cause of death in renal transplant patients, following cardiovascular disease and infectious complications with the peak incidence 3 to 5 years posttransplantation.[22,23] It is well-established that kidney graft recipients are at increased risk for malignancy, attributable to the effects of immunosuppression and unregulated oncogenic viral infections.[22,23] However, this increased risk is not evenly distributed over all types of cancers. Some cancer incidences are not increased (breast, prostate, ovarian, and cervical), whereas others are substantially increased (Kaposi's sarcoma, non-melanoma skin, lymphoma, colon, and liver).[24,25] Risk for lymphoma during the first year posttransplantation is 20-fold higher after kidney transplantation.[25,26] Hence, increased vigilence in cancer screening has become part of the routine management algorithm by transplant physicians.

Primary Renal Malignancy

The risk of primary renal malignancy involving the allograft as well as the native kidneys is increased in transplant kidney recipients.[22] There is an greater incidence of renal cell carcinoma in posttransplant patients. Primary malignancy in the renal allograft overall is elevated approximately six times more than the native kidney due to chronic immunosuppression.[7] This increased risk of malignancy is

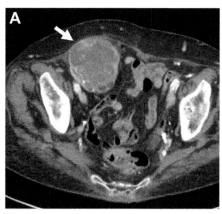 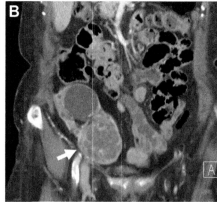

Fig. 12. A 72-year-old woman with a prior history of left native kidney renal cell carcinoma status post left nephrectomy now status post right iliac fossa deceased donor renal transplantation. (*A*) Axial and (*B*) coronal contrast-enhanced CT images demonstrate a large heterogeneously enhancing solid mass with necrotic center compatible with renal cell carcinoma (*arrow*).

thought to be multifactorial, including preexisting native renal disease, race, and gender.[9] Most renal cell carcinomas present as solid renal masses on imaging with variable enhancement features depending on the subtype. Infiltrative renal cell carcinomas can also occur (**Fig. 12**).

Posttransplantation Lymphoproliferative Disorder

Posttransplantation lymphoproliferative disorder (PTLD), a spectrum of uncontrolled lymphoid growth from hyperplasia to malignancy, is a well-known entity among solid organ transplant recipients.[26,27] For renal graft recipients, it is the most common malignancy after cutaneous malignancies, involving 0.8% to 2.5% of recipients with a bimodal distribution of 1 year and 10 to 14 years posttransplantation.[26,27] It arises in the setting of acquired or reactivated Epstein–Barr virus infection.

With different types of solid organ transplantation, there is a varied bodily distribution with nodal and extranodal involvement in those with kidney transplantation. The renal allograft is the most common site for renal graft recipients. Unlike lymphoma, PTLD tends to be more extranodal with the gastrointestinal system and liver being the next most common sites.[9]

In advanced stages of the disease, PTLD mimics lymphoma on imaging with homogenous soft tissue. On ultrasound, it will appear hypoechoic relative to the adjacent renal parenchyma. On contrast-enhanced CT and MR, lesions will appear as a hypoenhancing solid or infiltrative mass. The mass can involve the renal hilum, leading to renal outflow obstruction.[9] Nodal disease presents commonly as retroperitoneal lymphadenopathy. When bowel is involved, there is hypoenhancing, circumferential bowel wall thickening

of the mid to distal small bowel with generally no obstruction. Tissue diagnosis is the gold standard for diagnosis, with PET/CT being more sensitive and specific than CT for staging and assessing treatment response.

The mainstay of treatment is reduction of immunosuppression. The goal is to restore cellular immunity against the Epstein–Barr virus.[27] However, reduction of immunosuppression also increases the risk of graft loss and rejection. Thus, optimally minimizing immunosuppressive drugs as well as regular screening with noninvasive imaging is a key prevention strategy.

SUMMARY

Kidney grafts are the most common transplanted solid organs. As such, radiologists should be aware of the anatomy and potential complications unique to kidney grafts. Ultrasound plays the dominant role in diagnosing etiologies of kidney dysfunction, which include peritransplant collections, vascular and urologic complications, and malignancy. CT and MR imaging play a useful adjunctive role in diagnosing certain pathologies.

CLINICS CARE POINTS

- Duplex ultrasound is the modality of choice for routine surveillance and diagnostic evaluation of renal allografts.
- Allograft complications can be organized in a temporal distribution as well as by type of complication, thus helping narrow the differential diagnosis.

- An understanding of variations in vascular anatomy and surgical techniques are vital in evaluating allograft dysfunction.
- For vascular complications, time to diagnosis is critical for early intervention of potentially reversible diagnoses. MR and CT imaging can be used as adjunct imaging modalities.
- When pathologic diagnosis is necessary, ultrasound-guided biopsy and sampling is a relatively low risk and safe procedure.

DISCLOSURE

The authors have nothing to disclose.

REFERENCES

1. Sharfuddin A. Renal relevant radiology: imaging in kidney transplantation. Clin J Am Soc Nephrol 2014;9(2):416–29.
2. Friedewald SM, Molmenti EP, Friedewald JJ, et al. Vascular and nonvascular complications of renal transplants: sonographic evaluation and correlation with other imaging modalities, surgery, and pathology. J Clin Ultrasound 2005;33(3):127–39.
3. Kim N, Juarez R, Levy AD. Imaging non-vascular complications of renal transplantation. Abdom Radiol (NY) 2018;43(10):2555–63.
4. Akbar SA, Jafri SZ, Amendola MA, et al. Complications of renal transplantation. Radiographics 2005;25(5):1335–56.
5. Fananapazir G, Rao R, Corwin MT, et al. Sonographic Evaluation of Clinically Significant Perigraft Hematomas in Kidney Transplant Recipients. AJR Am J Roentgenol 2015;205(4):802–6.
6. Lockhart ME, Wells CG, Morgan DE, et al. Reversed diastolic flow in the renal transplant: perioperative implications versus transplants older than 1 month. AJR Am J Roentgenol 2008;190(3):650–5.
7. Sugi MD, Joshi G, Maddu KK, et al. Imaging of Renal Transplant Complications throughout the Life of the Allograft: Comprehensive Multimodality Review. Radiographics 2019;39(5):1327–55.
8. Aktas S, Boyvat F, Sevmis S, et al. Analysis of vascular complications after renal transplantation. Transplant Proc 2011;43(2):557–61.
9. Fananapazir G, Troppmann C. Vascular complications in kidney transplant recipients. Abdom Radiol (NY) 2018;43(10):2546–54.
10. Chen W, Kayler LK, Zand MS, et al. Transplant renal artery stenosis: clinical manifestations, diagnosis and therapy. Clin Kidney J 2015;8(1):71–8.
11. Fananapazir G, McGahan JP, Corwin MT, et al. Screening for Transplant Renal Artery Stenosis: Ultrasound-Based Stenosis Probability Stratification. AJR Am J Roentgenol 2017;209(5):1064–73.
12. Fananapazir G, Hannsun G, Wright LA, et al. Diagnosis and Management of Transplanted Kidney Extrarenal Pseudoaneurysms: A Series of Four Cases and a Review of the Literature. Cardiovasc Intervent Radiol 2016;39(11):1649–53.
13. Bhowmik DM, Dinda AK, Mahanta P, et al. The evolution of the Banff classification schema for diagnosing renal allograft rejection and its implications for clinicians. Indian J Nephrol 2010;20(1):2–8.
14. Naik R.H. and Shawar S.H., Renal Transplantation Rejection, In: StatPearls [Internet], 2023. Treasure Island (FL): StatPearls Publishing; 2023 Jan-. Available at: https://www.ncbi.nlm.nih.gov/books/NBK553074/
15. Fananapazir G, Navarro SM, Zhou C, et al. Sonographically Diagnosed Urothelial Thickening in Kidney Allografts: A Noninvasive and Clinically Highly Relevant Marker for the Detection of Acute Rejection. AJR Am J Roentgenol 2020;215(1):148–52.
16. Phillips CH, Malone FE, Biederman LE, et al. Clinical Significance of Renal Allograft Urothelial Thickening Identified by Ultrasound. J Ultrasound Med 2021;40(10):2173–9.
17. Fernandez CP, Ripolles T, Martinez MJ, et al. Diagnosis of acute cortical necrosis in renal transplantation by contrast-enhanced ultrasound: a preliminary experience. Ultraschall der Med 2013;34(4):340–4.
18. Shiekh Y, Ilyas M. Reverse rim sign: acute renal cortical necrosis. Abdom Radiol (NY) 2018;43(12):3507–8.
19. Siegelman SS, Goldman AG. The Trueta phenomenon. Angiographic documentation in man. Radiology 1968;90(6):1084–9.
20. Fishman JA. Infection in Organ Transplantation. Am J Transplant 2017;17(4):856–79.
21. Chuang P, Parikh CR, Langone A. Urinary tract infections after renal transplantation: a retrospective review at two US transplant centers. Clin Transplant 2005;19(2):230–5.
22. Manickavasagar R, Thuraisingham R. Post renal-transplant malignancy surveillance. Clin Med 2020;20(2):142–5.
23. Morath C, Mueller M, Goldschmidt H, et al. Malignancy in renal transplantation. J Am Soc Nephrol 2004;15(6):1582–8.
24. Sprangers B, Nair V, Launay-Vacher V, et al. Risk factors associated with post-kidney transplant malignancies: an article from the Cancer-Kidney International Network. Clin Kidney J 2018;11(3):315–29.
25. Kasiske BL, Snyder JJ, Gilbertson DT, et al. Cancer after kidney transplantation in the United States. Am J Transplant 2004;4(6):905–13.
26. Opelz G, Dohler B. Lymphomas after solid organ transplantation: a collaborative transplant study report. Am J Transplant 2004;4(2):222–30.
27. Abbas F, El Kossi M, Shaheen IS, et al. Post-transplantation lymphoproliferative disorders: Current concepts and future therapeutic approaches. World J Transplant 2020;10(2):29–46.

Pancreatic Transplantation
Surgical Anatomy and Complications

Benjamin M. Mervak, MD[a], Molly E. Roseland, MD[a,b], Ashish P. Wasnik, MD, FSAR, FSRU[a,*]

KEYWORDS

• Pancreas transplantation • Pancreas allograft • Imaging • Posttransplant complication

KEY POINTS

- An understanding of the complex, variable postsurgical anatomy of pancreatic transplants is essential to recognize normal imaging appearances and complications.
- Vascular complications (arterial and venous) are significant causes of morbidity and graft dysfunction. Critical diagnoses (thrombosis, stenosis, and pseudoaneurysm) have typical appearances on Doppler ultrasound (US) but computed tomography (CT)/MR imaging may be necessary if US is inconclusive.
- Complications associated with exocrine pancreatic drainage include bowel or bladder anastomotic leaks, which should be detectable by CT.
- Other important complications include pancreatitis, perigraft collections, rejection, and posttransplant lymphoproliferative disease, for which radiology plays a variable role in diagnosis.

INTRODUCTION

Pancreatic transplantation is a definitive surgical treatment of endocrine pancreatic insufficiency in severe insulin-dependent diabetes.[1] It is most commonly offered to patients with end-stage renal disease due to diabetic nephropathy and can be combined with a kidney transplant. These transplants are usually performed concurrently (simultaneous pancreas-kidney transplant) but may also be performed sequentially (pancreas-after-kidney transplants) or rarely in isolation (pancreas transplant alone [PTA], for brittle diabetics with preserved renal function). Pancreas transplants uniquely enable recipients to avert further diabetes-related complications, offering improved quality of life and long-term survival.[1]

After the first successful operation in 1966, pancreatic transplants have now been performed in nearly 50,000 patients.[2] However, the procedure remains less common and more technically challenging relative to other transplants. Despite evolving surgical techniques and novel immunosuppression leading to improved graft longevity, rates of pancreas transplantation have declined in the United States, with only 11 national centers in the United States performing more than 20 operations annually.[3] This rarity presents a challenge to radiologists who encounter pancreas transplants in practice because they may be unfamiliar with typical imaging appearances. Complex surgical anatomy also leads to frequent and distinct complications, which require an efficient and accurate radiologic diagnosis to preserve graft function. Therefore, in this review, we will describe common surgical methods and illustrate various imaging findings of pancreas transplant complications to improve diagnostic accuracy for such challenging cases.

PANCREAS TRANSPLANT SURGICAL ANATOMY

Nearly all (>99%) modern pancreatic transplants worldwide are whole-organ transplants harvested from deceased donors, although segmental

[a] Division of Abdominal Radiology, Department of Radiology, University of Michigan-Michigan Medicine, University Hospital, B1D502, 1500 East Medical Center Drive, Ann Arbor, MI 48109, USA; [b] Division of Nuclear Medicine, Department of Radiology, University of Michigan-Michigan Medicine, University Hospital, B1D502, 1500 East Medical Center Drive, Ann Arbor, MI 48109, USA
* Corresponding author.
E-mail address: ashishw@med.umich.edu

Radiol Clin N Am 61 (2023) 821–831
https://doi.org/10.1016/j.rcl.2023.04.005

radiologic.theclinics.com

pancreas transplantation has historically been performed.[4] After identification of a suitable donor, the pancreas is harvested en-bloc with the following components: a section of duodenum with the ampulla of Vater; the splenic artery and proximal superior mesenteric artery (SMA); a segment of the splenic vein, superior mesenteric vein (SMV), portal venous confluence, and main portal vein (MPV).[5,6] The donor common bile duct is divided and ligated. As part of the donor surgery, the distal donor common iliac artery (CIA)—including the bifurcation into the internal and external iliac arteries—is also harvested to provide a "Y-graft," as discussed below.

During transplantation, the pancreatic allograft is generally placed intraperitoneally in the recipient's right lower quadrant via a midline laparotomy. The head of the donor pancreas and duodenal segment is usually directed cranially (for portal venous drainage and/or exocrine drainage to bowel) but may also be caudally directed (for systemic venous drainage and/or exocrine drainage to the urinary bladder).[7,8] Retroperitoneal placement of the pancreatic allograft has been described with either portal venous or systemic drainage, although these remain less frequent.[9–11] The recipient's native pancreas is generally not resected.[12]

Arterial Supply

The head of the pancreatic allograft is normally supplied by the inferior pancreaticoduodenal artery originating from the SMA, whereas the body and tail are perfused from branches of the splenic artery. To allow for only one arterial anastomosis in the recipient, a "Y-graft" is created by harvesting a donor CIA bifurcation. The donor SMA and splenic artery stumps are then individually anastomosed with an end-to-end technique onto the limbs of the Y-graft in back-bench preparation. During transplantation in the right hemipelvis, the stem of the Y-graft is then anastomosed in an end-to-side fashion, most commonly to the recipient's right common or external iliac artery (EIA; Fig. 1A, B). Retroperitoneal placement of the pancreas also typically uses a Y-graft anastomosed to the common or EIA, although is disadvantaged by a technically complex arterial anastomosis with a need for a long Y-graft that traverses the ileal mesentery.[11]

Venous Outflow

Venous drainage of the pancreatic allograft is via the donor MPV, which drains the pancreatic head via the donor SMV and body/tail via the donor splenic vein. The donor MPV is often anastomosed in an end-to-side fashion to the recipient's inferior vena cava for systemic drainage. However, at some centers, the donor MPV is anastomosed to the recipient's external iliac vein (potentially necessitating a conduit of donor iliac vein), or can be anastomosed to the recipient SMV for portal drainage, particularly if the allograft is placed in the retroperitoneum.[5,6,11] Although portal drainage may more closely resemble the native drainage pathway of endocrine hormones, it has not been shown to improve long-term outcomes.[13]

Exocrine Secretions

During back-bench preparation, the donor duodenum is typically stapled proximally and distally to create a blind-ending conduit. Enteric drainage is currently the preferred for pancreatic exocrine secretions.[14] During transplantation, side-to-side anastomosis of this duodenal conduit is typically performed either directly to the patient's jejunum or ileum, or to a Roux limb of recipient jejunum.

A small number of pancreatic transplants (approximately 10%) have exocrine secretions managed by anastomosis to the urinary bladder[11] (Fig. 1C). This technique was commonly used until the 1990s because it enabled easy monitoring of pancreatic function (via urinary amylase levels).[14] However, this nonphysiologic configuration was later shown to lead to a higher rate of complications, including reflux pancreatitis, hematuria, urethral stricture, and urinary tract infections.[15,16] Despite its rarity, this alternative configuration is essential to recognize in older or PTA allografts.

IMAGING AND NORMAL PANCREAS GRAFT

Due to its widespread availability, low cost, and lack of radiation, ultrasound (US) is a mainstay for imaging evaluation of pancreatic transplants, used for baseline assessment and routine follow-up, as well as for the evaluation of potential complications. However, sonographic evaluation may be challenging due to graft positioning in the right lower quadrant, where shadowing from overlying bowel gas may obscure the graft, and where variable transplant configurations may make normal anatomy difficult to identify.

A complete US examination of a pancreatic transplant includes a combination of grayscale, color, and spectral Doppler images and cines. Both static and cine grayscale images of the entire allograft should be obtained in both transverse and longitudinal plane. Color Doppler images and spectral Doppler waveforms should be obtained of intraparenchymal venous and arterial segments

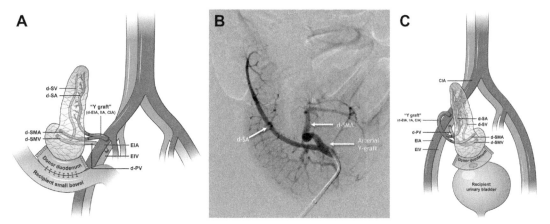

Fig. 1. Pancreas transplant anatomy. (*A*) Right lower quadrant pancreas graft. Arterial "Y graft" from donor external (d-EIA), internal (d-IIA), and common iliac artery (d-CIA) anastomosed to the donor superior mesenteric artery (d-SMA) and splenic artery (d-SA). The stem of "Y graft" is anastomosed to the recipient EIA. The donor portal vein (d-PV) is anastomosed to recipient external iliac vein (EIV). The donor duodenum is anastomosed to recipient ileal loop. (*B*) Transplant pancreas arteriogram showing the vascular anatomy. (*C*) Pancreas graft with enterovesical drainage, the donor duodenum is anastomosed to recipient urinary bladder.

in the head, body, and tail, as well as the Y graft and vascular anastomoses.

A normal pancreatic graft should have a homogeneous echotexture and attenuation similar to native pancreas on US, computed tomography (CT), or magnetic resonance (MR) (**Fig. 2**A, B). On grayscale and Doppler US, the pancreatic graft vasculature should appear patent without evidence for echogenic clot or lack of flow, and no aliasing/turbulence or elevated peak systolic velocity should be seen at the arterial anastomosis. Arterial spectral Doppler waveforms should show a brisk upstroke without reversal of diastolic flow (**Fig. 2**C). Notably, arterial resistive indices are not useful indicators of parenchymal impedance to flow due to the lack of a pancreatic capsule and are not routinely measured at our institution.[17]

CT and MR imaging also play a role in the evaluation of pancreatic transplants and complications, and can be used for more definitive diagnosis after a technically limited or equivocal US. A common dilemma encountered among patients undergoing pancreatic transplant is impaired renal function. Low glomerular filtration rate, either acute or chronic, may increase the risk of complications associated with intravenous iodinated or gadolinium contrast material, such as contrast-induced acute kidney injury or nephrogenic systemic fibrosis (NSF), although the American College of Radiology acknowledges that gadolinium agents in group II have a sufficiently low or nonexistent risk of NSF so as to obviate screening for low renal function before administration.[18] Nonetheless, due to its availability,

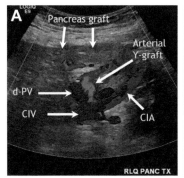
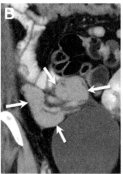
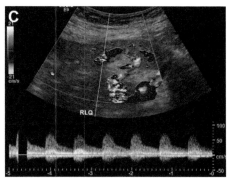

Fig. 2. (*A*) Normal pancreas graft on Doppler imaging with donor portal vein (d-PV) anastomosed to common iliac vein (CIV), arterial "Y-graft" anastomosed to CIA. (*B*) Coronal reformatted contrast-enhanced CT shows homogenously enhancing pancreatic graft in the right lower quadrant (*arrows*). (*C*) Normal arterial waveform on spectral Doppler imaging through the pancreatic graft.

noncontrast CT is frequently used to evaluate for perigraft hematomas or fluid collections. It may rarely enable diagnosis of a hyperattenuating acute vascular thrombosis. MR imaging can also assess for perigraft collections and vascular complications by using noncontrast MRA sequences such as time-of-flight or phase-contrast techniques. In patients with suspected vascular complications, a contrast-enhanced CT or MR imaging, including arterial and venous phase imaging, may ultimately be necessary to establish a critical diagnosis. A multidisciplinary conversation (including the patient, radiologist, nephrology team, and transplant team) is helpful in such settings to discuss the risks, benefits, and clinical necessity of contrast-enhanced imaging.

PANCREAS TRANSPLANT COMPLICATIONS
Vascular (Arterial or Venous) Thrombosis

Vascular thrombosis is the most common acute to subacute complication following pancreatic transplantation. It occurs in roughly 5% to 14% of patients[17,19–21] and is the second most common cause of graft failure after rejection.[21,22] Venous thrombosis occurs more commonly than arterial thrombosis, typically isolated to the ligated ends of the graft splenic vein or SMV, rather than extending into larger venous structures and preventing venous outflow. Venous thrombosis may be either partially or entirely occlusive. Although often multifactorial, venous thrombosis may occur secondary to slow flow rates caused by vascular kinking or twisting, a perigraft fluid collection, or graft pancreatitis (discussed below).[7,23]

Arterial thrombosis is a less common but more severe complication than venous thrombosis, leading to rapid graft dysfunction and necrosis. Arterial thrombosis frequently occurs within the first 3 months of transplantation, with risk factors including prolonged cold ischemic time, poor surgical technique, vessel caliber mismatch, small caliber arteries, arterial kinking, or acute rejection.[23] After 3 months, arterial thrombosis may be caused by chronic rejection.[7]

Imaging plays a critical role in the evaluation for vascular complications, as clinical and laboratory findings are generally nonspecific, and transplant failure can rapidly occur if a diagnosis is not made. US is typically the first-line imaging modality but may be limited by artifact or limited sonographic windows. When visualized, intravascular thrombus seems as a hyperechoic or hypoechoic intravascular filling defect on grayscale images (**Fig. 3**). Other indirect signs of vascular thrombosis and impaired graft perfusion include incomplete/absent intravascular flow on color Doppler

imaging, a heterogeneous graft with decreased or absent intraparenchymal color/power Doppler flow, low intraparenchymal arterial resistive indices, and/or a parvus-tardus waveform (low-velocity, delayed systolic upstroke) on spectral Doppler[17,24] (**Fig. 4**). A high-resistance arterial waveform with pandiastolic reversal of flow in the acute postoperative setting is both sensitive and specific for venous thrombosis.[21] A distended vein may also suggest thrombophlebitis or graft edema related to outflow obstruction.[17]

Contrast-enhanced CT or MR imaging is used secondarily to confirm vascular thromboses or when US is indeterminate. Multiphasic (arterial and venous) postcontrast imaging is preferred to fully evaluate both the arterial and venous structures and delineate the extent of thrombosis, seen as low-attenuation or low signal intensity filling defects within affected vessels. In patients with comorbid renal failure who cannot receive intravascular contrast material, noncontrast time-of-flight MR imaging may also show filling defects within vessels, and high signal thrombus on T1-weighted sequences. CT and MR imaging may further be useful to evaluate for portions of the graft, which are edematous or hypoenhancing, potentially indicating graft pancreatitis or developing necrosis (see **Fig. 4**).

Arterial Stenosis

Arterial stenosis in pancreatic transplants is uncommon. When present, it typically occurs at 1 of the 3 anastomoses, and can be a result of surgical technique, vessel trauma, or rejection.[23] As with arterial thrombosis, early recognition is vital to direct timely interventions, including angioplasty or stenting due to the high risk of graft failure.

Pancreatic graft arterial stenosis can be challenging to diagnose on US due to adjacent bowel limiting the ability to identify and interrogate the arterial anastomosis. Perhaps due to the rarity of arterial stenosis in pancreatic transplants, much of the literature on US findings in posttransplant arterial stenosis has been conducted on hepatic and renal allografts,[25–28] although general concepts would be expected to apply to pancreatic transplants as well. Specifically, color and spectral Doppler US may be used to evaluate for aliasing near the anastomosis; measure peak systolic velocities upstream of, at, and beyond the anastomoses; and evaluate spectral Doppler waveforms. Indirect signs of stenosis with US include turbulent flow with aliasing at the anastomosis, elevated peak systolic flow velocities (initial flow rates >400 cm/s or persistent flow rate faster than 300 cm/s), a 2-fold (or more) increase of flow

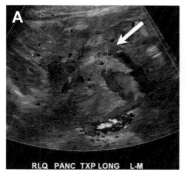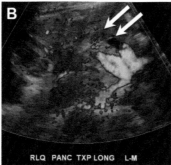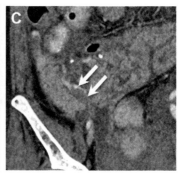

Fig. 3. A 36-year-old woman with pancreas graft segmental venous thrombosis. (*A*) Color Doppler image of the pancreas graft shows echogenic thrombus in the graft vein in the proximal body (*arrows*). (*B*) Power Doppler confirms segmental occlusion (*arrows*). (*C*) Coronal reformat CECT shows hypodense thrombus in the pancreas graft vein (*arrows*).

velocity in the stenotic segment versus the prestenotic segment, and/or a tardus-parvus waveform with low-resistive indices beyond the anastomosis[25,26,29] (**Fig. 5A**). CT angiography (CTA), MR angiography (MRA), or conventional angiography can be used to confirm anastomotic narrowing, although MRA in particular may overestimate or underestimate the severity in low-flow states or if there is substantial artifact from adjacent surgical material[30,31] (**Fig. 5B**).

Arterial Pseudoaneurysm

Arterial pseudoaneurysms can occur within pancreas transplants secondary to injury to an arterial wall from pancreatitis, infection, or biopsy.[29,32] Prompt identification and reporting are important due to the risk of rupture and hemorrhage. Although difficult to evaluate with US, the expected appearance would be a focal outpouching with turbulent bidirectional internal blood flow ("yin–yang" sign).[17] CTA or MRA can provide more definitive evaluation and localization of a pseudoaneurysm, showing a focal rounded outpouching mirroring the attenuation or signal intensity of the aorta and arterial vasculature on all postcontrast phases (**Fig. 6**). Catheter angiography remains the gold standard for both diagnosis and treatment of pseudoaneurysms.

Arteriovenous Fistula

Arteriovenous fistulas (AVFs) represent another uncommon vascular complication after pancreatic transplantation and are most often the result of iatrogenic injury during surgery or following biopsy. Most AVFs are small and managed conservatively, often resolving spontaneously. Larger fistulas resulting in hemodynamic changes may require surgical or endovascular repair. US findings are limited to observations on color and spectral Doppler imaging, where a focus of rapid flow and wrap-around artifact (aliasing) can be seen due to high-velocity flow from an artery into an

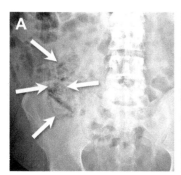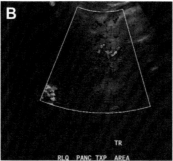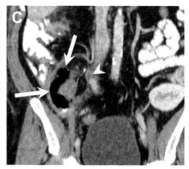

Fig. 4. A 42-year-old woman with pancreas graft necrosis secondary to arterial thrombosis. (*A*) Frontal abdominal radiograph for abdominal pain shows an oblong area of mottled gas in the expected location of right lower quadrant pancreas transplant (*arrows*). (*B*) Right lower quadrant abdominal Doppler US was gassed out without delineation of the pancreas graft prompting CT. (*C*) Coronal reformat CECT shows a necrosed pancreas graft with gas in the right lower quadrant (*arrows*) and abrupt occlusion from graft artery thrombus (*arrowhead*).

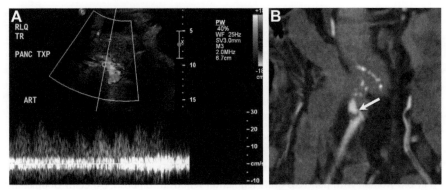

Fig. 5. A 48-year-old man with pancreas graft arterial anastomosis stenosis. (*A*) Doppler spectral imaging of the RLQ transplant pancreas shows delayed upstroke with significant low PSV (20 cm/s) in the graft segmental artery suggestive of significant upstream stenosis. (*B*) Coronal reformat CTA shows significant stenosis at the pancreatic graft arterial anastomosis to EIA (*arrow*).

adjacent draining vein with low resistance to flow. Flow within the draining veins may also appear "arterialized" and pulsatile on spectral Doppler.[27] Contrast-enhanced CT or MR imaging can also show early opacification of a draining vein during arterial phase images.[23,24,33]

Pancreas Graft Rejection

Graft rejection is the most common cause of pancreatic transplant failure, with the International Pancreas Transplant Registry attributing up to 40% of graft loss to immunologic causes.[2,34] Rejection can be categorized as hyperacute (within minutes to hours), acute (between 1 week and 3 months posttransplant), and chronic (after 6 months). Hyperacute rejection is now extremely

uncommon due to robust crossmatching and antibody screening before transplantation but occurs rarely due to preexisting antidonor antibodies in the recipient.[35] Acute rejection is thought to be most often due to immune-mediated small vessel arteritis and vessel occlusion. If recurrent, this can lead to fibrosis, atrophy, and chronic rejection.[7,35]

Imaging has limited specificity for diagnosing pancreatic graft rejection, and an image-guided biopsy is often necessary. Although US may be ordered as a screening modality, findings of rejection are nonspecific and are generally limited to graft enlargement and heterogeneity.[7,35] Similarly, CT and MR imaging may only show pancreatic parenchymal edema and surrounding inflammation, which can also be seen with pancreatitis. Imaging remains primarily valuable to exclude other

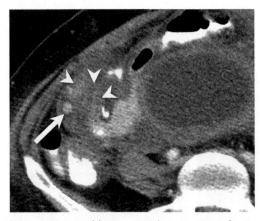

Fig. 6. A 39-year-old woman with pancreas graft arterial pseudoaneurysm. Axial CECT shows right lower quadrant graft pancreatitis and patchy necrosis in the pancreatic body (*arrowhead*) and a small round hyperdense focus (*arrow*) representing a pseudoaneurysm in the setting of pancreatitis.

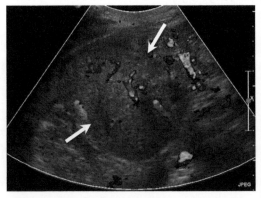

Fig. 7. A 41-year-old woman with acute graft pancreatitis with significantly elevated serum lipase and amylase. US with color Doppler showing an enlarged and edematous pancreas graft (*arrows*) with mild peripancreatic fluid.

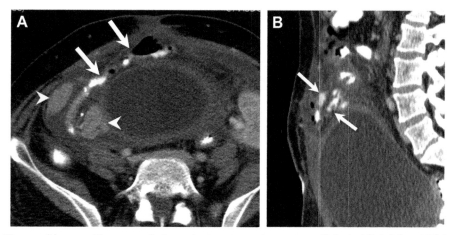

Fig. 8. A 47-year-old man with pancreatic transplant and enteric anastomotic leak. (*A*) Axial and (*B*) Saggital reformat CECT shows right lower quadrant pancreas graft (*arrowhead*) and extraluminal positive enteric contrast (*arrow*).

acute, surgical causes for graft failure, such as large vessel occlusion.[35]

Graft Pancreatitis

Graft pancreatitis is common in the immediate postoperative period. It is classically attributed to reperfusion injury,[7] although other risk factors for early pancreatitis have been suggested, including delays between organ procurement and transplantation, use of histidine-tryptophan-ketoglutarate solution during organ storage/transport, pancreatic duct obstruction, and bladder drainage of exocrine secretions. Although most cases are mild and subclinical/self-limited, severe pancreatitis occurs in roughly 10% of patients, and necrotizing pancreatitis in 2% to 4%; the latter can result in the subsequent need for surgical debridement or graft explant.[29] Clinical classification of severity can be difficult because traditional serum markers of native pancreatitis (eg, lipase) are unreliable in graft pancreatitis, and hyperamylasemia is common in the immediate posttransplant setting, even in the absence of pancreatitis.[20]

Similar to native pancreatitis, imaging evaluation for graft pancreatitis may be difficult because the disease can be radiologically occult or show nonspecific findings. US may show graft enlargement, heterogeneity, and edema, with or without surrounding free fluid. Contrast-enhanced CT and MR imaging may be useful as an adjunct to evaluate the possibility of graft necrosis, seen as nonenhancing areas of parenchyma and possible acute necrotic collections (**Fig. 7**). Notably, pancreatitis can also predispose to vascular thrombosis (due to local intimal injury), and vascular thromboses can also lead to graft inflammation ("secondary" pancreatitis). Therefore, contrast-enhanced CT/MR imaging is valuable to confirm vascular patency, which may otherwise be clinically indistinguishable from simple pancreatitis.

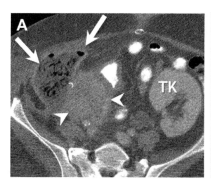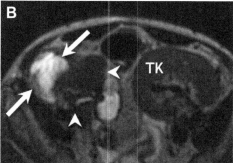

Fig. 9. Peripancreatic graft abscess. (*A*) Axial CECT showing a right lower quadrant pancreatic transplant (*arrowheads*) with a perigraft gas and fluid collection (*arrows*) (*B*) Axial T2-weighted MR image with right lower quadrant graft pancreas (*arrowheads*) and peripancreatic fluid collection (*arrows*), confirmed to be an abscess after drainage. TK, transplant kidney.

Table 1
Pancreas transplant complications

Complication	Timing	US Features	CT/MR Imaging Features
Arterial thrombosis	Usually early	Absence of flow in artery/Y-graft and parenchyma (often heterogeneous)	Nonopacification of artery or absent parenchymal enhancement/necrosis on postcontrast imaging
Venous thrombosis	Early or late	Filling defect on grayscale/color Doppler; absent venous waveforms; pandiastolic reversal of arterial flow	Filling defect or nonopacification of transplant veins on postcontrast images (variable); hyperdense clot on noncontrast CT
Arterial stenosis	Uncommon, late	Focal aliasing and high-velocity flow at the area of stenosis (usually the anastomosis); downstream tardus-parvus waveforms	Focal arterial narrowing at iliac or Y-graft anastomosis
Pseudoaneurysm	Postbiopsy, postpancreatitis	Focal hypoechoic structure with internal "yin–yang" Doppler flow, "to-and-fro" spectral waveform	Focal arterial outpouching
AVF	Postbiopsy	High-velocity, low-resistance arterial waveform, "arterialized" venous flow	Focal arterial–venous connection; early venous opacification on arterial phase postcontrast imaging
Pancreatitis	Early but can occur anytime	Graft enlargement, heterogeneity, perigraft fluid	Graft enlargement, heterogeneity, perigraft fluid
Rejection	Early or late, more common later	Graft enlargement, heterogeneity, perigraft fluid	Graft enlargement, heterogeneity, perigraft fluid
Anastomotic leak	Early	Perigraft fluid collection	Perigraft fluid/gas collection with extravasation of enteric or bladder contrast
Perigraft collection (hematoma, seroma)	Usually early	Perigraft collection, hypoanechoic if seroma, heterogeneously hyperechoic with reticular echoes if a hematoma	Perigraft collection of simple fluid density if seroma; high density or T1 hyperintense if hematoma, with or without active extravasation on postcontrast images
PTLD	Late	May be occult; pancreatic mass or lymphadenopathy	Lymphadenopathy and possible abdominal visceral masses

Pancreas Graft Enteric Anastomotic Leak

Exocrine anastomotic leaks occur in roughly 10% of pancreas transplants. Outcomes vary depending on the type of anastomosis; leak of bowel contents puts patients at increased risk for peritonitis or sepsis and can increase the potential for secondary graft loss. US is of limited utility in the evaluation for a leak, although may identify a nonspecific peri-transplant fluid collection. CT or fluoroscopy with ingested oral contrast material is generally the modalities of choice to evaluate for a leak if the graft is drained via bowel because they can visualize extraluminal enteric contrast (**Fig. 8**). In a graft drained via the urinary bladder, a CT cystogram or fluoroscopic cystogram can be used to identify a bladder wall defect and extravasation. Management can range from conservative treatment to surgical repair, depending on the site of the leak.

Peripancreatic Graft Collection

Fluid collections adjacent to pancreas transplants are most common in the early postoperative setting and are typically either hematomas or seromas. Following an episode of graft pancreatitis, acute peripancreatic collections and pseudocysts may also develop. Large collections may require image-guided drainage, particularly if there are clinical signs of infection.

Imaging evaluation of perigraft collections may include US, CT, or MR imaging, which can all be used to define the size and characteristics of the collection (Fig. 9). By US, an acute or subacute hematoma seems as a heterogeneous, variably echogenic collection, whereas a chronic maturing hematoma is often more hypoechoic. An enlarging hematoma or rapidly declining hemoglobin may warrant further evaluation with CT or MR imaging to identify the extent and source of bleeding. Acute hematoma is seen as a hyperdense collection on noncontrast CT, or as a heterogeneously T1 hyperintense collection on MR imaging. If there is active bleeding, contrast-enhanced imaging may also identify a culprit vessel or pseudoaneurysm, associated with progressive extravascular pooling/extravasation of contrast. Conversely, postsurgical seroma is typically anechoic on US and fluid attenuation/signal (without enhancement) on CT and MR imaging.

Posttransplant Lymphoproliferative Disorder

Posttransplant lymphoproliferative disorder (PTLD) is an uncommon late complication following pancreatic transplant, occurring in roughly 2% to 6% of patients and can result in patient mortality. PTLD is not specific to pancreatic transplant and is often seen among other organ transplant recipients requiring significant immunosuppression but is thought to be more common in patients negative for Epstein-Barr virus virologic surveillance is important.[36]

Diagnosis of PTLD depends on a combination of clinical, laboratory, imaging, and pathologic findings. Imaging is specifically necessary to identify sites of disease for tissue sampling and diagnostic confirmation. CT, MR imaging, or PET/CT are generally used because of the need to evaluate multiple organ systems and lymph nodes, which is challenging with US alone. Common findings revealed by CT and MR imaging include regional and/or nonregional lymphadenopathy or hepatosplenomegaly. Other organ involvement is somewhat less common in PTLD but can manifest as variably as other lymphomas, potentially with focal liver, splenic, or renal masses, focal bowel wall thickening, or focal mass/infiltration of the pancreatic graft itself.[29,37] Of note, the survival rate for PTLD after pancreatic transplant is lower than hepatic or renal transplants because it tends to present with more widespread disease.[36]

SUMMARY

Pancreas transplantation is an uncommon, complex, curative operation for severe insulin-dependent diabetes. Transplants have unique and variable surgical anatomy, which can influence the types, timing, and imaging appearances of postoperative complications.

Arterial anastomosis is typically to the recipient's right iliac system using a Y-graft to perfuse the donor SMA and splenic artery. Venous anastomosis may be performed to either the recipient's iliac or SMV. Imaging is essential for early and accurate diagnosis of associated vascular complications, first with Doppler US, and potentially with CT/MR imaging as necessary. Notable diagnoses include arterial thrombosis, venous thrombosis, arterial stenosis, AVFs, and pseudoaneurysms (Table 1).

Exocrine anastomosis is now generally performed to the small bowel, although previous surgical technique used the urinary bladder for exocrine drainage. This anastomosis may be complicated by early leaks, best detected by CT.

Finally, pancreatitis, peritransplant collections, rejection, and PTLD may occur over a large timeframe posttransplant; despite their nonspecific appearances, imaging may be used to exclude associated complications and/or guide biopsy. Altogether, an understanding of these significant transplant pathologic conditions and their imaging is essential for interpreting radiologists to improve patient outcomes.

CLINICS CARE POINTS

- Pancreatic transplants have intricate arterial anastomoses, with donor SMA/splenic artery connected to a donor Y-graft and then to recipient iliac artery. Doppler US is useful to identify arterial occlusion (absent parenchymal flow), narrowing (high-velocity flow at stenosis; downstream tardus-parvus waveform), pseudoaneurysm (yin-yang, to-and-fro waveform), or AVF (high-velocity, low-resistance waveform).

- Pancreatic transplant venous anastomoses are variable, with donor portal-splenic confluence connected to either systemic or portal veins of recipient. Grayscale and Doppler US are essential to diagnose thrombosis, which may seem as an intravenous filling defect, or, if hemodynamically significant, pandiastolic flow reversal in the arterial system.

- Contrast-enhanced CT/MR imaging (or non-contrast MRA/MRV) is important supplemental imaging tool for diagnosing vascular transplant complications if US is nondiagnostic.

- Exocrine anastomotic leaks are morbid early pancreas transplant complications that may require drainage or surgical revision. CT is best to identify extravasation of enteric contrast (if bowel anastomosis) or urine (if bladder anastomosis).

- Pancreatitis and rejection are common transplant complications with similar imaging appearances, including graft edema and perigraft fluid. Imaging is primarily helpful to exclude associated vascular thromboses or drainable collections.

- Posttransplant lymphoproliferative disease is a rare, late complication, manifesting as intra-abdominal masses and lymphadenopathy, potentially involving the graft. Imaging may suggest this diagnosis but biopsy is essential for confirmation.

DISCLOSURE

A.P. Wasnik: No disclosures related to this article. Unrelated disclosures include book royalty, Elsevier Inc.; royalty, intellectual property (IP), licensed by the University of Michigan to Applied Morphomics, Inc; and research support, Sequana Medical, NV, through the University of Michigan.

REFERENCES

1. Boggi U, Vistoli F, Marchetti P, et al. World Consensus Group on Pancreas Transplantation. First world consensus conference on pancreas transplantation: Part I-Methods and results of literature search. Am J Transplant 2021;21(Suppl 3): 1–16.
2. Gruessner AC, Gruessner RWG. The 2022 International Pancreas Transplant Registry Report—A Review. Transplant Proc 2022. https://doi.org/10.1016/j.transproceed.2022.03.059.
3. Stratta RJ, Gruessner AC, Odorico JS, et al. Pancreas Transplantation: An Alarming Crisis in Confidence. Am J Transplant 2016;16(9):2556–62.
4. Sutherland DER, Radosevich D, Gruessner R, et al. Pushing the envelope: living donor pancreas transplantation. Curr Opin Organ Transplant 2012;17(1): 106–15.
5. Chandra J, Phillips RR, Boardman P, et al. Pancreas transplants. Clin Radiol 2009;64(7):714–23.
6. Hampson FA, Freeman SJ, Ertner J, et al. Pancreatic transplantation: surgical technique, normal radiological appearances and complications. Insights Imaging 2010;1(5–6):339–47.
7. O'Malley RB, Moshiri M, Osman S, et al. Imaging of Pancreas Transplantation and Its Complications. Radiol Clin 2016;54(2):251–66.
8. Freund MC, Steurer W, Gassner EM, et al. Spectrum of Imaging Findings After Pancreas Transplantation with Enteric Exocrine Drainage: Part 1, Posttransplantation Anatomy. Am J Roentgenol 2004;182(4): 911–7.
9. Boggi U, Vistoli F, Signori S, et al. A Technique for Retroperitoneal Pancreas Transplantation with Portal-Enteric Drainage. Transplantation 2005;79(9):1137.
10. Ferrer J, Molina V, Rull R, et al. Pancreas transplantation: Advantages of a retroperitoneal graft position. Cir Esp 2017;95(9):513–20.
11. Rogers J, Farney AC, Orlando G, et al. Pancreas transplantation with portal venous drainage with an emphasis on technical aspects. Clin Transplant 2014;28(1):16–26.
12. França M, Certo M, Martins L, et al. Imaging of pancreas transplantation and its complications. Insights Imaging 2010;1(5–6):329–38.
13. Bazerbachi F, Selzner M, Marquez MA, et al. Portal Venous Versus Systemic Venous Drainage of Pancreas Grafts: Impact on Long-Term Results. Am J Transplant 2012;12(1):226–32.
14. Ferrer-Fàbrega J, Fernández-Cruz L. Exocrine drainage in pancreas transplantation: Complications and management. World J Transplant 2020;10(12): 392–403.
15. Baktavatsalam R, Little DM, Connolly EM, et al. Complications relating to the urinary tract associated with bladder-drained pancreatic transplantation. Br J Urol 1998;81(2):219–23.
16. Hickey DP, Bakthavatsalam R, Bannon CA, et al. Urological Complications of Pancreatic Transplantation. J Urol 1997;157(6):2042–8.
17. Wasnik AP, Aslam AA, Millet JD, et al. Multimodality imaging of pancreas-kidney transplants. Clin Imag 2021;69:185–95.
18. American College of Radiology - Committee on Drugs and Contrast Media. ACR Manual on Contrast Media.; 2022. Available at: https://www.acr.org/-/media/ACR/Files/Clinical-Resources/Contrast_Media.pdf. Accessed November 22, 2022.

19. Norton PT, DeAngelis GA, Ogur T, et al. Noninvasive Vascular Imaging in Abdominal Solid Organ Transplantation. Am J Roentgenol 2013;201(4):W544–53.

20. Troppmann C. Complications after pancreas transplantation. Curr Opin Organ Transplant 2010;15(1): 112–8.

21. Foshager MC, Hedlund LJ, Troppmann C, et al. Venous thrombosis of pancreatic transplants: diagnosis by duplex sonography. Am J Roentgenol 1997;169(5):1269–73.

22. Humar A, Ramcharan T, Kandaswamy R, et al. Technical Failures after Pancreas Transplants: Why Grafts Fail and the Risk Factors—A Multivariate Analysis. Transplantation 2004;78(8):1188–92.

23. Low G, Crockett AM, Leung K, et al. Imaging of Vascular Complications and Their Consequences Following Transplantation in the Abdomen. Radiographics 2013;33(3):633–52.

24. Heller MT, Bhargava P. Imaging in pancreatic transplants. Indian J Radiol Imag 2014;24(04):339–49.

25. Taylor KJ, Morse SS, Rigsby CM, et al. Vascular complications in renal allografts: detection with duplex Doppler US. Radiology 1987;162(1):31–8.

26. Snider JF, Hunter DW, Moradian GP, et al. Transplant Renal Artery Stenosis: Evaluation with Duplex Sonography. Radiology 1989;172(3):1027–30.

27. Brown ED, Chen MYM, Wolfman NT, et al. Complications of Renal Transplantation: Evaluation with US and Radionuclide Imaging. Radiographics 2000; 20(3):607–22.

28. Dodd GD, Memel DS, Zajko AB, et al. Hepatic artery stenosis and thrombosis in transplant recipients: Doppler diagnosis with resistive index and systolic acceleration time. Radiology 1994;192(3):657–61.

29. Sandrasegaran K, Lall C, Berry WA, et al. Enteric drainage pancreatic transplantation. Abdom Imaging 2006;31(5):588–95.

30. Zamboni GA, Pedrosa I, Kruskal JB, et al. Multimodality postoperative imaging of liver transplantation. Eur Radiol 2008;18(5):882–91.

31. Ishigami K, Stolpen AH, Al-kass FMH, et al. Diagnostic Value of Gadolinium-Enhanced 3D Magnetic Resonance Angiography in Patients With Suspected Hepatic Arterial Complications After Liver Transplantation. J Comput Assist Tomogr 2005;29(4):464–71.

32. Dillman JR, Elsayes KM, Bude RO, et al. Imaging of Pancreas Transplants: Postoperative Findings With Clinical Correlation. J Comput Assist Tomogr 2009; 33(4):609–17.

33. Hagspiel KD, Nandalur K, Pruett TL, et al. Evaluation of Vascular Complications of Pancreas Transplantation with High-Spatial-Resolution Contrast-enhanced MR Angiography. Radiology 2007;242(2):590–9.

34. Pozniak MA, Propeck PA, Kelcz F, et al. Imaging of Pancreas Transplants. Radiol Clin 1995;33(3): 581–94.

35. Vandermeer FQ, Manning MA, Frazier AA, et al. Imaging of Whole-Organ Pancreas Transplants. Radiographics 2012;32(2):411–35.

36. Paraskevas S, Coad JE, Gruessner A, et al. Posttransplant Lymphoproliferative Disorder in Pancreas Transplantation: A Single-Center Experience. Transplantation 2005;80(5):613–22.

37. Liong SY, Dixon RE, Chalmers N, et al. Complications following pancreatic transplantations: imaging features. Abdom Imaging 2011;36(2):206–14.

Imaging in Lung Transplantation
Surgical Techniques and Complications

Jiyoon Kang, DO[a,b], Subba R. Digumarthy, MD[a,b],*

KEYWORDS

- Lung transplant • Acute lung rejection • Chronic allograft dysfunction
- Posttransplant lymphoproliferative disease • Bronchiolitis obliterans syndrome
- Restrictive allograft syndrome

KEY POINTS

- A lung transplant is the definitive treatment of end-stage lung disease and there are different types of lung transplants.
- Surgical and nonsurgical complications after lung transplant are unique and are related to surgical technique, immune suppression, and allograft rejection.
- Knowledge of potential complications and imaging appearances are important for monitoring these patients.

INTRODUCTION

A lung transplant is the definitive treatment of end-stage lung disease. As a result, there is increased demand for transplants. According to the Organ Procurement and Transplantation Network/Scientific Registry of Transplant Recipients 2019 annual data, there were 2759 lung transplants in the United States.[1] The Organ Procurement and Transplantation Network uses lung allocation score to match donors' lungs to transplant candidates for optimal outcomes. There are four primary indications for a lung transplant: (1) obstructive lung disease, (2) pulmonary vascular disease, (3) infectious disease (including cystic fibrosis) and immunodeficiency disorders, and (4) restrictive lung disease.

Despite improvements in pretransplant evaluation, surgical techniques, and postsurgical care, the average posttransplant life expectancy is only around 6.5 years.[2] Therefore, early recognition of complications on imaging and treatment can improve survival.

This review covers surgical techniques and imaging appearance of postsurgical and nonsurgical complications, including allograft dysfunction, infections, neoplasms, and recurrence of primary lung disease.

SURGICAL TECHNIQUES

There are three main types of lung transplants: (1) bilateral lung, (2) single lung, and (3) lobar transplant. The approach for bilateral lung transplantation is bilateral anterior thoracotomy and transversal sternotomy with a clamshell incision. After resection of the native lung, the right lung is implanted first because of straightforward and quicker anatomic access. Bronchial anastomosis is first performed using three primary techniques: (1) continuous suturing of the entire circumference, (2) separate suturing for posterior membranous and anterior cartilaginous walls, and (3) telescopic suture for the size discrepant donor and recipient bronchi.[3] Ischemic complications are reduced by wrapping anastomosis with recipient fat, intercostal muscle, or donor pericardium (**Fig. 1**). Arterial end-to-end anastomosis is performed second, avoiding the excessive length of the artery to prevent obstructive plication at the

[a] Division of Thoracic Imaging and Intervention, Massachusetts General Hospital, 55 Fruit Street, Founders 202, Boston, MA 02114, USA; [b] Harvard Medical School, Boston, MA, USA
* Corresponding author. 55 Fruit Street, Founders 202, Boston, MA 02114.
E-mail address: sdigumarthy@mgh.harvard.edu

Radiol Clin N Am 61 (2023) 833–846
https://doi.org/10.1016/j.rcl.2023.04.006
0033-8389/23/© 2023 Elsevier Inc. All rights reserved.

radiologic.theclinics.com

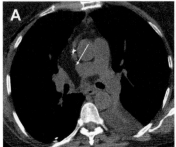
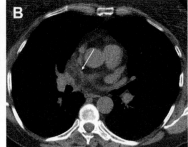
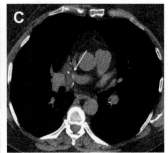

Fig. 1. Bronchial anastomotic wrapping with fat. Normal postoperative appearance (A). Evolving fat necrosis with fat stranding (B) and calcification (C) of the fat flap at the anastomosis (arrow).

anastomosis. Bronchial artery anastomosis to promote healing of anastomosis has been described in the past but has yet to be routinely performed because of time constraints and lack of clear advantages.[4] Atrial anastomosis is performed last by making end-to-end anastomosis after dividing the raphe of tissue between each native pulmonary vein, creating an atrial cuff. A single lung transplant is performed similarly, except the initial approach involves either a posterolateral or anterolateral thoracotomy (Fig. 2). The transplant can be performed without a cardiopulmonary bypass using a double-lumen endotracheal tube to isolate a lung. Lobar lung transplant generally involves the implantation of a single lobe from each large-sized donor's lungs into small-sized adult or pediatric patients. This technique requires accurate size matching after calculating total lung capacity using bronchopulmonary segments to choose the correct lobes for the patient.[5] Large grafts can cause recurrent atelectasis because of increased airway resistance and elevated pulmonary vascular resistance. Conversely, excessively smaller grafts increase pulmonary arterial pressure and pulmonary edema. Lower lobar transplants are preferred because of their larger vascular supply.

Patients with infectious or vascular diseases typically require bilateral lung transplants because native lung serves as a source of infection and hemodynamic instability, respectively. Patients who are critically ill and not expected to survive the wait time are suitable living lobar transplants.

POSTSURGICAL COMPLICATIONS

The bronchi receive half the blood flow through bronchial arteries, typically not anastomosed during surgery. The bronchi derive collateral blood supply from the pulmonary arteries, which can take up to 4 weeks to develop fully. Bronchial anastomotic complications range from 2% to 33%, with the mortality rate reaching 4%.[6] Severe bronchial anastomotic dehiscence has an incidence of up to 2% during the intermediate post-transplant period,[6] mostly from mucosal necrosis. Risk factors include ischemia, and immunosuppression, particularly sirolimus inhibiting granulation tissue and cell proliferation for wound healing.[7] The telescoping suture technique reduces the risk of dehiscence, and the resultant endoluminal flap and adjacent air at the site of the anastomosis should not be confused with

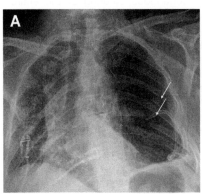
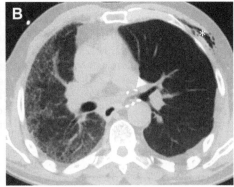

Fig. 2. Single left lung transplant. Chest radiograph (A) and computed tomography (B) show postthoracotomy rib changes (arrow), surgical clips at the left main stem bronchus (arrowhead), and subcutaneous emphysema (asterisk). Note fibrotic changes in the native right lung.

dehiscence (**Fig. 3**). The imaging findings of dehiscence are extraluminal air near bronchial anastomosis and focal defects within the bronchial walls (**Fig. 4**). Small, less than 4 mm bronchial defects with small extraluminal air generally do not require intervention.[8] Delayed-onset pneumothorax or pneumomediastinum with subcutaneous emphysema are other imaging features raising suspicion of dehiscence. Bronchial stenosis is seen in the late posttransplant period with an incidence of up to 10%[6] and is defined as greater than 70% luminal stenosis.[9] Bronchial narrowing is seen in inspiratory and expiratory images or can cause bronchial obliteration in severe cases (**Fig. 5**).[6] Bronchomalacia secondary to cartilage weakness narrows the anteroposterior lumen during expiration, leading to dynamic airway obstruction. It most commonly occurs within 4 months, with an incidence of 1% to 4%.[6] Dynamic bronchoscopy is the gold standard for definitive diagnosis, but dynamic inspiratory and expiratory imaging is also suitable. In imaging, bronchomalacia has greater than 70% luminal narrowing during expiration with flattening of the anterolateral cartilages (**Fig. 6**).

Vascular complications, specifically stenosis and thrombosis of pulmonary arteries and veins, are associated with high morbidity and mortality, and fibrotic interstitial disease increases the risk.[10] Pulmonary artery stenosis typically occurs within 2 weeks of transplant with an incidence of 2%.[10] Pulmonary venous stenosis and thrombosis occur in the perioperative period of 24 to 48 hours, with an incidence of 1% to 15%.[11] Imaging findings of stenosis include focal narrowing, sometimes with poststenotic dilation. Thrombosis has intraluminal filling defects (**Fig. 7**) with indirect

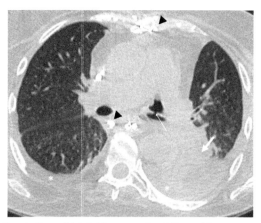

Fig. 4. Bronchial dehiscence after bilateral lung transplant. Extraluminal air and focal defect in the anterior wall of left bronchial anastomosis (*arrow*). Note surgical clips, sternotomy wires (*arrowheads*), pleural effusions (*asterisk*), and left lower lobe consolidation (*bold arrow*).

parenchymal findings, which may include ground-glass or consolidative opacities with interlobular septal thickening.[11] Of note, folds of vascular walls measuring 1 to 2 mm at the site of anastomosis should not be confused with stenosis.[11]

Primary Graft Dysfunction

Primary graft dysfunction, also referred to as reimplantation edema or ischemic reperfusion injury, usually occurs within the first 24 to 72 hours, peaks on Day 5, and typically resolves by the end of the first week. The incidence is 20% of double lung transplants and up to 60% of single transplants.[12] It is a form of acute lung injury from increased vascular permeability and inflammatory reaction to ischemia and reperfusion. The causes include lymphatic interruption, donor lung denervation, ischemia, decreased surfactant production, and preexisting donor lung injury. Risk factors include the smoking history in the donor, pulmonary hypertension, use of cardiopulmonary bypass, sarcoidosis in the recipient, increased Fio_2 during lung perfusion, and single lung transplant.[13] The imaging findings are airspace or reticular opacities worse in the perihilar and mid to lower lungs. Patchy peripheral distribution of opacities is specific to noncardiogenic reperfusion edema. Other findings include subpleural septal lines, indistinct pulmonary vasculature, and peribronchial cuffing, similar to cardiogenic edema (**Fig. 8**).

Allograft Rejection

The allograft rejection is hyperacute, acute, or chronic based on the time since the transplant.

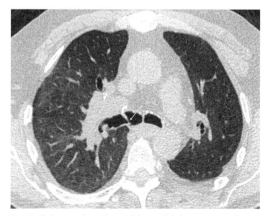

Fig. 3. Telescoping sign of bronchial anastomosis. Endoluminal flap from telescoping suturing for the discrepant size of recipient and donor bronchi (*arrow*). Adjacent air to the flap should not be confused with dehiscence.

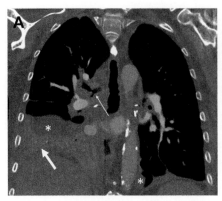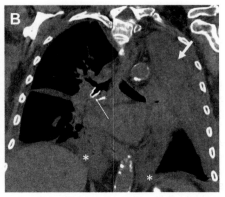

Fig. 5. Bronchial stenosis. Right bronchial stenosis (*arrow*) distal to the anastomosis site after bilateral lung transplant before (*A*) and after stent placement (*B*). Note bilateral pleural effusions (*asterisk*) and consolidation (*bold arrow*).

Hyperacute rejection occurs within 24 hours after the lung transplant from preformed recipient antibodies against the donor's HLA. This complication characterized by rapid allograft deterioration is rare because of improvements in screening and presents with rapid-onset respiratory distress with severe hypoxia. The pathology is acute pulmonary edema, diffuse alveolar damage, and multiorgan failure secondary to coagulopathy. The imaging findings are nonspecific and similar to pulmonary edema with diffuse homogeneous consolidation, ground-glass opacities, and septal thickening.

Acute Allograft Rejection

Acute allograft rejection can occur at any time after lung transplant but typically occurs 5 days after transplant and during the first 3 weeks, with a peak incidence in the second week. The International Society of Heart and Lung Transplantation noted that 28% of lung transplant recipients have at least one acute rejection within the first year.[14] Patients are asymptomatic or present with fever, cough, dyspnea, worsening gas exchange, and pulmonary function tests. Acute rejections are of two types: cellular rejection and antibody-mediated rejection. Acute cellular rejection is more common and mediated by T-lymphocyte response against histocompatibility complex antigens of the donor's lung and typically occurs within the first year of transplant. The histologic grading of cellular rejection is further categorized based on the severity of inflammation in the vascular component from no rejection (A0) to severe rejection (A4) and the airway component from no airway inflammation (B0) to high-grade small airway inflammation (B2R).[15] Acute antibody rejection is also caused by a response against HLA antigens in the donor's lung and occurs within a few weeks to months after surgery. Histologically, peribronchial and perivascular inflammatory infiltrates with lymphocytes and immunoblasts are seen with more pulmonary vein involvement than arterioles. Alveolar edema followed by hyaline membranes and desquamation of alveolar lining cells ultimately leads to necrosis of alveolar walls, bronchi, and vessels. The imaging is nonspecific,

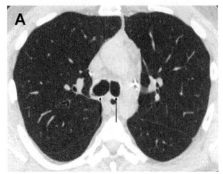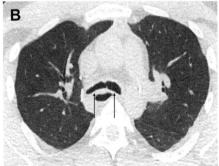

Fig. 6. Bronchomalacia. Greater than 70% luminal narrowing in main stem bronchi in inspiratory (*A*) and expiratory (*B*) computed tomography after bilateral lung transplant (*arrow*).

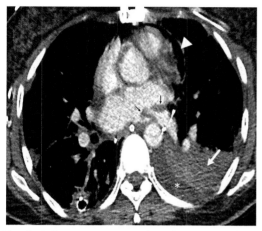

Fig. 7. Pulmonary venous thrombosis. Hypodense filling defect at the ostium of the left inferior pulmonary vein (*arrows*). Note pneumopericardium (*arrowhead*), pleural effusion (*asterisk*), and left lower lobe consolidation (*bold arrow*).

and findings include air-space, reticular, ground-glass, and consolidative opacities; basilar interlobular septal thickening; and new or increasing pleural effusions (**Fig. 9**). It is often difficult to differentiate acute rejection from primary graft dysfunction and infection. Consequently, transbronchial biopsy remains the most specific method for diagnosis.

Chronic Lung Allograft Dysfunction

Chronic lung allograft dysfunction (CLAD) typically occurs 1 year after the transplant, characterized by an irreversible decline of lung function (FEV$_1$ of 20% less than transplant baseline) lasting more than 3 weeks.[16] CLAD is the most common chronic complication of lung transplant and a major limiting factor for long-term survival. Major risk factors are recurrent episodes of primary graft dysfunction, acute rejection, infections, gastroesophageal reflux, and noncompliance with medications.[16] The International Society of Heart and Lung Transplantation reports CLAD in approximately 50% of patients at 5 years and in 76% of patients at 10 years after the transplant.[17] CLAD has two major distinctive phenotypes that can evolve interchangeably: bronchiolitis obliterans syndrome (BOS) associated with obstructive disease, and restrictive allograft syndrome (RAS) associated with restrictive disease. BOS is the most common subtype of CLAD, accounting for up to 70%,[16] characterized by fibrotic scarring, stenosis, and obliteration of the terminal and respiratory bronchioles. FEV$_1$ spirometry values do the severity grading of BOS. The imaging features are mosaic attenuation of the lung parenchyma, air trapping on expiratory computed tomography (CT), bronchial wall thickening, and bronchiectasis (**Fig. 10**). Air trapping is often the earliest and most specific CT finding.[18] The lucent lungs have smaller vessels because of hypoxemic vasoconstriction. CT findings can suggest BOS but may not correlate with the stage or degree of obstructive disease observed with pulmonary function tests. RAS is a more recently recognized form of CLAD and is associated with a poorer prognosis than BOS. The hallmark of RAS is a restrictive pattern of decline in pulmonary function, including a greater than 10% decline in total lung capacity from the transplant baseline.[19] Histologically, RAS is pleuroparenchymal fibroelastosis of upper lobes caused by damaged alveoli and fibrosis in the alveolar interstitium, visceral pleura, and interlobular septae.[19] The imaging findings closely resemble idiopathic pleuroparenchymal fibroelastosis, with upper lobe predominant apical fibrosis, central or peripheral consolidations/ground-glass opacities, reticulations, architectural distortion with volume

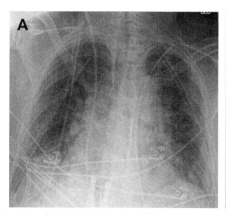
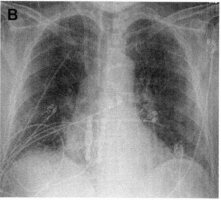

Fig. 8. Primary graft dysfunction after bilateral lung transplantation. Day 1 postoperative chest radiograph shows findings of pulmonary edema (*A*) with near-complete resolution on Day 5 (*B*).

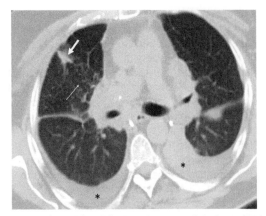

Fig. 9. Acute allograft rejection. Interlobular septal thickening (*arrow*), right middle lobe nodular consolidation (*arrowhead*), and bilateral pleural effusions (*asterisk*) 3 weeks after bilateral lung transplant and confirmed by biopsy.

loss and hilar retraction, honeycombing, traction bronchiectasis, and apical pleural thickening (**Fig. 11**). Similar to BOS, the radiologic findings of RAS might not directly correlate with the degree and severity of the disease and even precede the clinical symptoms.

Infections

Infection is the most common cause of perioperative mortality and the second most common cause of late mortality following chronic allograft dysfunction. Because of immunosuppression, opportunistic infection incidence ranges from 34% to 59%.[20] The other factors are impaired mucociliary transport from loss of cough reflex in denervated transplant; altered phagocytosis in alveolar macrophages; interrupted lymphatic drainage; and continuous, direct communication to the external environment.[20] The risk of infections is highest in the first month and 6 to 12 months of transplant.[21] Therefore, successful management of lung

transplant patients requires a balance between immunosuppression to control rejection while minimizing infections. The types of infection depend on the time interval from the transplant. Bacterial infections are common in the first month of transplant and include hospital- and community-acquired organisms. Hospital-acquired organisms include *Pseudomonas aeruginosa*, Enterobacteriaceae, *Klebsiella pneumoniae*, and methicillin-resistant *Staphylococcus aureus*.[21] Typical community-acquired organisms include *Streptococcus pneumonia*, *Haemophilus influenzae*, and *S aureus*, and atypical organisms include *Legionella*, *Mycoplasma pneumoniae*, and *Chlamydia pneumoniae*.[22] Opportunistic infections include *Burkholderia*, *Nocardia*, and tuberculous and nontuberculous mycobacterium.[22] *P aeruginosa* infection (**Fig. 12**) is associated with BOS and humoral rejection and is a significant cause of morbidity and mortality.[23,24] The imaging features are listed in **Table 1**.

The leading opportunistic viral infection is cytomegalovirus (CMV), ranging between 54% and 92% without prophylaxis and commonly occurs 1 to 4 months after transplant.[27] CMV is associated with BOS, and most transplant centers implement prophylaxis with 6 to 12 months of oral valganciclovir and closely monitor for CMV viremia in patients with CMV-seropositive donors.[28] Epstein-Barr virus (EBV) is a significant infection associated with posttransplant lymphoproliferative disease (PTLD). Transplant patients from seropositive donors and infected during the pretransplant period have uninhibited growth of EBV-infected B cells, leading to PTLD and possibly graft loss. Other opportunistic viruses include herpes simplex virus, which can cause a disseminated form of Kaposi sarcoma, and varicella-zoster virus.[29] Lung transplant patients are also vulnerable to common community-acquired respiratory viruses, such as respiratory syncytial virus, parainfluenza virus, rhinovirus,

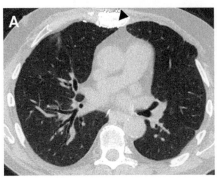
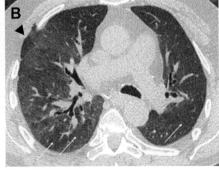

Fig. 10. Bronchiolitis obliterans syndrome. Inspiratory (*A*) and expiratory (*B*) CT show mosaic attenuation because of air trapping (*arrow*). Clamshell sternotomy and focal lung herniation are seen (*arrowheads*).

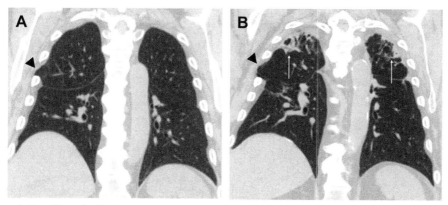

Fig. 11. Restrictive allograft syndrome. Baseline postoperative CT (*A*). CT 6 years later (*B*) shows upper lung predominant reticulation and traction bronchiectasis (*arrow*). Note focal lung herniation (*arrowhead*).

influenza, enterovirus, human metapneumovirus, and coronavirus (COVID-19), all reported to cause severe infection. These infections can quickly progress into lower respiratory involvement and the development of BOS in respiratory syncytial virus and parainfluenza virus infections.[30] A multicenter study of 30 lung transplant patients with COVID-19 infection showed a 28-day mortality rate of 20.5% (**Fig. 13**).[31] Viral infections are less likely to have lobar or sublobar consolidation than bacterial infections (see **Table 1**).[32] CMV typically has a more diffuse pattern with nodular, consolidative, and ground-glass opacities than herpes simplex virus and varicella-zoster virus (**Fig. 14**).[33] Varicella-zoster virus has a classic pattern of halo sign with 5 to 10 mm ill-defined or confluent nodules, which calcifies after healing.[33]

Fungal infections are invasive among transplant patients and typically occur between 1 and 6 months posttransplant. Although less common than bacterial or viral infections, an incidence of 15% to 35% carries a higher mortality rate reaching up to 80%.[34] Patients with frequent viral and bacterial infections with airway colonization and chronic rejections are more prone to fungal infections.[23] Because of insufficient blood supply and subsequent epithelial sloughing, the anastomotic sites serve as a nidus for fungal hyphae.[35] Invasive aspergillosis is the commonest infection and can cause airway colonization and tracheobronchitis to life-threatening lower airway infections and the angioinvasive form causes nodules with halo that can lead to infarcts and necrotizing pneumonia (**Fig. 15**).[36] Invasive candidiasis, attributed to the colonization of the explanted native lungs,[37] is more common in combined heart and lung transplantation and has a prevalence of 11% in lung transplants.[38] *Pneumocystis jirovecii*, a ubiquitous fungus, has infections in up to 10% to 40% without prophylaxis but less than 6% after using trimethoprim/sulfamethoxazole prophylaxis.[39] Some transplant centers use universal antifungal prophylaxis for several months; however, there are no established guidelines because of long-term toxicity. The imaging appearance is specific depending on the organisms (see **Table 1**).

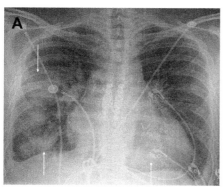
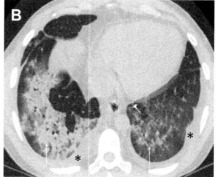

Fig. 12. Pseudomonas pneumonia. Multilobar bilateral lobar consolidation 6 months after a bilateral lung transplant in chest radiograph (*A*) and CT (*B*) (*arrows*). Note small pleural effusions (*asterisk*).

Table 1
Imaging patterns of bacterial, viral, and fungal infections after lung transplant

Types of Infections	Organism	Imaging Features	Timing	References
Bacterial				
Hospital acquired	*Pseudomonas aeruginosa* Methicillin-resistant *Staphylococcus aureus* *Klebsiella pneumoniae*	Cavitation Bronchopneumonia Bulging fissure Lobar consolidation Cavitation	Within first month	21–26
Community acquired	*Streptococcus pneumoniae* *Haemophilus influenzae* *S aureus* *Legionella* *Mycoplasma pneumoniae* *Chlamydia pneumoniae*	Lobar consolidation Bronchopneumonia Bronchopneumonia with cavitation Interstitial opacities, bronchial wall thickening, and bronchopneumonia	Anytime	
Opportunistic	*Burkholderia* *Nocardia* Tuberculous mycobacterium Nontuberculous mycobacterium	Consolidation and cavitation Upper lung consolidation and cavitation	Weeks to months	
Viral				
Nonopportunistic	RSV PIV Rhinovirus Coronavirus Enterovirus	Bronchial wall thickening, ground-glass opacities, interlobular septal thickening	Anytime	30–32
Opportunistic	CMV VZV HSV	Ground-glass opacities Multifocal ground-glass and consolidative opacities, tiny nodules Multifocal ground-glass and consolidative opacities	Weeks to months	27,29,33
Fungal				
	Aspergillus *Candida* PJP	Upper lung consolidation, cavitation, bronchopneumonia, halo sign Multiple nodules, consolidation, mililary pattern Upper lung central ground-glass opacities, cysts	Months	36–40

Abbreviations: CMV, cytomegalovirus; HSV, herpes simplex virus; PIV, parainfluenza virus; PJP, *Pneumocystis jirovecii*; RSV, respiratory syncytial virus; VZV, varicella-zoster virus.

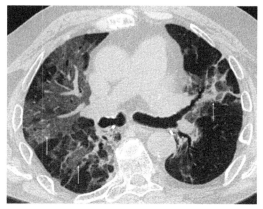

Fig. 13. COVID-19 pneumonia. Bilateral multifocal ground glass opacities (*arrows*) 2 months after bilateral lung transplant.

Neoplasms

The malignancy risk is two to four times higher in solid organ transplant patients because of chronic immunosuppression.[41] PTLD associated with EBV is the second most common malignancy in solid organ transplantation. The cumulative incidence of PTLD in adult lung transplant recipients is up to 10%, higher than in other commonly transplanted organs.[42] PTLD in lung transplant patients has a mortality rate of up to 50% because of treatment failures or chemotherapy complications.[43] PTLD commonly occurs within the first year of transplant, with peak incidence at 4 months. Intrathoracic allograft involvement is more common within the first year of transplant, and extrathoracic involvement is more common in later years.[44] Major risk factors for developing PTLD are EBV status mismatch, CMV seronegativity, and intense immunosuppression.[45] Diagnosis of PTLD requires a tissue diagnosis, immunophenotype, clonality presence, and EBV testing.[45] The World Health Organization categorizes PTLD into benign early

lesions, polymorphic PTLD, monomorphic PTLD including B and T cells, and Hodgkin disease.[45] The two most common forms found after lung transplant are polymorphic B-cell lymphoma and monomorphic diffuse large B-cell lymphoma.[45] Rituximab, an anti-CD20 monoclonal antibody, is the standard therapy along with chemotherapy regimens, such as CHOP (cyclophosphamide, doxorubicin, vincristine, and prednisone).[46] On imaging, solitary homogeneous or multiple pulmonary nodules are seen in up to 50% of patients[47] and are fluorodeoxyglucose avid on PET. Other findings include peribronchovascular and septal thickening, multifocal consolidation, and lymphadenopathy.[47] Less common features include pleural effusion and thickening, pericardial effusion, chest wall nodules and masses, and thymic enlargement or necrosis (**Fig. 16**).[47]

Nonmelanoma skin cancers are the commonest malignancies and account for up to 50% of cancers.[48] Squamous cell carcinoma is the most common, with up to 200-fold higher prevalence, followed by up to 24-fold increase for Merkel cell carcinoma, a 10-fold increase for basal cell carcinoma, and up to a three-fold increase for melanoma.[48] Because of the high level of immunosuppression in the posttransplant period, skin cancers can progress quickly and aggressively, with frequent recurrences and metastases. Risk factors include male sex, increased age, high sun exposure, human papilloma virus infection, and use of antifungal medication voriconazole specifically for squamous cell carcinoma.[49]

There is a five-fold higher risk of lung cancer after a lung transplant, with a prevalence of 1% to 9%.[50] The incidence after single and double lung transplants is 6.9% to 9.8% and 0% to 1.8%, respectively.[51] Risk factors include smoking, male gender, long-term immunosuppression, increased age, longer life expectancy after transplant, emphysema, and idiopathic pulmonary

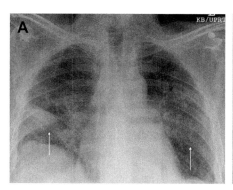
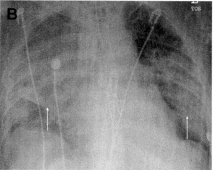

Fig. 14. Cytomegalovirus pneumonia after double lung transplantation. Notice progressive bilateral consolidative and interstitial opacities (*arrows*) on chest radiograph at admission (*A*) and 3 days later (*B*).

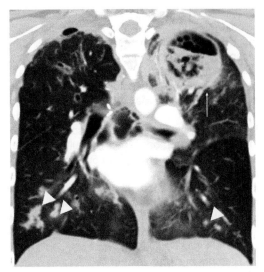

Fig. 15. Invasive aspergillus infection after double lung transplantation. Necrotizing pneumonia with cavitation in the left upper lobe (*arrow*) and multiple bilateral lung nodules (*arrowheads*).

fibrosis in the native lung.[51] The outcomes are worse because prolonged immune suppression leads to an aggressive course. Although most lung cancers arise in the native lung of single lung transplant recipients, other less common scenarios can also occur, including incidental lung cancer in the explanted lung, lung cancer in the allograft, or de novo malignancy.[52] Lung cancer often starts as nodules and rapidly progress into masses (**Fig. 17**), demonstrating fluorodeoxyglucose avidity in PET scan.

Recurrence of Primary Lung Disease

Primary lung disease can recur after a lung transplant at any time but most commonly after

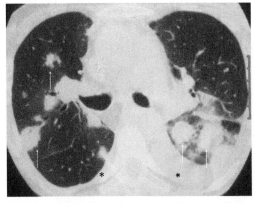

Fig. 16. Posttransplant lymphoproliferative disease. Bilateral lung nodules, masses (*arrows*), and pleural effusions (*asterisk*).

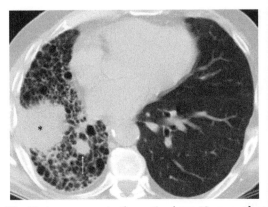

Fig. 17. Lung cancer in the native lung 12 years after single lung transplantation. Mass (*asterisk*) and nodule (*arrow*) in the native right lung with idiopathic pulmonary fibrosis.

months to years.[53] The recurrent disease has similar signs, symptoms, and morphology to the original disease. The conditions likely to recur are sarcoidosis, idiopathic pulmonary fibrosis, fibrosing nonspecific interstitial pneumonia, other interstitial lung diseases, pulmonary hypertension, α_1-antitrypsin deficiency, lymphangioleiomyomatosis (LAM), pulmonary alveolar proteinosis, pulmonary Langerhans cell histiocytosis (PLCH), and obliterative bronchiolitis.[54] Sarcoidosis accounts for 35% of recurrent primary diseases,[54] but the prognosis is generally good, with few progressing into end-stage lung disease, possibly related to an antirejection regimen.[54] A heterogeneous group of interstitial lung diseases can recur, with idiopathic pulmonary fibrosis having the poorest prognosis. However, the most common recurrent disease among interstitial lung diseases is desquamative interstitial pneumonia and smoking-related interstitial fibrosis, with recurrence occurring as early as 1-month posttransplant mainly related to smoking.[54] α_1-Antitrypsin deficiency leading to early onset panlobular emphysema, bronchiectasis with bronchial wall thickening, and bulla formation can have similar imaging manifestations on recurrent disease.[55] Only two case reports showed recurrent emphysema after the lung transplant; the most common reason was smoking.[56] LAM is caused by abnormal smooth muscle–like cell proliferation causing cystic lung disease, either sporadic or related to tuberous sclerosis.[57] Recurrence of LAM is rare, around 7% after transplant, with a favorable prognosis and long-term survival.[57] Imaging features of LAM are scattered numerous thin-walled rounded cysts, opacities related to hemorrhage, small nodules, and pneumothorax (**Fig. 18**). PLCH is another disease that can rarely

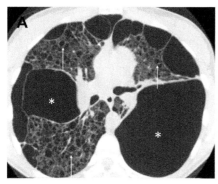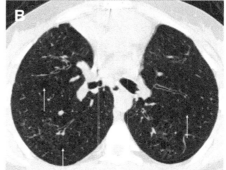

Fig. 18. Recurrent lymphangioleiomyomatosis after bilateral lung transplantation. Notice the extensive cysts (*arrows*) and bullae (*asterisk*) before lung transplant (*A*) with recurrence of cysts years after transplant (*B*).

recur after a lung transplant, and most cases of PLCH recur within 5 to 60 months with good prognosis.[58]

SUMMARY

Lung transplant is an established treatment of patients with end-stage lung disease, and there is an increase in transplant surgeries. Therefore, knowledge of surgical techniques and imaging findings of surgical and nonsurgical complications is essential.

CLINICS CARE POINTS

- Lung transplants are bilateral, unilateral, or lobar. Lobar transplantation is usually performed in small-sized adults and pediatric patients. Single lung transplantation is not performed for an end-stage lung disease associated with infection.

- The telescoping type of bronchial anastomosis can cause an endobronchial flap that should not be mistaken for dehiscence. The presence of extraluminal and focal defect in the bronchial wall are signs of bronchial dehiscence.

- Primary graft dysfunction is a common self-limiting condition that usually resolves by the end of the first week. This is related to increased vascular permeability and resembles pulmonary edema.

- Acute allograft rejection is cellular or humoral mediated, which is seen after the fifth postoperative day with a peak incidence in the second week. However, acute rejection can develop at any time. The imaging findings are nonspecific and can have airspace, reticular opacities, and pleural effusions. The diagnosis is made by transbronchial biopsy.

- Chronic allograft dysfunction is of two types: bronchiolitis obliterans syndrome (BOS) and restrictive allograft syndrome (RAS). The air trapping on expiratory CT image is the most sensitive sign for BOS. The findings of RAS resemble pleuroparenchymal fibroelastosis with fibrotic changes in the lung apices.

- Infections are a common cause of mortality in lung transplants and can start from the immediate postoperative period. Opportunistic infections are common because of immunosuppression. The disease patterns are specific for certain organisms. For example, aspergillus infection has nodules with surrounding halo; pneumocystis has perihilar ground-glass opacity, and interstitial thickening and bacterial pneumonia can present with lobar consolidation. Infections related to cytomegalovirus and aspergillus can predispose to BOS.

- Malignancies are significantly increased after transplant because of chronic immunosuppression. Posttransplant lymphoproliferative disease is associated with Epstein-Barr virus infection and is the second most common malignancy. The imaging features are in the thorax or outside the thorax. The common findings in the lungs are nodules, masses and pleural effusions.

- Skin malignancies are the most common neoplasms after lung transplant, squamous cell carcinoma being the commonest. The skin malignancy tends to be more aggressive and can have metastasis.

- Recurrence of primary lung disease can occur after transplantation. Generally, the recurrent disease tends to have a milder course. The common diseases that recur after transplant are sarcoidosis, interstitial lung diseases, and lymphangioleiomyomatosis. The imaging findings are similar to the primary disease.

DISCLOSURES

S.R. Digumarthy provides independent image analysis for hospital-contracted clinical research trials programs for Merck, Pfizer, Bristol Myers Squibb, Novartis, Roche, Polaris, Cascadian, Abb-Vie, Gradalis, Bayer, Zai laboratories, Biengen, Resonance, and Analise; has received research grants from Lunit Inc, South Korea, GE, United States, Qure AI, Vuno Inc; and honorarium from Siemens.

REFERENCES

1. Valapour M, Lehr CJ, Skeans MA, et al. OPTN/SRTR 2019 Annual Data Report: Lung. Am J Transplant 2021;21(Suppl 2):441–520.

2. Chambers DC, Cherikh WS, Goldfarb SB, et al. The International Thoracic Organ Transplant Registry of the International Society for Heart and Lung Transplantation: Thirty-Fifth Adult Lung and Heart-Lung Transplant Report-2018; Focus Theme: Multiorgan Transplantation. J Heart Lung Transplant 2018; 37(10):1169–83.

3. Gust L, D'Journo XB, Brioude G, et al. Single-lung and double-lung transplantation: technique and tips. J Thorac Dis 2018;10(4):2508–18.

4. Yacoub M, Al-Kattan KM, Tadjkarimi S, et al. Medium term results of direct bronchial artery revascularisation using IMA for single lung transplantation (SLT with direct revascularisation). Eur J Cardio Thorac Surg 1997;11:1030–6.

5. Nakajima D, Date H. Living-donor lobar lung transplantation. J Thorac Dis 2021;13(11):6594–601.

6. Mahajan AK, Folch E, Khandhar SJ, et al. The diagnosis and management of airway complications following lung transplantation. Chest 2017;152(3): 627–38.

7. Tejwani V, Panchabhai TS, Kotloff RM, et al. Complications of lung transplantation: a roentgenographic perspective. Chest 2016;149(6):1535–45.

8. Schlueter FJ, Semenkovich JW, Glazer HS, et al. Bronchial dehiscence after lung transplantation: correlation of CT findings with clinical outcome. Radiology 1996;199(3):849–54.

9. Amadi CC, Galizia MS, Mortani Barbosa EJ Jr. Imaging evaluation of lung transplantation patients: a time and etiology-based approach to high-resolution computed tomography interpretation. J Thorac Imaging 2019;34(5):299–312.

10. Siddique A, Bose AK, Özalp F, et al. Vascular anastomotic complications in lung transplantation: a single institution's experience. Interact Cardiovasc Thorac Surg 2013;17(4):625–31.

11. Batra K, Chamarthy MR, Reddick M, et al. Diagnosis and interventions of vascular complications in lung transplant. Cardiovasc Diagn Ther 2018;8(3): 378–86.

12. Snell GI, Yusen RD, Weill D, et al. Report of the ISHLT Working Group on Primary Lung Graft Dysfunction, part I: definition and grading—a 2016 Consensus Group statement of the International Society for Heart and Lung Transplantation. J Heart Lung Transplant 2017;36(10):1097–103.

13. Diamond JM, Lee JC, Kawut SM, et al, Lung Transplant Outcomes Group. Clinical risk factors for primary graft dysfunction after lung transplantation. Am J Respir Crit Care Med 2013;187(5): 527–34.

14. Chambers DC, Yusen RD, Cherikh WS, et al. The Registry of the International Society for Heart and Lung Transplantation: Thirty-fourth Adult Lung And Heart-Lung Transplantation Report-2017; Focus Theme: Allograft ischemic time. J Heart Lung Transplant 2017;36:1047–59.

15. Stewart S, Fishbein MC, Snell GI, et al. Revision of the 1996 working formulation for the standardization of nomenclature in the diagnosis of lung rejection. J Heart Lung Transplant 2007;26:1229–42.

16. Parulekar AD, Kao CC. Detection, classification, and management of rejection after lung transplantation. J Thorac Dis 2019 Sep;11(Suppl 14):S1732–9.

17. Yusen RD, Edwards LB, Kucheryavaya AY, et al. The Registry of the International Society for Heart and Lung Transplantation: Thirty-second Official Adult Lung and Heart-Lung Transplantation Report–2015; Focus Theme: Early Graft Failure. J Heart Lung Transplant 2015;34(10):1264–77.

18. Knollmann FD, Ewert R, Wündrich T, et al. Bronchiolitis obliterans syndrome in lung transplant recipients: use of spirometrically gated CT. Radiology 2002;225(3):655–62.

19. Glanville AR, Verleden GM, Todd JL, et al. Chronic lung allograft dysfunction: definition and update of restrictive allograft syndrome: a consensus report from the Pulmonary Council of the ISHLT. J Heart Lung Transplant 2019;38(5):483–92.

20. Speich R, van der Bij W. Epidemiology and management of infections after lung transplantation. Clin Infect Dis 2001;33(Suppl 1):S58–65.

21. van Delden C, Stampf S, Hirsch HH, et al. Burden and timeline of infectious diseases in the first year after solid organ transplantation in the Swiss transplant cohort study. Clin Infect Dis 2020. https://doi.org/10.1093/cid/ciz1113.

22. Remund KF, Best M, Egan JJ. Infections relevant to lung transplantation. Proc Am Thorac Soc 2009;6(1): 94–100.

23. Botha P, Archer L, Anderson RL, et al. Pseudomonas aeruginosa colonization of the allograft after lung transplantation and the risk of bronchiolitis obliterans syndrome. Transplantation 2008;85(5): 771–4.

24. Kulkarni HS, Tsui K, Sunder S, et al. Pseudomonas aeruginosa and acute rejection independently increase the risk of donor-specific antibodies after lung transplantation. Am J Transplant 2020;20(4): 1028–38.

25. Walker CM, Abbott GF, Greene RE, et al. Imaging pulmonary infection: classic signs and patterns. AJR Am J Roentgenol 2014;202(3):479–92.

26. Nambu A, Ozawa K, Kobayashi N, et al. Imaging of community-acquired pneumonia: roles of imaging examinations, imaging diagnosis of specific pathogens and discrimination from noninfectious diseases. World J Radiol 2014;6(10):779–93.

27. Azevedo LS, Pierrotti LC, Abdala E, et al. Cytomegalovirus infection in transplant recipients. Clinics 2015;70(7):515–23.

28. Kotton CN, Kumar D, Caliendo AM, et al. Updated international consensus guidelines on the management of cytomegalovirus in solid-organ transplantation. Transplantation 2013;96(4):333–60.

29. Rossetti V, Morlacchi L, Rosso L, et al. Kaposi's sarcoma in lung transplantation: a decade's single-centre case series. J Heart Lung Transplant 2019; 38(4):S313–4.

30. Peghin M, Los-Arcos I, Hirsch HH, et al. Community-acquired respiratory viruses are a risk factor for chronic lung allograft dysfunction. Clin Infect Dis 2019;69(7):1192–7.

31. Kates OS, Haydel BM, Florman SS, et al. COVID-19 in solid organ transplant: a multi-center cohort study. Clin Infect Dis 2020. https://doi.org/10.1093/cid/ciaa1097.

32. Miller WT Jr, Mickus TJ, Barbosa E Jr, et al. CT of viral lower respiratory tract infections in adults: comparison among viral organisms and between viral and bacterial infections. AJR Am J Roentgenol 2011;197(5):1088–95.

33. Koo HJ, Lim S, Choe J, et al. Radiographic and CT features of viral pneumonia. Radiographics 2018; 38(3):719–39.

34. Solé A, Salavert M. Fungal infections after lung transplantation. Curr Opin Pulm Med 2009;15(3): 243–53.

35. Krenke R, Grabczak EM. Tracheobronchial manifestations of Aspergillus infections. Sci World J 2011; 11:2310–29.

36. Burguete SR, Maselli DJ, Fernandez JF, et al. Lung transplant infection. Respirology 2013;18(1):22–38.

37. Schulman LL, Htun T, Staniloae C, et al. Pulmonary nodules and masses after lung and heart-lung transplantation. J Thorac Imaging 2000;15(3):173–9.

38. Baker AW, Maziarz EK, Arnold CJ, et al. Invasive fungal infection after lung transplantation: epidemiology in the setting of antifungal prophylaxis. Clin Infect Dis 2019;70(1):30–9.

39. Fishman JA, Gans H. Pneumocystis jiroveci in solid organ transplantation: guidelines from the American Society of Transplantation infectious diseases community of practice. Clin Transplant 2019;33(9): e13587.

40. Hussien A, Lin CT. CT findings of fungal pneumonia with emphasis on aspergillosis. Emerg Radiol 2018; 25(6):685–9.

41. Engels EA, Pfeiffer RM, Fraumeni JF Jr, et al. Spectrum of cancer risk among US solid organ transplant recipients. JAMA 2011;306(17):1891–901.

42. Kumarasinghe G, Lavee O, Parker A, et al. Post-transplant lymphoproliferative disease in heart and lung transplantation: defining risk and prognostic factors. J Heart Lung Transplant 2015;34: 1406–14.

43. Kremer BE, Reshef R, Misleh JG, et al. Post-transplant lymphoproliferative disorder after lung transplantation: a review of 35 cases. J Heart Lung Transplant 2012;31:296–304.

44. Paranjothi S, Yusen RD, Kraus MD, et al. Lymphoproliferative disease after lung transplantation: comparison of presentation and outcome of early and late cases. J Heart Lung Transplant 2001;20(10): 1054–63.

45. Isabel P. Posttransplant lymphoproliferative disease after lung transplantation. Journal of Immunology Research 2013. https://doi.org/10.1155/2013/430209.

46. Trappe R, Oertel S, Leblond V, et al. Sequential treatment with rituximab followed by CHOP chemotherapy in adult B-cell post-transplant lymphoproliferative disorder (PTLD): the prospective international multicentre phase 2 PTLD-1 trial. Lancet Oncol 2012;13:196–206.

47. Borhani AA, Hosseinzadeh K, Almusa O, et al. Imaging of posttransplantation lymphoproliferative disorder after solid organ transplantation. RadioGraphics 2009;29(4):981–1000 [discussion: 1000–1002].

48. Rashtak S, Dierkhising RA, Kremers WK, et al. Incidence and risk factors for skin cancer following lung transplantation. J Am Acad Dermatol 2015;72: 92–8.

49. Grager N, Leffler M, Gottlieb J, et al. Risk factors for developing nonmelanoma skin cancer after lung transplantation. J Skin Cancer 2019;2019:7089482.

50. Pérez-Callejo D, Torrente M, Parejo C, et al. Lung cancer in lung transplantation: incidence and outcome. Postgrad Med J 2018;94(1107):15–9.

51. Yserbyt J, Verleden GM, Dupont LJ, et al. Bronchial carcinoma after lung transplantation: a single-center experience. J Heart Lung Transplant 2012;31: 585–90.

52. Shtraichman O, Ahya VN. Malignancy after lung transplantation. Ann Transl Med 2020;8(6):416.

53. Collins J, Hartman MJ, Warner TF, et al. Frequency and CT findings of recurrent disease after lung transplantation. Radiology 2001;219(2):503–9.

54. Rama Esendagli D, Ntiamoah P, Kupeli E, et al. Recurrence of primary disease following lung transplantation. ERJ Open Res 2022;8(2):00038–2022.

55. Ranes J, Stoller J. A review of alpha-1 antitrypsin deficiency. Semin Respir Crit Care Med 2005;26(2):154–66.

56. Mal H, Guignabert C, Thabut G, et al. Recurrence of pulmonary emphysema in an α-1 proteinase inhibitor-deficient lung transplant recipient. Am J Respir Crit Care Med 2004;170:811–4.

57. Benden C, Rea F, Behr J, et al. Lung transplantation for lymphangioleiomyomatosis: the European experience. J Heart Lung Transplant 2009;28:1–7.

58. Gabbay E, Dark JH, Ashcroft T, et al. Recurrence of Langerhans' cell granulomatosis following lung transplantation. Thorax 1998;53:326–7.

Heart Transplantation
Indications, Surgical Techniques, and Complications

Markus Y. Wu, MD*, Ranish Deedar Ali Khawaja, MD, Daniel Vargas, MD

KEYWORDS

- Heart transplantation • Surgical technique • Complications • Acute allograft rejection
- Cardiac allograft vasculopathy

KEY POINTS

- Heart transplantation has been increasingly performed for patients with end-stage heart failure most commonly related to ischemic and non-ischemic cardiomyopathies.
- The major complications are procedure-related complications, infection, acute rejection, cardiac allograft vasculopathy, and malignancy.
- Radiologists have an important role in the evaluation of transplant candidates and early detection of postoperative complications.

INTRODUCTION

Since the first successful human heart transplant (HT) performed in 1967, HT has become the standard treatment of patients with end-stage heart failure.[1] In more recent years, the annual number of HTs has been relatively stable at 4000 to 5000 globally and approximately 131,249 adult HTs have been performed through June 2018, according to the International Society for Heart and Lung Transplantation.[2] Although substantial progress in immunosuppression and patient management has been made over the past few decades, complications such as acute and chronic rejections still pose obstacles to long-term survival after HT. Both non-invasive and invasive imaging play a crucial role in identifying post-transplantation complications early. Radiologists must be knowledgeable about typical and abnormal post-transplant imaging features. This article covers the surgical methods of HT, preoperative evaluation, expected post-surgical imaging findings, and post-transplantation complications.

INDICATIONS

The most common diagnoses for patients receiving an HT are non-ischemic cardiomyopathy (50.8% of adult recipients from 2010 to 2018) and ischemic cardiomyopathy (32.4% of adult recipients from 2010 to 2018). Other less common causes in the adult population include restrictive cardiomyopathy, hypertrophic cardiomyopathy, congenital heart disease, and valvular cardiomyopathy, each accounting for less than 4% of transplants.[3] Repeat HTs for graft failure, rejection, and cardiac allograft vasculopathy (CAV) represented nearly 3% of all transplants between 2010 and 2018.[2]

For HTs performed between January 1985 and June 2017, the median 1-year survival was >80%. For recipients who survived in the past 1 year, the median survival after adult HTs performed between 2002 and 2009 was 14.8 years.[3] Improvements in immunosuppression techniques and the widespread use of endomyocardial biopsy to diagnose rejection account for most of the improvement in early survival statistics.[3]

Department of Radiology, University of Colorado, 12401 East 17th Avenue, Aurora, CO 80045, USA
* Corresponding author.
E-mail address: markus.wu@cuanschutz.edu
Twitter: @WuMarkusY (M.Y.W.); @RanishKhawaja (R.D.A.K.); @DanielVargasMD (D.V.)

Radiol Clin N Am 61 (2023) 847–859
https://doi.org/10.1016/j.rcl.2023.04.011
0033-8389/23/© 2023 Elsevier Inc. All rights reserved.

PREOPERATIVE EVALUATION OF HEART TRANSPLANT RECIPIENTS

Preoperative evaluation of HT recipients focuses on selection of appropriate candidates given the limited number of available donor organs. Radiologic imaging is used primarily to screen for contraindications to transplantation. The most important contraindications are active infections and malignancy, as the risk of infection, tumor progression, or recurrence increases with the use of immunosuppression. Other contraindications that could be evaluated by imaging include cirrhosis, pulmonary parenchymal disease, pulmonary artery hypertension, and pulmonary embolism.[4] Preoperative chest computed tomography (CT) also allows the radiologist to examine the chest for conditions that might increase the technical difficulty of the transplantation or increase the surgical risk. Such conditions include extensive mediastinal fibrosis or adhesions from previous coronary artery bypass surgery; pathology of the thoracic aorta (aneurysms, severe atherosclerosis, or dissection); and anomalies of the superior vena cava (SVC) (left-sided or duplicated superior vena cava) and pulmonary artery, because these structures will serve as sites of anastomosis between donor and recipient.[5]

SURGICAL TECHNIQUES

The majority of HTs in recent years are orthotopic transplants, in which the recipient's heart is removed through a median sternotomy and replaced by the donor heart. There has been a transition over the years from the biatrial technique to the current standard of bicaval anastomosis[6,7] (Fig. 1).

The biatrial method entails the removal of the native heart while leaving behind a cuff of the right and left atrium as well as the aorta and pulmonary artery. The donor heart is then anastomosed to the native left and right atrial cuffs. The native SVC and inferior vena cava (IVC) drain blood into the donor heart.[8] The donor aorta above the aortic valve is attached to the recipient's ascending aorta stump and the donor and recipients' pulmonary arteries are anastomosed end to end. The benefit of the biatrial technique is its straightforward approach requiring only four anastomoses—the two atria, the aorta, and the pulmonary trunk. The faster approach allows for less allograft ischemic time. However, the suture lines along the right atrium become sites of incisional atrial arrhythmias, with a higher rate of sinoatrial node injury from the right atrial anastomosis and permanent pacemaker implantation.[9]

These limitations led to the development of the newer bicaval technique in 1991, and is now the

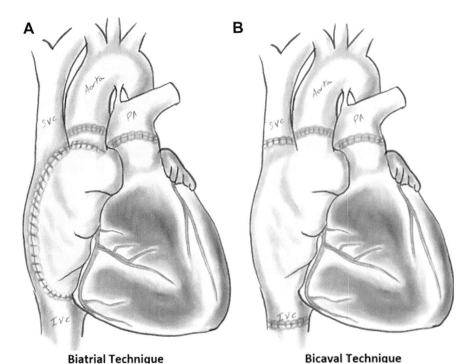

Biatrial Technique   **Bicaval Technique**

Fig. 1. Two different approaches for anastomosis during orthotropic HT (*A*) biatrial technique and (*B*) bicaval technique. (*From* Falls C, Kolodziej AR. Surgical Approaches in Heart Failure. Crit Care Nurs Clin North Am. 2019;31(3):267-283.)

most frequently used orthotopic transplant procedure.[10] This approach involves individual anastomoses of the SVC and IVC, in place of the right atrial cuff anastomosis used in the biatrial method. Therefore, there is no injury to the donor right atrium, avoiding sinoatrial node injury and atrial tissue redundancy, with lower permanent pacemaker implantation rates, and a slightly improved 30-day survival compared to the biatrial technique.[9]

In heterotopic HT, the recipient's heart remains. The donor heart is placed to the right of the native heart and connected to it so that the donor left ventricle provides the majority of left-sided cardiac output and the native right ventricle provides the right-sided cardiac output. This is reserved for patients who have high pulmonary vascular resistance, who receive a small donor organ, or who have acute or potentially reversible myocardial dysfunction.[11] Heterotopic HT was used primarily in the 1970s and 1980s, but it is rarely used today because of inferior long-term survival.[6]

NORMAL POSTOPERATIVE IMAGING FINDINGS
Orthotopic Transplant

The cardiac silhouette usually appears enlarged on the radiograph mainly due to the discrepancy in sizes between the transplanted heart and the native pericardium.[12] A double right atria contour can be seen, secondary to the overlap of donor and recipient right atria.[13] A constriction or waist may be noted in the posterior atrial contour because of the anastomosis of the donor and recipient atria (Fig. 2). Enlargement of the left atrium in the anteroposterior dimension with an angulation toward the left is an expected appearance and should not be mistaken for abnormal atrial dilatation.

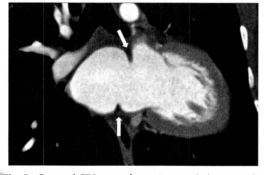

Fig. 2. Coronal CT image shows a constriction or waist (white arrows) at the anastomosis along the left atrium in a 28-year-old woman after HT, which is an expected postoperative finding.

Heterotopic Transplant

The cardiac silhouette usually appears markedly enlarged on the radiograph as the heterotopic donor heart is placed in the right hemithorax, lateral to the patient's native heart. Significant right lower lobe atelectasis may be seen secondary to the position of the heterotopic donor heart.[14]

COMPLICATIONS
Chest Wall, Mediastinal, and Procedure-Related Complications

Post-transplant patients may develop complications associated with sternotomy, with the complication rates after sternotomy ranging from 2% to 5%.[15] Sternal dehiscence may manifest as migration or rotation of sternal wires on radiograph (Fig. 3). Other signs of sternal dehiscence on CT include increased sternal gap (>3 mm), retrosternal fluid or air, and abscess formation.[16] Acute mediastinitis appears as mediastinal widening or pneumomediastinum on radiography, and on CT as obliteration of fat planes, localized fluid collections, and abscess formation. Differentiating expected post-surgical changes from infection can be challenging based on imaging alone.[17] On a timeline, mediastinal fluid collections that persist or increase 3 weeks postoperatively, with or without intrinsic air, are concerning for infection[18] (Fig. 4). Infected mediastinal fluid collections may demonstrate rim enhancement with intravenous contrast. Chronic sternal and mediastinal infections can develop into draining sinus tracts and mediastinal-cutaneous fistulae.

Postoperative bleeding complications include hemothorax, hemopericardium, and mediastinal bleeding (Fig. 5). Mediastinal hematoma typically occurs at the site of sternotomy or vascular anastomosis. CT is necessary for diagnosis if mediastinal bleeding is suspected clinically as this can be challenging to detect on the radiograph as the cardiac silhouette remains enlarged. Additionally, increased thrombogenicity during the perioperative periods increases the risk for cerebral infarction, deep venous thrombosis, and pulmonary embolism[19] (Figs. 6 and 7).

The prevalence of aortic dissection and pseudoaneurysm after HT is less than 1%.[20] Aortic wall incision and mediastinal infection increase the risk for aortic dissection or pseudoaneurysm, particularly at the site of bypass cannulation.[16] These complications can occur weeks or years after surgery. On a radiograph, aortic dissection or pseudoaneurysm manifests as a widened mediastinum or enlarged aorta. On CT,

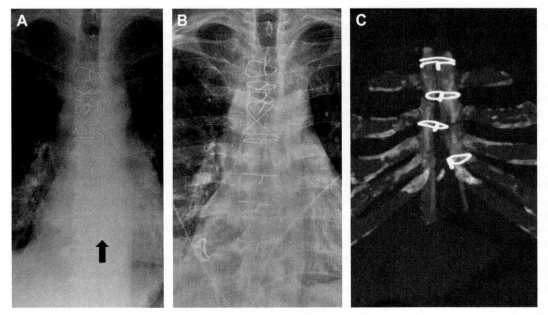

Fig. 3. Sternal dehiscence in a 65-year-old man 1 month after HT. Chest radiograph performed 1 month after HT (*A*) shows leftward shift of the inferior-most sternal wire (*black arrow*) compared to the immediate postoperative radiograph (*B*). Coronal maximum intensity projection reformatted image (*C*) confirms slipping of the inferior-most sternal wire in the left inferior sternal halve with increased sternal gap.

pseudoaneurysm manifests as a focal contrast-enhanced outpouching along the cannulation site or at anastomotic sites. Aortic dissection presents as two contrast-enhanced channels separated by an intimomedial flap.

As with other cardiothoracic surgeries, evaluation of the positioning of various life-support devices is important. These devices usually include endotracheal and enteric tubes, central venous catheters, pulmonary artery catheter, mediastinal drains and chest tubes, as well as epicardial pacing wires. Postoperative chest radiographs should be scrutinized and timely detection of malpositioned lines and catheters is crucial for decreasing morbidity postoperatively[21] (**Fig. 8**).

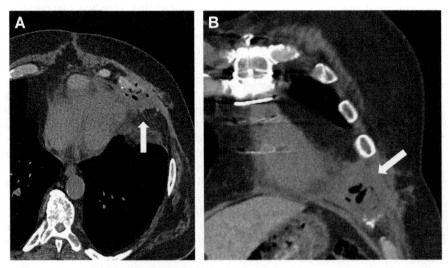

Fig. 4. Axial (*A*) and coronal (*B*) CT images in a 61-year-old man 2 months after HT show a fluid collection (*white arrows*) with internal gas and adjacent stranding in the previous left ventricular assist device pocket, concerning for a superimposed infection and abscess formation.

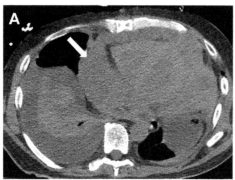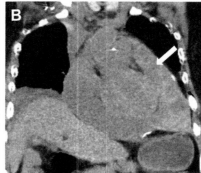

Fig. 5. Axial (*A*) and coronal (*B*) CT images in a 61-year-old man 2 months after HT presenting with cardiogenic shock show a large heterogeneously attenuating pericardial effusion (*white arrows*) with mass effect on the cardiac chambers, consistent with hemopericardium with possible tamponade physiology.

Infection

Although the HT recipient is continually at risk for infection due to life-long immunosuppression, most severe infections occur during the first 3 months post-transplantation when rejection risk is highest and the degree of immunosuppression is greatest.[22] Infection that occurs within the first month is often bacterial or fungal in etiology and the lungs are the most common site of infection.[23] Opportunistic infections caused by *Aspergillus*, cytomegalovirus (CMV), *Legionella*, protozoa, and other fungal species can occur at any time, but peak in incidence between 2 and 6 months posttransplantation[24] (**Fig. 9**). After the first 6 months, community acquired pneumonias become more common, but patients are still at risk for opportunistic infections.[24]

Bacterial pneumonias are the most common bacterial infection and may be caused by single or multiple pathogens, including *Staphylococcus aureus*, and gram-negative organisms, such as *Escherichia coli, Pseudomonas aeruginosa* or *Klebsiella pneumoniae*.[23] Imaging manifestations of bacterial pneumonia are similar to those that occur in the general population including consolidation and bronchocentric nodules. Nocardia infection affects less than 4% of HT recipients and may arise as a coinfection with *Aspergillus* species. Pulmonary infection is the most common site and is occasionally complicated by hematogenous

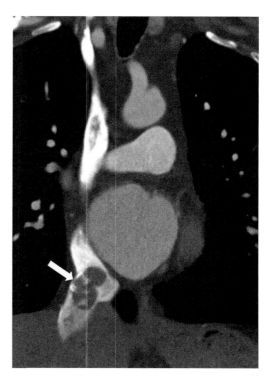

Fig. 7. Coronal CT image shows a heterogeneous thrombus (*white arrow*) in the right atrium and IVC in a 61-year-old man 6 months after HT.

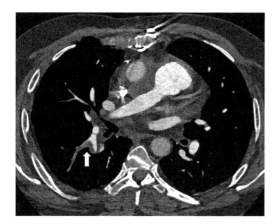

Fig. 6. Axial CTA image in a 54-year-old man 1 month after HT shows acute pulmonary embolism in the right lower lobe segmental and subsegmental pulmonary arteries (*white arrow*). Note the sternotomy wires and anastomosis in the main pulmonary artery.

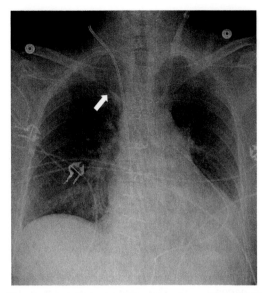

Fig. 8. Frontal chest radiograph in a 22-year-old woman after HT shows the left internal jugular catheter crossing midline and terminating in the right brachiocephalic vein (*white arrow*).

spread to skeletal structures, soft tissue, and the central nervous system[25] (**Fig. 10**).

The Aspergillus infection in HT recipients remains a frequent and dreaded complication with the highest mortality rate among opportunistic pathogens in the first 90 days following transplant.[26] Angioinvasive aspergillosis usually presents with inflammatory pulmonary nodules or mass-like consolidation. Larger lesions may demonstrate a surrounding halo of ground glass opacity (CT halo sign)[27] (**Fig. 11**). Airway-invasive aspergillosis portends a higher mortality rate than angioinvasive aspergillosis and manifests with

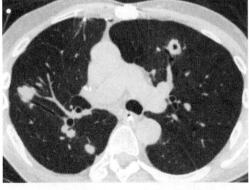

Fig. 9. Axial CT image in a 56-year-old man 5 months after HT shows multiple irregular solid pulmonary nodules, some of which demonstrate cavitation. The biopsy showed mucormycosis.

peribronchial consolidations and tree-in-bud centrilobular nodules.[28]

The CMV infection is associated with significant morbidity and mortality in HT recipients.[29] It can cause myocarditis, pneumonia, hepatitis, and gastrointestinal ulceration. The CMV infection is also associated with the development of CAV, post-transplant lymphoproliferative disease, and compromised immunity, resulting in additional opportunistic infections and malignancy.[30] Imaging findings of CMV pneumonitis are nonspecific including consolidations, ground-glass opacities, or centrilobular tree-in-bud nodules (**Fig. 12**).

Acute Allograft Rejection

Acute allograft rejection remains a major complication despite the development of new immunosuppressive therapies over the decades. The risk of allograft rejection is greatest during the 1st year, with peak rates between weeks 2 and 12, but can be seen at any time after transplantation.[3] Most acute rejections are cellular and caused by a T-cell-mediated inflammatory response.[31] The symptoms and signs of acute rejection are often nonspecific and may only manifest late. Therefore, the definitive diagnosis is made by routine endomyocardial biopsies. Biopsy samples are usually taken from the right ventricular septal wall. Complications include right bundle branch block, tricuspid regurgitation, right ventricular perforation, pericardial tamponade, rarely pneumothorax, and hemothorax.[32] Radiographic manifestations of cardiac allograft rejection are nonspecific and include cardiomegaly and pulmonary edema.

Features of acute rejection that can be identified on echocardiography include increased wall thickness, myocardial echogenicity, pericardial effusion, and a decrease in left ventricular ejection fraction.[21] However, these findings are not sensitive enough to replace endomyocardial biopsy.[1] A more recent echocardiographic feature that has shown correlation with acute cellular rejection is left ventricular global longitudinal strain, now commonly used in most centers during post-transplant surveillance.[33]

Cardiac MR imaging can provide detailed and complex information on anatomy, morphology, and functional parameters of the transplanted heart, as seen with traditional echocardiography, with the added benefit of improved myocardial tissue characterization. Findings of rejection on MR imaging include T2 signal hyperintensity (related to myocardial edema), increased left ventricular myocardial mass, and delayed myocardial contrast enhancement (**Fig. 13**).[16,34] Quantitative T2 mapping can be used to improve myocardial

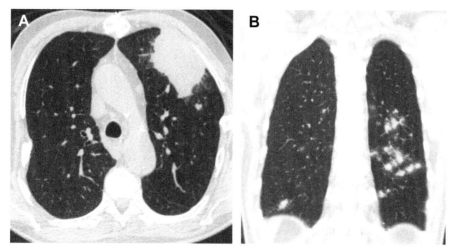

Fig. 10. Nocardiosis in a 64-year-old man 1 year after HT. Axial CT image (*A*) shows a large spiculated mass-like consolidation in the left upper lobe. Coronal reformat image (*B*) shows additional multifocal bronchocentric nodular opacities bilaterally.

T2 signal detection and to provide a quantitative value.[35] In addition, as cardiac MR imaging can assess the entire myocardial wall, it can detect areas of rejection that could have been missed in a random endomyocardial biopsy sample.

Cardiac Allograft Vasculopathy

Chronic rejection often manifests as CAV, one of the main long-term complications after HT. About half of the recipients develop CAV within 10 years after HT, and its detection more than doubles the risk of death the following year, accounting for 18% and 33% of deaths after 5 and 10 years, respectively.[36] CAV is characterized by diffuse intimal hyperplasia, smooth muscle proliferation, lipid deposition, and inflammatory cell accumulation in the walls of coronary arteries.[37] Luminal narrowing typically begins in the distal small coronary arteries and progresses proximally to the epicardial vessels. Vessels are affected diffusely and concentrically while not disrupting the internal elastic lamina and are generally devoid of calcium[38] (**Fig. 14**). Treatment of CAV focuses on the use of proliferation signal inhibitors such as everolimus and sirolimus to decrease progression, statin therapy for long-term survival benefit, antiplatelet therapy, and percutaneous revascularization, although the benefit may be limited because of the diffuse nature of the disease.[39]

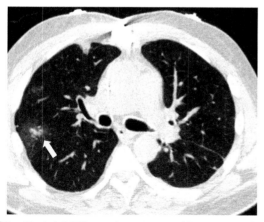

Fig. 11. Axial CT image in a 57-year-old man 3 months after HT shows multiple pulmonary nodules and masses, some with surrounding ground-glass opacity (CT halo sign, *white arrow*), biopsy proven to be *Aspergillosis*.

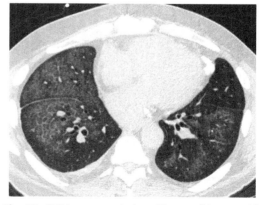

Fig. 12. CMV pneumonia in a 63-year-old man with remote history of HT. Axial CT image shows bilateral patchy ground-glass opacities with interlobular septal thickening (crazy—paving pattern) and relative subpleural sparing.

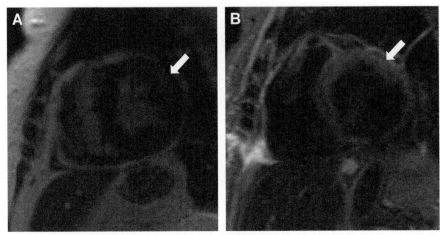

Fig. 13. Short-axis myocardial delayed-enhancement (*A*) and T2-weighted (*B*) cardiac MR imaging in a 69-year-old woman 12 months after HT shows subtle mid-myocardial enhancement and ill-defined increased T2 signal in the anterolateral wall (*white arrows*), nonspecific and could represent rejection and/or myocarditis. Endomyocardial biopsy demonstrates moderate acute cellular rejection.

Coronary angiography is the gold standard in routine CAV surveillance (**Fig. 15**). The guidelines recommend a baseline angiographic screening for donor-transmitted coronary artery disease 4 to 6 weeks after transplantation. Afterward, annually or biannually angiographic screening is recommended for the first 3 to 5 years post-transplant. If CAV is not present at this time point, the time interval between angiographic surveillance may be extended.[40] Although angiography is a widely available diagnostic modality and provides valuable prognostic data, there are limitations including its invasiveness, complication risk of 1% to 2%, and underestimation of early CAV. Angiography assesses the lumen of epicardial coronary arteries but cannot evaluate for intimal hyperplasia or wall thickness. Early accelerated CAV is more likely to result in diffuse intimal hyperplasia with concentric epicardial disease and negative remodeling and thus may not be recognized on angiography.[41]

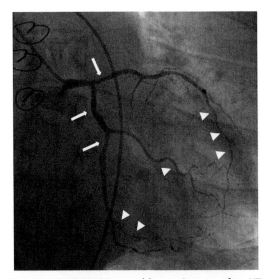

Fig. 14. CAV in a 67-year-old man 9 years after HT. Left coronary angiogram (right anterior oblique projection) shows mild stenosis (*white arrows*) in the proximal left anterior descending artery, circumflex artery, and obtuse marginal branch, as well as distal pruning (*arrowheads*) in the distal left anterior descending artery and circumflex branches.

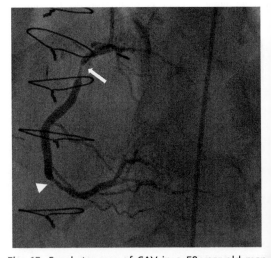

Fig. 15. Focal stenoses of CAV in a 59-year-old man 10 years after HT. The right coronary angiogram (left anterior oblique projection) shows focal severe stenoses in the proximal (*white arrow*) and distal (*white arrowhead*) right coronary artery.

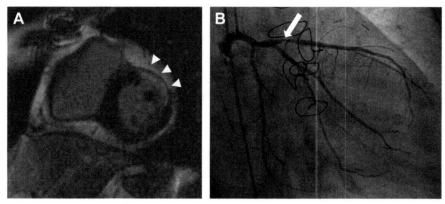

Fig. 16. Severe CAV in a 61-year-old man after HT. Short-axis myocardial delayed-enhancement cardiac MR imaging (A) shows a moderately sized transmural delayed myocardial enhancement in the anterior and anterolateral walls of the left ventricle (*white arrowheads*), consistent with a nonviable myocardium. Left coronary angiogram (right anterior oblique projection) (B) shows high-grade stenosis of the proximal left anterior descending coronary artery (*white arrow*).

Intravascular ultrasound (IVUS) has increasingly been used as an adjunct to coronary angiography following HT, as it provides greater sensitivity for early CAV diagnosis. IVUS can detect early intimal thickening and negative remodeling that is often not yet detectable by conventional coronary angiography.[42] Another novel emerging imaging technique is optical coherence tomography (OCT), an intravascular imaging modality that employs near-infrared light to evaluate the coronary vessel wall, with reported spatial resolution of 10 μm, a 10-fold increase over IVUS.[43] However, current consensus does not recommend routine use of these methods for CAV monitoring in spite of angiography, because of their cost and the lack of evidence that IVUS or OCT-triggered interventions may improve patient prognosis.[4]

Coronary computed tomography angiography (CTA) is a non-invasive modality that offers the advantage of evaluating the coronary artery lumen as well as the wall. Studies have shown that 30%–50% of coronary segments classified as normal with conventional angiography show wall thickening at CTA.[44] A handful of studies with limited number of patients suggested comparable accuracy of CTA for CAV diagnosis to that of conventional angiography.[41] Limitations of CTA include suboptimal visualization of distal small coronary

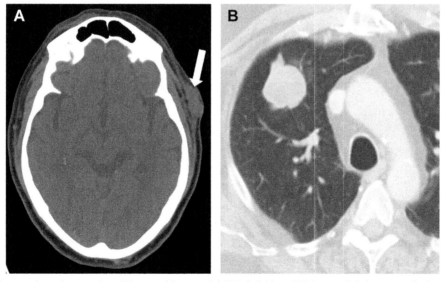

Fig. 17. Metastatic melanoma in a 65-year-old man with HT. Axial head CT image (A) shows a soft tissue lesion in the left frontotemporal scalp (*white arrow*). Axial chest CT image (B) shows a large mass in the right upper lobe.

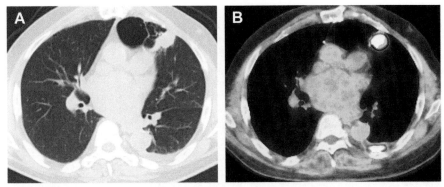

Fig. 18. Axial CT (*A*) and fused FDG PET/CT (*B*) images in a 70-year-old man with a history of HT 10 years ago show a spiculated left upper lobe mass with avid FDG uptake, which was proven to be squamous cell carcinoma. Note the FDG avid metastatic small left pleural effusion.

arteries (where CAV predominates), motion artifacts due to tachycardia (common in recipients of HT due to denervation and loss of vagal tone), beam attenuation artifact due to patient body habitus, and radiation dose.[16]

Cardiac MR imaging may provide indirect evidence of silent myocardial infarctions by identifying areas of subendocardial late gadolinium enhancement (LGE)[45] (**Fig. 16**). Stress perfusion cardiac MR imaging can estimate myocardial perfusion reserve for detecting microvascular disease.

Diffuse CAV can manifest in the microvasculature independent of lesions in the epicardial vessels. Therefore, CAV may be more advanced than suggested by intravascular imaging modalities such as angiography or IVUS.[46]

Malignancy

Malignancies are a major long-term complication in patients with HT. The cumulative prevalence of malignancy (all types combined) at 1 year is 2.8% and

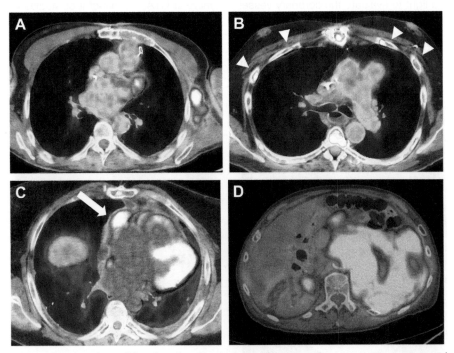

Fig. 19. Post-transplant lymphoproliferative disorders in four different patients status post-HT. Fused axial FDG PET/CT images show (*A*) left axillary lymphadenopathy; (*B*) diffuse lymphoproliferative disease involving the entire skeleton (*white arrowheads*); (*C*) an enlarged right paracardiac mass (*white arrow*); (*D*) a large ill-defined left retroperitoneal mass.

at 10 years is 30.6%.[36] The risk of malignancy has been reported to be higher in HT candidates than in other solid organ recipients due to the greater intensity of immunosuppressive agents.[47] The majority of these malignancies are skin cancers (Fig. 17), lymphomas, visceral tumors, and Kaposi's sarcoma. Squamous cell carcinoma of the skin is the most common malignancy reported in around 10% of 5-year survivors and 18% of 10-year survivors.[36] These can be detected by physical examination and confirmed with excision biopsy; however, imaging with CT or fluorodeoxyglucose (FDG) PET/CT is often required to evaluate the extent of disease, nodal involvement, and distant metastases. Other common visceral tumors include lung cancer and gastrointestinal malignancies (Fig. 18).

The reported incidence of lymphoproliferative disorders in HT patients is 2% to 6%.[48] This includes lymphoid hyperplasia, post-transplantation lymphoproliferative disorder (PTLD), and malignant lymphoma. PTLD may affect any organ with a diverse spectrum of histologic manifestations, ranging from low-grade lymphoma to high-grade diffuse large B-cell lymphoma. Common intrathoracic manifestations of PTLD include single or multiple pulmonary nodules and/or masses and mediastinal and hilar lymphadenopathy. The distribution of PTLD in the abdomen is often extranodal including bowel and hepatic involvement. FDG PET/CT is more sensitive than conventional CT in the detection of extranodal disease and is vital to the diagnosis, staging, and monitoring of PTLD[49] (Fig. 19).

SUMMARY

Heart transplantation has been increasingly performed for patients with end-stage heart failure most commonly related to ischemic and non-ischemic cardiomyopathies. The major complications are procedure-related complications, infection, acute rejection, CAV, and malignancy. Radiologists have an important role in the evaluation of transplant candidates and early detection of postoperative complications.

CLINICS CARE POINTS

- Preoperative chest CT allows examination of the chest for conditions that might increase the technical difficulty of the surgery including extensive mediastinal fibrosis or adhesions from previous coronary artery bypass surgery; pathology or anomalies of the thoracic aorta, SVC, and pulmonary artery.

- Infection that occurs within the first-month post-transplantation is often bacterial or fungal in etiology. Opportunistic infections caused by *Aspergillus*, CMV, and other fungal species can occur at any time, but peak between 2 and 6 months. After the first 6 months, community acquired pneumonias become more common.

- Chronic rejection manifests as CAV, characterized by luminal narrowing starting in the distal small coronary arteries and progressing proximally to the epicardial vessels. The CAV lesions affect the vessels diffusely and concentrically while not disrupting the internal elastic lamina and are generally devoid of calcium.

- The risk of malignancy is higher in HT recipients than in other solid organ recipients due to the greater intensity of immunosuppressive agents. The majority of these malignancies are skin cancers, lymphomas, visceral tumors, and Kaposi's sarcoma.

DISCLOSURE

The authors have nothing to disclose.

REFERENCES

1. Estep JD, Shah DJ, Nagueh SF, et al. The role of multimodality cardiac imaging in the transplanted heart. JACC Cardiovasc Imaging 2009;2(9): 1126–40.

2. Khush KK, Hsich E, Potena L, et al. The International Thoracic Organ Transplant Registry of the International Society for Heart and Lung Transplantation: Thirty-eighth adult heart transplantation report - 2021; Focus on recipient characteristics. J Heart Lung Transplant 2021;40(10):1035–49.

3. Khush KK, Cherikh WS, Chambers DC, et al. The International Thoracic Organ Transplant Registry of the International Society for Heart and Lung Transplantation: Thirty-sixth adult heart transplantation report - 2019; focus theme: Donor and recipient size match. J Heart Lung Transplant 2019;38(10): 1056–66.

4. Mehra MR, Canter CE, Hannan MM, et al. The 2016 International Society for Heart Lung Transplantation listing criteria for heart transplantation: A 10-year update. J Heart Lung Transplant 2016;35(1):1–23.

5. Kuhlman JE. Thoracic imaging in heart transplantation. J Thorac Imag 2002;17(2):113–21.

6. Stehlik J, Kobashigawa J, Hunt SA, et al. Honoring 50 Years of Clinical Heart Transplantation in Circulation: In-Depth State-of-the-Art Review. Circulation 2018;137(1):71–87.

7. Falls C, Kolodziej AR. Surgical Approaches in Heart Failure. Crit Care Nurs Clin North Am 2019;31(3):267–83.

8. Arora S, Attawar S. Current Status of Cardiac Transplantation in the 21st Century. Indian Journal of Clinical Cardiology 2022;3(2):94–102.

9. Davies RR, Russo MJ, Morgan JA, et al. Standard versus bicaval techniques for orthotopic heart transplantation: an analysis of the United Network for Organ Sharing database. J Thorac Cardiovasc Surg 2010;140(3):700–8.

10. Sievers HH, Weyand M, Kraatz EG, et al. An alternative technique for orthotopic cardiac transplantation, with preservation of the normal anatomy of the right atrium. Thorac Cardiovasc Surg 1991;39(2):70–2.

11. Copeland J, Copeland H. Heterotopic Heart Transplantation: Technical Considerations. Operat Tech Thorac Cardiovasc Surg 2016;21(3):269–80.

12. Guthaner DF, Schnittger I, Wright A, et al. Diagnostic challenges following cardiac transplantation. Radiol Clin North Am 1987;25(2):367–76.

13. Shirazi KK, Amendola MA, Tisnado J, et al. Radiographic findings in the chest of patients following cardiac transplantation. Cardiovasc Intervent Radiol 1983;6(1):1–6.

14. Adey CK, Nath PH, Soto B, et al. Heterotopic heart transplantation: a radiographic review. RadioGraphics 1987;7(1):151–60.

15. Templeton PA, Fishman EK. CT evaluation of post-sternotomy complications. AJR Am J Roentgenol 1992;159(1):45–50.

16. Smith JD, Stowell JT, Martinez-Jimenez S, et al. Evaluation after Orthotopic Heart Transplant: What the Radiologist Should Know. RadioGraphics 2019;39(2):321–43.

17. Jolles H, Henry DA, Roberson JP, et al. Mediastinitis following median sternotomy: CT findings. Radiology 1996;201(2):463–6.

18. Knisely BL, Mastey LA, Collins J, et al. Imaging of cardiac transplantation complications. RadioGraphics 1999;19(2):321–39. discussion 340-1.

19. Elboudwarej O, Patel JK, Liou F, et al. Risk of deep vein thrombosis and pulmonary embolism after heart transplantation: clinical outcomes comparing upper extremity deep vein thrombosis and lower extremity deep vein thrombosis. Clin Transplant 2015;29(7):629–35.

20. Henry DA, Corcoran HL, Lewis TD, et al. Orthotopic cardiac transplantation: evaluation with CT. Radiology 1989;170(2):343–50.

21. Chughtai A, Cronin P, Kelly AM. Heart Transplantation Imaging in the Adult. Semin Roentgenol 2006;41(1):16–25.

22. Clauss HE, Bettiker RL, Samuel R, et al. Infections in Heart and Lung Transplant Recipients. Clin Microbiol Newsl 2012;34(3):19–25.

23. Montoya JG, Giraldo LF, Efron B, et al. Infectious complications among 620 consecutive heart transplant patients at Stanford University Medical Center. Clin Infect Dis 2001;33(5):629–40.

24. Thaler SJ, Rubin RH. Opportunistic infections in the cardiac transplant patient. Curr Opin Cardiol 1996;11(2):191–203.

25. Roberts SA, Franklin JC, Mijch A, et al. Nocardia infection in heart-lung transplant recipients at Alfred Hospital, Melbourne, Australia, 1989-1998. Clin Infect Dis 2000;31(4):968–72.

26. Montoya JG, Chaparro SV, Celis D, et al. Invasive aspergillosis in the setting of cardiac transplantation. Clin Infect Dis 2003;37(Suppl 3):S281–92.

27. Kousha M, Tadi R, Soubani AO. Pulmonary aspergillosis: a clinical review. Eur Respir Rev 2011;20(121):156–74.

28. Kim JH, Lee HL, Kim L, et al. Airway centered invasive pulmonary aspergillosis in an immunocompetent patient: case report and literature review. J Thorac Dis 2016;8(3):E250–4.

29. Mendez-Eirin E, Paniagua-Martín MJ, Marzoa-Rivas R, et al. Cumulative incidence of cytomegalovirus infection and disease after heart transplantation in the last decade: effect of preemptive therapy. Transplant Proc 2012;44(9):2660–2.

30. Rubin RH. Prevention and treatment of cytomegalovirus disease in heart transplant patients. J Heart Lung Transplant 2000;19(8):731–5.

31. Olymbios M, Kwiecinski J, Berman DS, et al. Imaging in Heart Transplant Patients. JACC (J Am Coll Cardiol): Cardiovascular Imaging 2018;11(10):1514–30.

32. From AM, Maleszewski JJ, Rihal CS. Current status of endomyocardial biopsy. Mayo Clin Proc 2011;86(11):1095–102.

33. Clemmensen TS, Eiskjær H, Løgstrup BB, et al. Left ventricular global longitudinal strain predicts major adverse cardiac events and all-cause mortality in heart transplant patients. J Heart Lung Transplant 2017;36(5):567–76.

34. Vermes E, Pantaléon C, Auvet A, et al. Cardiovascular magnetic resonance in heart transplant patients: diagnostic value of quantitative tissue markers: T2 mapping and extracellular volume fraction, for acute rejection diagnosis. J Cardiovasc Magn Reson 2018;20(1):59.

35. Usman AA, Taimen K, Wasielewski M, et al. Cardiac magnetic resonance T2 mapping in the monitoring and follow-up of acute cardiac transplant rejection: a pilot study. Circ Cardiovasc Imaging 2012;5(6):782–90.

36. Lund LH, Khush KK, Cherikh WS, et al. The Registry of the International Society for Heart and Lung Transplantation: Thirty-fourth Adult Heart Transplantation Report-2017; Focus Theme: Allograft ischemic time. J Heart Lung Transplant 2017;36(10):1037–46.

37. Mitchell RN, Libby P. Vascular remodeling in transplant vasculopathy. Circ Res 2007;100(7):967–78.
38. Mehra MR, Ventura HO, Smart FW, et al. New developments in the diagnosis and management of cardiac allograft vasculopathy. Tex Heart Inst J 1995; 22(2):138–44.
39. Schmauss D, Weis M. Cardiac allograft vasculopathy: recent developments. Circulation 2008; 117(16):2131–41.
40. Costanzo MR, Costanzo MR, Dipchand A, et al. The International Society of Heart and Lung Transplantation Guidelines for the care of heart transplant recipients. J Heart Lung Transplant 2010;29(8):914–56.
41. Wever-Pinzon O, Romero J, Kelesidis I, et al. Coronary computed tomography angiography for the detection of cardiac allograft vasculopathy: a meta-analysis of prospective trials. J Am Coll Cardiol 2014;63(19):1992–2004.
42. Tuzcu EM, Kapadia SR, Sachar R, et al. Intravascular ultrasound evidence of angiographically silent progression in coronary atherosclerosis predicts long-term morbidity and mortality after cardiac transplantation. J Am Coll Cardiol 2005;45(9): 1538–42.
43. Hou J, Lv H, Jia H, et al. OCT assessment of allograft vasculopathy in heart transplant recipients. JACC Cardiovasc Imaging 2012;5(6):662–3.
44. Miller CA, Chowdhary S, Ray SG, et al. Role of noninvasive imaging in the diagnosis of cardiac allograft vasculopathy. Circ Cardiovasc Imaging 2011; 4(5):583–93.
45. Steen H, Merten C, Refle S, et al. Prevalence of different gadolinium enhancement patterns in patients after heart transplantation. J Am Coll Cardiol 2008;52(14):1160–7.
46. Erbel C, Mukhammadaminova N, Gleissner CA, et al. Myocardial Perfusion Reserve and Strain-Encoded CMR for Evaluation of Cardiac Allograft Microvasculopathy. JACC Cardiovasc Imaging 2016; 9(3):255–66.
47. Collett D, Mumford L, Banner NR, et al. Comparison of the Incidence of Malignancy in Recipients of Different Types of Organ: A UK Registry Audit. Am J Transplant 2010;10(8):1889–96.
48. Armitage JM, Kormos RL, Stuart RS, et al. Posttransplant lymphoproliferative disease in thoracic organ transplant patients: ten years of cyclosporine-based immunosuppression. J Heart Lung Transplant 1991;10(6):877–86. discussion 886-7.
49. Metser U, Lo G. FDG-PET/CT in abdominal posttransplant lymphoproliferative disease. Br J Radiol 2016;89(1057):20150844.

Intestinal and Multivisceral Transplantation
Indications and Surgical Techniques

Rosa Alba Pugliesi, MD[a], Anil K. Dasyam, MD[b], Amir A. Borhani, MD[a],*

KEYWORDS

- Intestinal transplantation • Multivisceral transplantation • Transplantation • Intestinal failure
- Postsurgical anatomy

KEY POINTS

- Short gut syndrome is the most common indication for intestinal transplantation.
- Isolated small bowel transplant, combined liver–intestine transplant, and multivisceral transplant are the three main types of intestinal transplantation.
- Increasingly, organs besides small intestines (such as liver, pancreas, duodenum, stomach, and colon) are included in the allograft. Simultaneous liver transplant (in form of combined liver-intestine or multivisceral transplant) is performed in patients with end-stage liver disease.
- Postoperative visceral and vascular anatomy is complex.

INTRODUCTION

Intestinal transplantation (IT) is a technically challenging procedure which has evolved over years to become an established treatment of patients with irreversible end-stage intestinal failure. Several iterations of this technique have been introduced over the years to address individual patient's needs, such as inclusion of liver in the allograft for patients with end-stage liver failure. Given its inherent technical and medical challenges, very selective institutions perform this procedure with only less than 3500 cases performed in the United States since inception of this technique in 1989.[1]

In this article, the authors review the indications and the most commonly performed surgical techniques for IT with emphasis on the surgical and vascular anatomy. The authors also review the common imaging workup of these patients in preparation for transplant surgery.

ETIOLOGIES OF INTESTINAL FAILURE AND INDICATIONS FOR INTESTINAL TRANSPLANT
Intestinal Failure: Definition and Pathogenesis

Irreversible end-state intestinal failure is the most common indication for IT both adult and pediatric populations.[2,3] Intestinal failure is defined as inability of native bowel to adequately absorb fluid, electrolytes, and major nutrients as a result of decreased absorptive surface and/or impaired function of small bowel.[4] This can be caused by enterocyte dysfunction, intestinal dysmotility, acute or chronic loss of the majority of the small intestine (short gut syndrome), or a combination thereof. The likelihood of end-stage intestinal failure is highly determined by the length and functional capacity of the remaining small intestine. Short gut syndrome is the most common indication in both pediatric and adult population, followed by malabsorption and motility disorders

a Department of Radiology, Northwestern University Feinberg School of Medicine, 676 North St. Claire Street, Suite 800, Chicago, IL 60611, USA; b Department of Radiology, University of Pittsburgh School of Medicine, 200 Lothrop Street, Pittsburgh, PA 15213, USA
* Corresponding author.
E-mail address: amir.borhani@northwestern.edu

Radiol Clin N Am 61 (2023) 861–870
https://doi.org/10.1016/j.rcl.2023.04.007
0033-8389/23/© 2023 Elsevier Inc. All rights reserved.

and tumors (**Table 1**).[5] In adult population, approximately 100 cm of small bowel (or 60 cm when there is a functioning colon) is needed to provide minimal required intestinal absorption.[6] Patients with shorter length of intestine are considered to have short gut syndrome and will be parenteral nutrition-dependent. The most common causes of short gut syndrome in adult are bowel ischemia and Crohn's disease.[7] In pediatric population, congenital conditions (including gastroschisis, malrotation, and necrotizing enterocolitis) are the leading causes of short gut syndrome.[8]

Indications for Intestinal Transplant

Most patients with end-stage intestinal failure are managed medically with special feeding formulations and/or parenteral nutrition. Medical management however is not always successful and can result in complications. Several surgical reconstruction techniques have been introduced to lengthen small bowel based on longitudinal division or transverse division enteroplasty.[9] Other surgical techniques have also been invented to slow the intestinal transit time, such as antiperistaltic segment insertion or isoperistaltic colon segment insertion.[10] All these surgical options should be carefully studied before considering the patient for IT.

The subset of patients with irreversible intestinal failure who can be considered for IT are (1) patients with impending or overt liver failure related to long-term total parenteral nutrition (TPN), (2) patients without suitable vascular access for TPN secondary to catheter-related thrombosis of central veins, (3) patients with recurrent episodes of sepsis secondary to central line infection, (4) patients in whom medical management fails (such as frequent episodes of dehydration), (5) patients with congenital mucosal disorders, and (6) patients unwilling to tolerate long-term TPN.[11] In addition, patients with aggressive desmoid tumors in setting of familial adenomatous polyposis maybe considered for intestinal transplant to adequately remove the tumor(s), despite the preserved intestinal function. Thrombosis of at least two major venous access routes (such as the subclavian or femoral veins), at least two episodes of catheter-related sepsis, and the onset of associated cholestatic liver disease are the most common indications for IT in adult patients receiving TPN.[12] About 15% to 20% of patients receiving chronic TPN are thought to be potential candidates for IT.[13] However, only a small percentage of these individuals ultimately receive transplants due to a lack of donor organs or lack of access to centers with required surgical expertise. The most common indications for intestinal transplant in adult and pediatric population are listed in **Table 1**.

SURGICAL TECHNIQUES AND DIFFERENT TYPES OF SMALL BOWEL TRANSPLANTATION

Numerous factors, mainly the recipient's underlying disease, influence the choice of transplanted organs. In patients receiving long-term TPN, for instance, liver is commonly included in the allograft to address the TPN-associated liver disease. The small intestine, stomach, colon, and liver are typically transplanted in patients with abdominal catastrophes caused by extensive portal and mesenteric venous system thrombosis. The simultaneous transplantation of multiple organs is becoming more common. When organs besides small bowel are included in the allograft (such as liver, stomach, duodenum, and pancreas), the term "composite intestinal allograft" is used.[14] The three main iterations of small-bowel-containing allografts are reviewed here.

Isolated Small Bowel Transplantation

In isolated small bowel transplant, the allograft only contains the donor jejunum and ileum (**Fig. 1**). In this technique, the native distal duodenum or proximal jejunum is connected with donor jejunum in a side-to-side fashion. Distal donor ileum is anastomosed with the native colon, usually using a side-to-end anastomosis. Commonly, an ileostomy (so-called "chimney" ileostomy) is also created to

Table 1
Common indications for small bowel transplant in adult and pediatric populations

Indications for Intestinal Transplantation	
Adult Population	**Pediatric Population**
Short gut syndrome • Ischemia • Volvulus • Trauma • Crohn's disease	Short gut syndrome • Midgut volvulus • Necrotizing enterocolitis • Gastroschisis
Tumor	Intestinal motility disorders Hirschsprung disease Pseudo-obstruction syndromes
Motility disorders	Disorders of the intestinal mucosa Microvillus inclusion disease Malabsorption
Retransplant	Tumor Retransplant

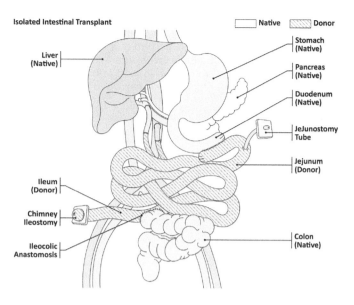

Isolated Intestinal Transplant

Native   Donor

Liver (Native)

Stomach (Native)

Pancreas (Native)

Duodenum (Native)

JeJunostomy Tube

Jejunum (Donor)

Ileum (Donor)

Chimney Ileostomy

Ileocolic Anastomosis

Colon (Native)

Fig. 1. Schematic of common postsurgical anatomy of isolated intestinal transplant. Chimney ileostomy allows access for surveillance ileoscopy.

allow access for endoscopic biopsies, which is an essential part of postoperative surveillance for early detection of rejection and other complications.[15] In addition, a percutaneous proximal enteric access, usually via a jejunostomy, is created to allow early feeding.[16] In a variation of isolated intestinal transplant, which is more commonly performed, part of donor colon is included in the graft.[7] Isolated intestinal transplant is performed in patients with preserved liver function and intact porto-mesenteric venous circulation.

Combined Liver–Intestinal Transplantation

Liver failure is a common complication of chronic TPN and a common indication for IT in patients with intestinal failure.[15,17] These patients typically undergo simultaneous transplantation of liver and small intestine from the same donor. The techniques for this type of transplant have evolved over years to improve the outcome. In its initial form, the liver and small bowel allografts were harvested separately from the same donor and were transplanted separately. The respective transplantation techniques for individual grafts were similar to isolated small bowel transplant and isolated liver transplant. This technique was abandoned over time, mainly due to high rate of biliary complications.[18] With the current technique, the liver and small bowel along with donor duodenum and pancreas are retrieved as a single unit (Fig. 2). This allows for shorter harvest time and easier vascular anastomoses as there is a single outflow (hepatic veins). Also, there is no need for biliary reconstruction with this technique as the intact biliary tree and papilla are already contained within

the en bloc graft. Donor pancreas is serendipitously included in the graft as the resection of pancreas is associated with pancreatic leak.[19] It is important to emphasize that the recipients of this type of transplant will have two duodena and two pancreata (Fig. 3). The radiologist should correctly recognize the native and transplanted pancreata, for accurate communication with the surgeons, and should evaluate them individually for possible complications.

Multivisceral Transplantation

Multivisceral transplantation is the technique invented to address both foregut and midgut failure in a single operation.[20] The stomach (or parts of stomach), pancreaticoduodenal complex, and small intestine are essential parts of en bloc allograft in this operation (Figs. 4 and 5). Other organs such as donor's liver, kidneys, and large intestine may or may not be transplanted at the same time. This technique is reserved for patients with complex abdominal conditions such as extensive portomesenteric venous thrombosis, extensive desmoid tumors or other locally aggressive neoplasms, multiple traumas, and generalized dysmotility disorders affecting both foregut and midgut.[21] When liver is included in the allograft, the term "full multivisceral transplant" is used. The term "modified multivisceral transplant" is reserved for the transplants not containing liver allograft (Fig. 6).

Arterial Anastomoses

Different types of arterial anastomoses are summarized in Fig. 7. In case of isolated intestinal

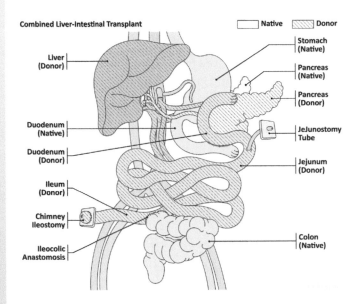

Fig. 2. Schematic of common postsurgical anatomy of combined liver–intestinal transplant. Different variations of this transplant with different vascular anastomoses exist. In most common technique, recipient will have two pancreata and two duodena.

allograft, donor's superior mesenteric artery (SMA) is the only arterial supply of the allograft, which is anastomosed to the recipient infrarenal aorta or iliac artery (**Fig. 8**). An interposition arterial graft (using iliac artery) may be used to lengthen the inflow. Carrel patch technique, that is, inclusion of rim of aorta surrounding the ostium of SMA, is used to increase the circumference of anastomosis and to decrease the risk of anastomotic stricture (see **Fig. 8**).[15]

In the setting of composite transplantation (ie, combined liver–intestinal transplant and multivisceral transplant), the allograft is supplied by SMA and celiac artery (as well as inferior mesenteric artery if distal colon is included in the allograft). In the common technique, instead of transecting these

arteries and creating separate small arterial anastomoses, a segment of donor's suprarenal aorta (which contains the ostia of SMA and celiac artery) is harvested along the visceral allograft and is anastomosed to the recipient aorta or iliac artery (**Fig. 9**).[22]

Venous Drainage

Outflow reconstruction and venous anastomoses have more variations based on the type of allograft and recipient anatomy. In case of isolated intestinal transplant, donor superior mesenteric vein (SMV) is the only drainage of the allograft which will be anastomosed to either recipient SMV, portal vein, splenic vein, inferior vena cava (IVC), or iliac vein

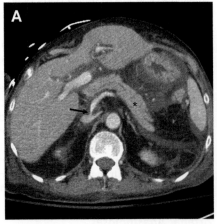
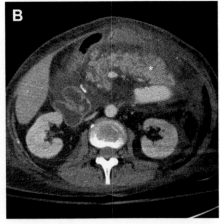

Fig. 3. Axial contrast-enhanced CT images in patient with a history of combined liver–intestinal transplant show native pancreas (*black asterisk* in *A*) and transplant pancreas (*white asterisk* in *B*). The native splenic vein is anastomosed to IVC (*arrow* in *A*) as native portal vein is removed as part of liver and intestinal explantation.

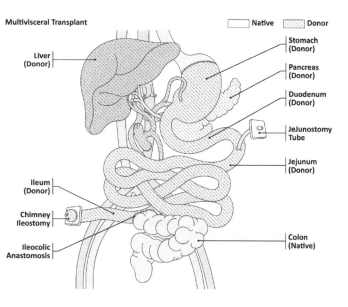

Multivisceral Transplant   ☐ Native ▨ Donor

Liver
(Donor)

Stomach
(Donor)

Pancreas
(Donor)

Duodenum
(Donor)

JeJunostomy
Tube

Jejunum
(Donor)

Ileum
(Donor)

Chimney
Ileostomy

Ileocolic
Anastomosis

Colon
(Native)

Fig. 4. Schematic of common postsurgical anatomy of full multivisceral transplant. Donor aorta (containing celiac artery and superior mesenteric artery) is anastomosed to infrarenal aorta to supply the liver, foregut, and midgut.

depending on the status of those veins in the recipient. Drainage of intestinal allograft into the portomesenteric system is more physiologic and is the preferred method if technically feasible.[23] Modified multivisceral transplant (when liver not included in the graft) has somewhat similar venous drainage via portal vein, which can be anastomosed to recipient portal vein, SMV, splenic vein, or IVC.[22]

When liver is included in the graft (full multivisceral transplant or en bloc liver–intestinal transplant), the entire graft drains via the donor hepatic veins. The outflow will be reconstructed by attaching donor suprahepatic IVC to recipient IVC using side-to-side (piggyback) or end-to-end cavocaval anastomoses, similar to one commonly performed for orthotopic liver transplant. In case of combined liver–intestinal transplant, drainage of native stomach, duodenum, and pancreas (which, unlike multivisceral transplant, are kept in place) should be restored by attaching native portal vein to IVC or donor portal vein.[15]

Other Technical Variations

Historically, colon was not included in the intestinal transplant due to concern for increased rate of rejection. Subsequent studies however showed benefits with inclusion of ileocecal valve and proximal colon without compromising graft survival and outcome.[24] As such, there has been an increasing trend in utilization of colon in intestinal grafts.[25,26]

In classic technique of multivisceral transplant, native spleen is removed along with the pancreas. Donor spleen is also not included in the graft, due to concern for increased risk of graft-versus-host disease (GVHD),[27] which leaves the recipient in asplenic state and prone to infection from encapsulated organisms especially in pediatric population. Later studies however did not show increased risk of GVHD and graft rejection when spleen was included in the allograft.[28] As such, some investigators advocate for preserving native spleen, when feasible, or including allogenic spleen in the allograft.[28,29] In the former-modified multivisceral transplant technique, native spleen, pancreas, and duodenum are preserved as a unit to ensure adequate splenic perfusion. The recipient will have two duodena and two pancreata in this scenario.

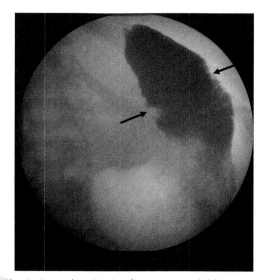

Fig. 5. Frontal projection from water-soluble contrast upper gastrointestinal fluoroscopic examination shows the gastro-gastric anastomosis (*arrows*) in patient with history of full multivisceral transplant.

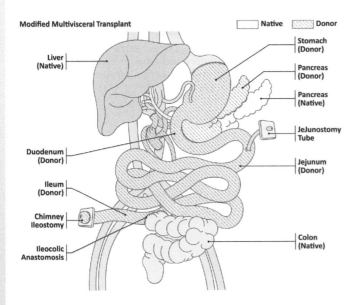

Fig. 6. Schematic of common postsurgical anatomy of modified multivisceral transplant.

In patients with concomitant end-stage renal failure, donor kidneys can be harvested and transplanted at the same time of intestinal transplant. If patient undergoing multivisceral or combined liver–IT, donor kidneys and other viscera are harvested en bloc and in continuity.[30]

Intestinal allografts are classically harvested from deceased donors. Utilization of segmental small bowel allografts from living donors has been proposed as a mean to increase the donor pool. There are also potential immunologic benefits to this approach. Very few cases of segmental living-related donors have been performed to this date with reported 3-year patient and graft survival of 82% and 75%, respectively.[31] In this method, a portion of donor distal small bowel (usually 200 cm in length) is retrieved electively. The graft is then transplanted in a similar way as deceased

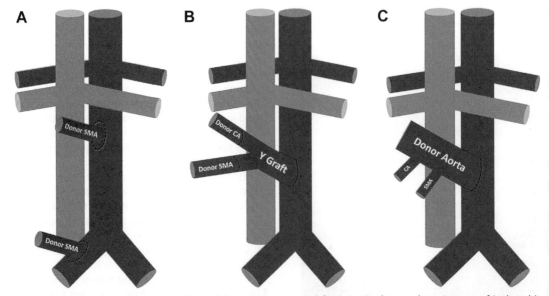

Fig. 7. Schematic of common types of arterial anastomoses used for intestinal transplant. In case of isolated intestinal transplant (*A*), donor SMA is usually anastomosed to either infrarenal aorta or iliac artery. When the allograft contains both SMA and celiac artery (in the case of multivisceral and combined liver–intestinal transplant), those arteries can be anastomosed to infrarenal aorta (*B*) via a cadaveric "Y" graft. Alternatively (and more commonly), donor aorta which contains both SMA and celiac artery is anastomosed to the native infrarenal aorta (*C*). CA, celiac artery; SMA, superior mesenteric artery.

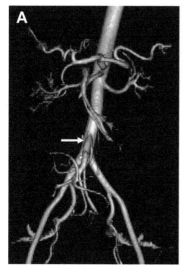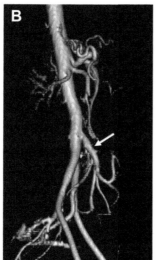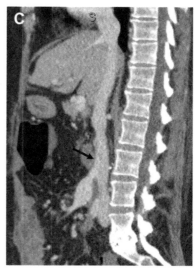

Fig. 8. Frontal (*A*) and lateral (*B*) projection volume-rendered reformats in patient with isolated intestinal transplant show the arterial anastomosis between the donor SMA and infrarenal aorta (*white arrows*). Sagittal contrast-enhanced CT (*C*) in the same patient shows anastomosis of donor SMV to infrarenal IVC (*black arrow*).

donor isolated small bowel transplant. As only a portion of small bowel is being transplanted, the inflow and outflow vessels are smaller branches (compared with SMA and SMV in case of deceased donor intestinal transplant) and might require more complex vascular reconstruction.

IMMUNOSUPPRESSION

The development and success of intestinal transplant is owing to advances in immunosuppression regimens. Mesenteric lymph nodes and gut-associated lymphoid tissues contain approximately 80% of total body immune cells. As such, IT delivers a significant load of donor immune cells

to the recipient.[23] Even after repopulation of the donor lymphoid content with native immune cells, the allograft epithelial cells remain highly immunogenic.[32] As a result, intestinal transplant recipients require stronger immunosuppression regimen. Compared with other types of transplants, intestinal transplants continue to have higher rate of graft rejection, GVHD, and posttransplant lymphoproliferative disorder.[14]

TRENDS AND OUTCOMES

Given its complexity and higher rates of postoperative complications compared with other forms of organ transplantation, fewer number of patients

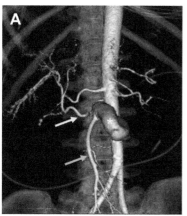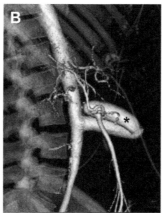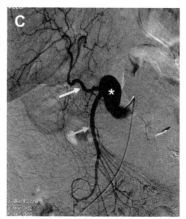

Fig. 9. Frontal (*A*) and lateral (*B*) volume-rendered reformats in patient with a history of multivisceral transplant show the donor aorta (*asterisks*) anastomosed to the infrarenal aorta. Frontal projection from catheter angiogram (*C*) better shows the vascular anatomy. Donor celiac artery and SMA are annotated by yellow and blue arrows, respectively.

receive intestinal transplant. Less than 3500 cases have been performed worldwide to this date.[3] The number of ITs performed in the United States is declining since 2007 (when it reached its highest annual record of 198 transplants), which is multifactorial and partly related to greater success of parenteral nutrition programs.[1]

Overall outcomes and survival have drastically improved over years, thanks to advancements in surgical techniques, immunosuppression regimens, and postoperative medical and surgical care for early detection and management of complications. The survival is affected by the type of transplantation (isolated vs composite transplants) and expertise of the center. Average survival rates at 1 year and 5 years are reported at 77% and 58%, respectively[14] with more experienced centers reporting much higher survival rates as high as greater than 90% at 1 year.[14] The Organ Procurement and Transplantation Network reported a 1-year graft survival rate of 93% for isolated intestinal transplants and 53% for multivisceral transplant for the 2016 to 2017 period.[33] The data from the largest single-center cohort at the University of Pittsburgh showed encouraging long-term outcome with graft survival of 59% and 50% at 10 years and 15 years, respectively.[34]

Acute rejection and GVHD remain high compared with other forms of organ transplant given the large volume of lymphoid tissue naturally found in the intestines. Recipients are also more prone to infection due to stronger immunosuppression and the nature of intestinal allograft (which is not sterile). In addition, the nutritional status of the recipients is generally poor which adversely affects wound and anastomotic healing. Despite all these shortcomings, IT remains the only hope and only curative treatment of certain patients such as the ones with history of intestinal catastrophes and those on chronic TPN who have life-threatening complications.[35]

PREOPERATIVE WORKUP

Intestinal transplant candidates undergo extensive medical, surgical, and psychosocial workup for optimal patient selection and optimal surgical planning. Bowel reconstruction surgeries, which are less invasive than intestinal transplant, are considered and offered to certain patients. Imaging is an essential part of preoperative workup, given the complexity of intestinal and multivisceral transplantation. The major objectives of preoperative imaging are (1) assessment of anatomy, length, and motility of native bowel; (2) assessment of status of liver; (3) evaluation of major visceral arterial and venous structures; (4) assessment of vascular accesses and central venous patency; and (5) excluding conditions that deem contraindications for intestinal transplant. Calculations of liver and spleen volumes and an examination for the presence of enterocutaneous fistulas are also performed in selected cases.[36,37]

Contrast-enhanced CT is the most commonly used imaging modality given its extended coverage and ability to assess the vasculature as well as the solid and hollow viscera all in one examination. Arterial phase (CT angiography, [CTA]) may be included in the protocol for optimal mapping of mesenteric arteries. Non-contrast phase may also be added to improve the sensitivity for detection of hepatic steatosis, if not already known based on biopsy or other modalities. MR imaging has the potential to provide comprehensive evaluation of liver parenchyma via dedicated sequences (such as proton density fat fraction and MR elastography) and should be considered in selected patients. Radiologists should pay special attention to subtle findings of fibrosis and early portal hypertension on imaging to prompt further workup. Although liver biopsy is performed in most candidates, MR imaging may provide additional information that is not captured on histology. MR imaging can also be used for general abdominopelvic imaging in patients with contraindication for iodinated contrast. Contrast-enhanced MR angiography/venography (or non-contrast angiography sequences, when there is contraindication to gadolinium-based contrast) can be added to the protocol for selected cases when optimum vascular mapping is needed.[7]

The visceral vasculature can be also be evaluated through conventional catheter angiography. In some institutions, catheter angiography is a standard part of presurgical workup. Abdominal aorta, iliac arteries, and major splanchnic arteries are assessed by angiography to give a roadmap to the surgeons. In addition, delayed images are obtained after injection of contrast into SMA and splenic artery to allow for opacification and assessment of splenic vain, SMV, and portal venous system. Transjugular cavogram and hepatic venogram ($\pm$ simultaneous transjugular liver biopsy) may be performed in certain cases, mainly to assess the central systemic veins. Carbon dioxide can be used as a contrast agent for central venographic studies (where lower spatial resolution does not affect the diagnostic performance of the study) to reduce the total amount of iodinated contrast and in patients with contraindications to iodine-based contrast. In pediatric population, Doppler ultrasound might be considered for vascular imaging to reduce exposure to ionizing radiation[38]

Fluoroscopic upper gastrointestinal study and small bowel follow through examination are routinely performed to assess the length and motility of the native bowel. Lower gastrointestinal study might be performed in certain cases, when the surgeons need to assess the hindgut. In most institutions, water-soluble contrast is used instead of barium.[7]

SUMMARY

IT, despite technical and postoperative challenges, is a viable curative option for selected number of patients with irreversible end-stage intestinal failure who have other organ failures or have severe complications of TPN. Increasingly, the allograft includes other organs besides small intestines, which results in complex postoperative anatomy. Familiarity with surgical techniques and postoperative anatomy is essential for accurate interpretation of imaging studies after transplant in these patients.

CLINICS CARE POINTS

- Several techniques are used for intestinal and multivisceral transplant, resulting in different post-surgical anatomies.
- Vascular anatomy after intestinal and multivisceral transplants is usually rather complex.

DISCLOSURE

None of the authors have relevant commercial or financial conflicts of interest to disclose.

ACKNOWLEDGMENTS

The authors would like to thank David C Botos for his help with illustrations.

REFERENCES

1. OPTN website. Available at: https://optn.transplant. hrsa.gov/patients/about-transplantation/. Accessed 1 April, 2023.
2. Martinez Rivera AWP. Intestinal transplantation in children: current status. Pediatr Surg Int 2016;32(6): 529–40. https://doi.org/10.1007/s00383-016-3885-2.
3. Matsumoto CS, Subramanian S, Fishbein TM. Adult Intestinal Transplantation. Gastroenterol Clin North Am 2018;47(2):341–54. https://doi.org/10.1016/j. gtc.2018.01.011.
4. Pironi L. Definitions of intestinal failure and the short bowel syndrome. Best Pract Res Clin Gastroenterol 2016;30(2):173–85. https://doi.org/10.1016/j.bpg. 2016.02.011.
5. Yildiz BD. Where are we at with short bowel syndrome and small bowel transplant. World J Transplant 2012;2(6):95–103. https://doi.org/10.5500/wjt. v2.i6.95.
6. Platell CF, Coster J, McCauley RD, et al. The management of patients with the short bowel syndrome. World J Gastroenterol 2002;8(1):13–20. https://doi. org/10.3748/wjg.v8.i1.13.
7. Rees MA, Amesur NB, Cruz RJ, et al. Imaging of Intestinal and Multivisceral Transplantation. Radiographics 2018;38(2):413–32. https://doi.org/10.1148/rg.20181 70086.
8. Amin SC, Pappas C, Iyengar H, et al. Short bowel syndrome in the NICU. Clin Perinatol 2013;40(1): 53–68. https://doi.org/10.1016/j.clp.2012.12.003.
9. Rege A. The Surgical Approach to Short Bowel Syndrome - Autologous Reconstruction versus Transplantation. Viszeralmedizin 2014;30(3):179–89. https:// doi.org/10.1159/000363589.
10. Sommovilla J, Warner BW. Surgical options to enhance intestinal function in patients with short bowel syndrome. Curr Opin Pediatr 2014;26(3):350–5. https://doi.org/10.1097/mop.0000000000000103.
11. Kaufman SS, Atkinson JB, Bianchi A, et al. Indications for pediatric intestinal transplantation: a position paper of the American Society of Transplantation. Pediatr Transplant. Apr 2001;5(2): 80–7. https://doi.org/10.1034/j.1399-3046.2001.005 002080.x.
12. Vianna RMMR, Tector AJ. Current status of small bowel and multivisceral transplantation. Adv Surg 2008 2008;42:129–50.
13. Kaufman SSAY, Beath SV, Ceulemans LJ, et al. New Insights Into the Indications for Intestinal Transplantation: Consensus in the Year 2019. Transplantation 2020;104(5):937–46. https://doi.org/10.1097/TP.000 0000000003065.
14. Abu-Elmagd K, Reyes J, Bond G, et al. Clinical intestinal transplantation: a decade of experience at a single center. Ann Surg 2001;234(3):404–16.
15. Nickkholgh A, Contin P, Abu-Elmagd K, et al. Intestinal transplantation: review of operative techniques. Clin Transplant 2013;27(suppl 25):56–65.
16. Mazariegos GVSD, Horslen S, Farmer D, et al. Intestine transplantation in the United States, 1999–2008. Am J Transpl 2010;10(4 Pt 2):1020–34.
17. Bueno JA-EK, Mazariegos G, Madariaga J, et al. Composite liver–small bowel allografts with preservation of donor duodenum and hepatic biliary system in children. J Pediatr Surg 2000;35(2):291–5. discussion 295–296.
18. Lauro A, Vaidya A. Role of "reduced-size" liver/bowel grafts in the "abdominal wall transplantation" era. World J Gastrointest Surg 2017;9(9):186–92.

19. Al-Adra D, McGilvray I, Goldaracena N, et al. Preserving the Pancreas Graft: Outcomes of Surgical Repair of Duodenal Leaks in Enterically Drained Pancreas Allografts. Transplant Direct 2017;3(7):e179.

20. Tzakis AG Kato T, Levi DM, et al. 100 multivisceral transplants at a single center. Ann Surg 2005; 242(4):480–90.

21. Canovai E, Ceulemans LJ, Gilbo N, et al. Multivisceral Transplantation for Diffuse Portomesenteric Thrombosis: Lessons Learned for Surgical Optimization. Front Surg 2021;8:645302.

22. Cruz RJ, Costa G, Bond G, et al. Modified "liver-sparing" multivisceral transplant with preserved native spleen, pancreas, and duodenum: technique and long-term outcome. J Gastrointest Surg 2010; 14(11):1709–21.

23. TM F. Intestinal transplantation. N Engl J Med 2009; 361(10):998–1008.

24. Grant D, Abu-Elmagd K, Reyes J, et al. 2003 Report of the intestine transplant registry: a new era has dawned. Ann Surg 2005;241(4):607–13.

25. Kato T, Selvaggi G, Gaynor JJ, et al. Inclusion of donor colon and ileocecal valve in intestinal transplantation. Transplantation 2008;86(2):293–7.

26. Matsumoto CSKS, Fishbein TM. Inclusion of the colon in intestinal transplantation. Curr Opin Organ Transplant 2011;16(3):312–5.

27. D S. The current state of intestine transplantation: indications, techniques, outcomes and challenges. Am J Transplant 2014;14(9):1976–84.

28. Kato T, Tzakis AG, Selvaggi G, et al. Transplantation of the spleen: effect of splenic allograft in human multivisceral transplantation. Ann Surg 2007; 246(3):436–44. discussion 445–446.

29. Preservation KMA-E. of the native spleen, duodenum, and pancreas in patients with multivisceral transplantation: nomenclature, dispute of origin, and proof of premise. Transplantation 2007;84(9): 1208–9. author reply 1209.

30. Hashimoto KCG, Khanna A, Fujiki M, et al. Recent advances in intestinal and multivisceral transplantation. Adv Surg 2015;49:31–63.

31. Benedetti E, Holterman M, Asolati M, et al. Living related segmental bowel transplantation: from experimental to standardized procedure. Ann Surg 2006;244(5):694–9.

32. Iwaki Y, Starzl TE, Yagihashi A, et al. Replacement of donor lymphoid tissue in small-bowel transplants. Lancet 1991;337(8745):818–9.

33. Abu-Elmagd KM, Costa G, Bond GJ, et al. Five hundred intestinal and multivisceral transplantations at a single center: major advances with new challenges. Ann Surg 2009;250(4):567–81.

34. Abu-Elmagd KM, Wu G, Costa G, et al. Preformed and de novo donor specific antibodies in visceral transplantation: long-term outcome with special reference to the liver. Am J Transplant 2012;12(11): 3047–60.

35. Sandrasegaran K, Lall C, Ramaswamy R, et al. Intestinal and multivisceral transplantation. Abdom Imaging 2011;36:382–9.

36. Swerdlow DRTA, Girlanda R, Matsumoto C, et al. Computed tomography (CT) colonography with CT arteriography and venography for the workup of intestinal transplant candidates. Clin Transplant 2013;27(1):126–31.

37. Tzakis AGTS, Starzl TE. Intestinal transplantation. Annu Rev Med 1994;45:79–91.

38. Phillips GSBP, Stanescu L, Dick AA, et al. Pediatric intestinal transplantation: normal radiographic appearance and complications. Pediatr Radiol 2011;41(8): 1028–39.

Intestinal and Multivisceral Transplantation: Complications

Anil K. Dasyam, MD[a],*, Amir A. Borhani, MD[b], Nikhil V. Tirukkovalur, MBBS[c], Ruy J. Cruz Jr, MD, PhD[d]

KEYWORDS

- Intestinal transplantation • Multivisceral transplantation • Liver–intestinal transplantation
- Complications • Rejection

KEY POINTS

- The outcomes of intestinal transplant patients have been improving in the last few decades, and transplant recipients are living longer.
- Intestinal transplant, being highly immunogenic and loaded with commensal flora, is prone for immunologic complications and infections.
- Different types of intestinal transplantation involve complex surgeries with multiple anastomoses and are susceptible to multiple complications including gastrointestinal, vascular, pancreaticobiliary, urologic, and neoplastic complications.
- Knowledge of normal posttransplantation anatomy and imaging appearance helps radiologists in prompt and accurate detection of several major postoperative complications.

Abbreviations	
ITx	Intestinal transplantation
IITx	Isolated intestinal transplantation
L-ITx	Liver-intestinal transplantation
MVTx	Modified multivisceral transplantation;
ACR	Acute cellular rejection
GVHD	Graft-versus-host disease
PTLD	Post-transplant Lymphoproliferative disorder

INTRODUCTION

As the first multivisceral transplantation performed nearly 4 decades ago, several advancements have been made with respect to immunosuppression protocols, surgical techniques, and postoperative care resulting in vastly improved outcomes for intestinal transplant (ITx) recipients. According to the recent report from the International Intestinal Transplant Registry, 50% (2060 of 4130) of all ITx

[a] Department of Radiology, University of Pittsburgh School of Medicine, 200 Lothrop Street, Pittsburgh, PA 15216, USA; [b] Department of Radiology, Northwestern University Feinberg School of Medicine, 676 North Street Claire Street, Suite 800, Chicago, IL 60611, USA; [c] Kamineni Academy of Medical Science and Research Centre, LB Nagar, Hyderabad, TG 500068, India; [d] Intestinal Rehabilitation and Multivisceral Transplant Program, Starzl Transplant Institute
* Corresponding author.
E-mail address: dasyamak@upmc.edu

Radiol Clin N Am 61 (2023) 871–887
https://doi.org/10.1016/j.rcl.2023.04.008
0033-8389/23/© 2023 Elsevier Inc. All rights reserved.

recipients since 1985 are alive.[1-3] Graft survival for ITx has progressively improved in the last 2 decades with only 6.7% graft failure by 1 year for transplants in 2019 versus 31.7% of transplants in 2009. Five-year graft survival, however, remains around 50%.[4] Depending on the allograft components included the three main types of ITx include isolated ITx (IITx), liver-ITx (L-ITx), and multivisceral transplantation (MVTx).[5]

ITx poses certain unique challenges. The organ is highly immunogenic as it is home for 80% of the immune cells. Unlike other transplant organs, it is loaded with commensal flora which can cause infection in the setting of immune suppression as breakdown of protective barriers from surgical alterations. The surgery is complex and can involve multiple organs and hence, multiple anastomoses, each of which is associated with risk of varied complications.[5,6] In this article, the authors discuss expected postoperative imaging appearances and the spectrum of complications relevant to radiologists.

ROLE OF IMAGING IN EVALUATION OF THE INTESTINAL TRANSPLANT RECIPIENT

The spectrum of organs included in the transplant, the complex nature of the surgery, and the multiple anastomoses created necessitate utilization of multiple imaging modalities for postoperative assessment of the ITx recipient. Intestinal allograft anatomy, mucosal fold pattern, function, and patency as well as anastomotic integrity are best assessed with fluoroscopic procedures such as upper gastrointestinal, small bowel follow-through, and lower gastrointestinal (GI) examination. Computed tomography (CT) scan, especially with intravenous contrast, remains the workhorse modality for more comprehensive imaging assessment of the intestinal allograft, other abdominal organs, vasculature, mesentery, peritoneal cavity, and abdominal wall. Ultrasound is commonly used for imaging of the hepatic allograft in the early postoperative setting and periodically thereafter. Other common indications for ultrasound include evaluation of genitourinary tract and hepatobiliary system. Magnetic resonance imaging (MRI)/magnetic resonance cholangiopancreatography (MRCP) is most commonly used for hepatobiliary and pancreatic assessment but can rival CT in assessment of vasculature and in fact is superior to CT when patient is unable to receive intravenous contrast. Ultrasound and CT scan are also commonly used for image-guided interventions such as biopsy and percutaneous drainage procedures. Catheter angiography and percutaneous biliary interventions are occasionally performed for diagnostic and therapeutic reasons.[7]

Normal Postoperative Findings

ITx recipients have extensively altered bowel and vascular anatomy, which vary based on the type of transplantation. A thorough knowledge of the operative technique and allograft components used is crucial for understanding normal postoperative anatomy and early detection of complications. Mild dilation and mural thickening of the intestinal allograft, small amount of peritoneal fluid, and mild enlargement of mesenteric lymph nodes are normal findings in the immediate postoperative setting due to the lack of normal innervation and lymphatic drainage. These findings often resolve spontaneously in a few weeks (**Fig. 1**). Mild biliary dilation involving the liver allograft, especially in the setting of biliary-enteric anastomosis, is also an expected early postoperative finding. Pneumatosis of the small bowel allograft, which in other settings is considered ominous, is a finding that is frequently seen in the early post-ITx setting, especially following ileoscopy and is generally of no clinical significance in the asymptomatic patient.[7,8]

Complications of Intestinal Transplantation

Collections

As with any major abdominal surgery, hematoma and seroma are commonly encountered in the early postoperative period after ITx and can be diagnosed based on their higher-than-water and near-water attenuation, respectively (**Fig. 2**). These collections resolve spontaneously when small. Diagnostic aspiration may be required when there is suspicion of superimposed infection. Larger collections when symptomatic or associated with significant mass effect may require percutaneous image-guided drainage. Unlike most other abdominal surgeries, chylous collections are also common in the setting of ITx due to disruption of the lymphatic drainage pathways in the mesentery. Chylous collections, such as seromas, are generally of water attenuation but can sometimes harbor focal areas of fat attenuation or fat-fluid levels, which is a strong diagnostic clue to the chylous nature of the collection. Chylous collections are often large and require percutaneous drainage as they usually do not resolve spontaneously. Bilomas can occur from bile leak when duct-to-duct or biliary-enteric anastomoses are involved in the transplantation.[7] Biliary complications are discussed in more detail below under the section on "Pancreaticobiliary complications."

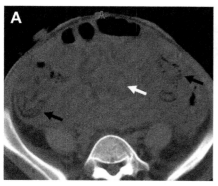
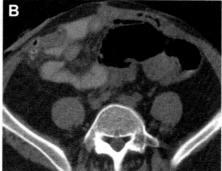

Fig. 1. Normal postoperative findings: Young man in his mid-30s with a history of Crohn's disease, status post isolated intestinal transplantation 3 weeks earlier and underwent ileoscopy earlier on the same day. Axial unenhanced CT image (*A*) demonstrates diffuse mesenteric edema, mesenteric lymph nodal enlargement (*white arrow*), and small bowel pneumatosis (*black arrow*), which subsequently resolved spontaneously. CT scan from a year later (*B*) was normal.

Infective Complications

Infection is the most common complication after ITx with an incidence of up to 93% with most patients developing more than one infection.[9] Infections are most common in the first month after transplantation and are most commonly bacterial in origin. Viral infections with an incidence of approximately 40% and invasive fungal infections with an incidence of approximately 20% are more common after the first month.[9,10] Infection is a major cause of morbidity and mortality in patients undergoing ITx, especially MVTx. Fatal infections are often either bacterial (61%) or fungal (31%).[11] The commonest sites of infection include abdomen, central venous catheters, lung, and genitourinary tract.[9] Imaging can help localize the site of clinically occult infections typically with CT scan of chest, abdomen, and pelvis. Abdominal abscess may be suspected based on the imaging studies, although their definite diagnosis requires fluid aspiration. Common clues on imaging include loculated collection with mass effect, enhancing

rim, adjacent fat stranding, and internal gas unrelated to an intervention. Similarly, though nonspecific, peritoneal thickening, enhancement, and loculated ascites are imaging features suggesting peritonitis in the appropriate clinical context. Bacterial seeding through portal circulation leads to liver being a common site of parenchymal abscess (**Fig. 3**).[12] When sufficiently large and accessible, image-guided percutaneous catheter drainage is widely used for management of abscesses. Infectious enteritis, especially of viral origin, is common after ITx, but imaging findings are nonspecific and overlap with those of rejection.[13] Bacteremia from enteric pathogens has been shown to be associated with intestinal rejection or gastrointestinal posttransplant lymphoproliferative disorder (PTLD), and corresponding imaging clues should be actively sought.[14]

Immunologic Complications

ITx is associated with a complex immunologic environment as it is lymphoid-rich prepopulated

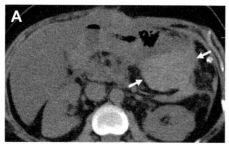
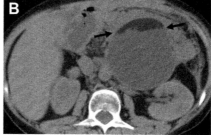

Fig. 2. Postoperative collections: Axial unenhanced CT (*A*) in a woman in her early 50s who underwent isolated intestinal transplantation 1 week earlier demonstrates an acute hyperdense retrogastric hematoma (*white arrows*). Axial unenhanced CT (*B*) in another boy in his late teens who underwent modified multivisceral transplantation 5 months earlier demonstrates a deep-seated loculated abdominal collection with nondependent layering fat (*black arrows*), which is a characteristic finding of chylous collection.

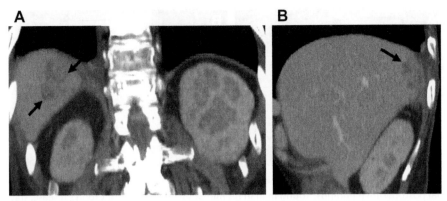

Fig. 3. Nearly 40-year-old man with a history of Factor V Leiden and Budd–Chiari syndrome, status post multivisceral transplantation 1 year earlier. Coronal (A) and sagittal (B) contrast-enhanced CT images demonstrate multiloculated hepatic abscess (*black arrows*) in posterior right hepatic lobe.

with donor immune cells, later becoming repopulated with recipient immune cells. The genotype of the allograft-enteric mucosal epithelium, however, remains that of the donor resulting in an immunogenic chimeric organ.[6] Immunologic complications of ITx include rejection, graft-versus-host disease (GVHD), and PTLD, all of which have a higher incidence than with other solid organ transplantations.[15–17]

Rejection
According to the most recent data, acute cellular rejection (ACR) of the intestinal allograft has an incidence of 41.2% in adult IITx patients and 35.4% in L-ITx patients among 2018 to 2019 recipients.[4] ACR is a major cause of intestinal allograft loss and patient death. Allograft loss is more likely in non-liver inclusive grafts than liver inclusive allografts. The first episode of ACR has a median time of 2.5 weeks, and most episodes occur in the first

year. The imaging findings of ACR are nonspecific and include diffuse bowel wall thickening, mucosal hyperenhancement, and ascites (**Fig. 4**).[7] Clinical manifestations of ACR are also nonspecific, and diagnosis is made by routine endoscopic surveillance and biopsy of allograft bowel mucosa initially via donor "chimney ileostomy" and later via lower or upper endoscopy.[18] Histologic findings suggestive of ACR include mucosal ulcerations, architectural distortion, greater than 6 apoptotic bodies/10 crypts, and diffuse inflammatory infiltrate. Chronic rejection has an incidence of 15% with affected patients presenting with chronic diarrhea, bloating, and protein-losing enteropathy. Chronic rejection is characterized by myointimal hyperplasia of medium-sized mesenteric, serosal, and submucosal arteries leading to ischemic injury to mucosa and fibrosis of the lamina propria. Endoscopic biopsies and imaging may not be diagnostic and may require enterectomy for a definitive diagnosis.

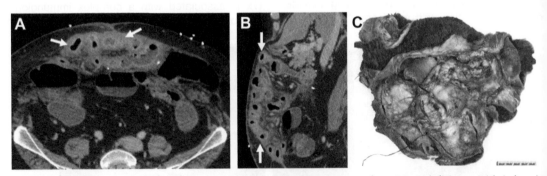

Fig. 4. Acute cellular rejection: Young man in his early 30s with a history of protein S deficiency with ischemic bowel and short gut syndrome, status post isolated intestinal transplantation, developed severe acute cellular rejection requiring allograft enterectomy. Axial (A) and coronal (B) contrast-enhanced CT images show circumferential allograft bowel wall thickening (*white arrows*), mucosal hyperenhancement, and mild adjacent mesenteric fat stranding. Allograft enterectomy specimen (C) on histopathology evaluation demonstrated extensive mucosal ulceration, mucosal necrosis, lamina propria granulation tissue, and increased apoptosis.

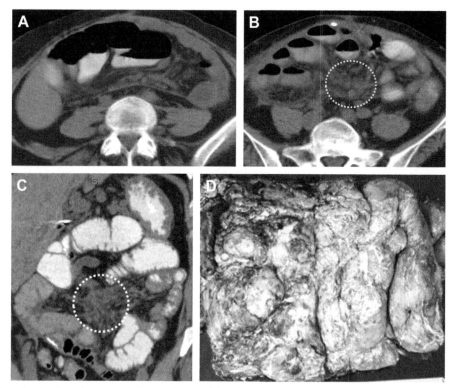

Fig. 5. Chronic rejection: A woman in her early 50s with isolated intestinal transplantation 7 years earlier for short gut syndrome secondary to superior mesenteric artery (SMA) thrombosis. On evaluation for recurrent small bowel obstruction, she was found to have chronic rejection requiring allograft enterectomy. Axial (*B*) and coronal (*C*) unenhanced CT images showed persistent mild small bowel dilation, but the mesenteric stranding and soft tissue (*white circle*) was new from a CT from 1 year earlier (*A*). Allograft enterectomy specimen (*D*) on histopathology evaluation demonstrated severe obliterative arteriopathy of the medium and large mesenteric arteries and extensive serosal adhesions and "sclerotic change of mesenteric soft tissue."

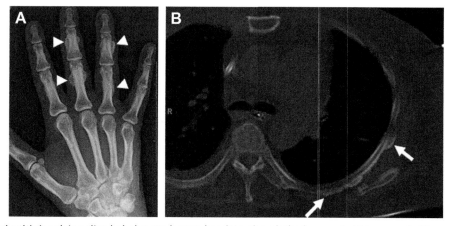

Fig. 6. Periostitis involving distal phalanges (*arrow heads* in *A*) and ribs (*arrows* in *B*) in a nearly 50-year-old man history of isolated intestinal transplantation. This patient experienced episodes of acute cellular rejection and was also on long-term voriconazole therapy, both of which have been implicated in periostitis/hypertrophic osteoarthropathy.

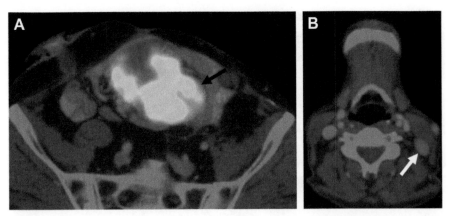

Fig. 7. PTLD in a middle-aged man in his early 60s who underwent multivisceral transplantation nearly 10 years earlier. During workup for small bowel obstruction, a conglomerate mesenteric lymph nodal mass was found, and FDG PET/CT (*A* and *B*) was performed for further evaluation. The mesenteric nodal mass was intensely FDG-avid (*black arrow*) and proven to be diffuse large B-cell lymphoma subtype on biopsy. Another enlarged mildly FDG-avid lower left cervical node (*white arrow*) was also noted which interestingly on biopsy proved to be a synchronous classic Hodgkin lymphoma subtype of PTLD.

Imaging findings are nonspecific and may include changes of chronic ischemia, sclerosing peritonitis, or loss of mucosal fold pattern (**Fig. 5**). Loss of mucosal fold pattern can also be seen with ACR.[7,19–21] Hypertrophic osteoarthropathy, presenting as periosteal reaction involving extremity bones and axial skeleton, has been reported in a few ITx recipients with ACR. However, similar findings of periostitis can be seen with patients on long-term antifungal therapy with voriconazole, which is commonly used in transplant patients (**Fig. 6**).[7,22,23]

Graft-versus-host disease GVHD is a dreaded complication of ITx with a relatively high mortality of 40% to 77%. Its incidence of 5% to 16% in ITx patients, although significantly lower than the reported 40% to 50% incidence after hematopoietic stem cell transplantation, is higher when compared with other types of solid organ transplantation. The incidence is higher in adults, with liver-included allografts, and in asplenic patients. Most common presenting symptom is symmetric erythematous skin rashes which usually raises the initial clinical suspicion. Other manifestations include mucosal ulcers, lymphadenopathy, bone marrow suppression, and liver dysfunction. Diagnosis is confirmed by skin biopsy.[16,24] Imaging findings are nonspecific and variable but commonly included segmental or diffuse bowel wall thickening, mucosal enhancement, mesenteric stranding, and ascites.[25]

Posttransplant lymphoproliferative disease PTLD continues to be a major cause of morbidity and mortality in ITx recipients, but with improved immunosuppression regimes, the incidence has steadily declined from 19.2% between 1985 and 1995 to 8.7% between 2008 and 2018. Although PTLD comprises of a heterogeneous group of lymphoid disorders, most are associated with Epstein–Barr virus and are of B-cell origin.[4,17] PTLD is more common in children, and the incidence is highest within a few months to the first-year posttransplant when the level of immunosuppression is highest.[11] However, in patients surviving more than 10 years after Itx, a later peak incidence may be seen with one study demonstrating 19% incidence in such cohort with median time of 5.6 years for development of PTLD.[26] Imaging cannot distinguish between monomorphic PTLD, which is the most common subtype, from other subtypes such as polymorphic and classic Hodgkin lymphoma but can categorize them into nodal and extranodal patterns based on the primary disease burden (**Fig. 7**). Evaluation can be performed with CT scan or MR enterography. The lesions are fluorodeoxyglucose (FDG)-avid and PET/CT scan is helpful in defining the disease burden and for longitudinal assessment of treatment response.[27,28] Allograft intestine is the most common primary site of PTLD, followed by nodal involvement and involvement of other organs.[17] The distal small bowel and proximal colon are the most common sites of intestinal involvement by PTLD. Intestinal involvement can lead to mural thickening and luminal obstruction or can be associated with mucosal ulceration resulting in gastrointestinal bleed. Alternatively, PTLD can lead to aneurysmal dilation of bowel, which occurs secondary to either necrosis within the thickened

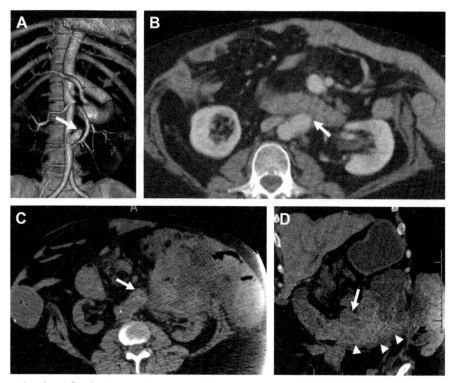

Fig. 8. Aortoduodenal fistula in a nearly 40-year-old woman with initial modified multivisceral transplantation followed by full multivisceral transplantation around 10 years earlier. Baseline CT angiogram images (*A* and *B*) show oversewn aortic graft stump (*white arrows*) from an initial modified multivisceral transplantation, in close proximity to D3 segment of duodenum. Note the longer, patent aortic graft from subsequent multivisceral transplantation (*red arrow*). Axial (*C*) and coronal (*D*) images from a subsequent unenhanced CT performed for gastrointestinal bleed demonstrate new extensive hyperdense blood products in distal duodenum (*white arrow heads*) contiguous with hyperdensity in the tip of the oversewn aortic graft stump. Aortoduodenal fistula was identified at surgery.

wall or as a result of infiltration and destruction of myenteric plexus leading to the loss of contractility. Nodal involvement can be seen as enlargement of multiple individual nodes or may result in formation of a conglomerate mass. The disease can be unifocal or multifocal. With visceral involvement, lesions are usually seen as low-attenuation masses on CT scan and tend to be hypointense on both T1- and T2-weighted images at MR imaging. Enhancement is variable, but the lesions are often hypoenhancing.[7,28,29]

Vascular Complications

Vascular complications are dreaded due to the associated risk for morbidity, allograft loss, and mortality. In a large study of 500 ITx s, Abu-Elmagd and colleagues reported vascular complications including thromboses and pseudoaneurysms in 3.8% of their patients. When bleeding is also included in the complications, some studies with smaller cohorts have reported up to 19% complications.[11,30,31] Vascular complications can occur at any time after transplantation and include hemorrhage, vascular stenosis, pseudoaneurysm, thrombosis, arteriovenous fistula, and aortoenteric fistula. Knowledge of the allograft vascular anatomy and any surgical alterations in native vascular structures is critical in planning appropriate imaging and prompt recognition of assessment of vascular complications. Catheter angiogram offers excellent diagnostic imaging but is invasive and usually considered when therapeutic interventions such as thrombolysis, stenting, balloon dilation, or coil embolization are warranted. CT angiogram is the best noninvasive imaging modalities for assessing the allograft vasculature. MR angiogram rivals CT in assessment of allograft vasculature but is generally not considered as the first-line imaging modality as the prolonged imaging times and motion-related artifacts make it less than ideal for the potentially sick patients with vascular complications. When intravenous contrast is

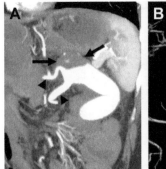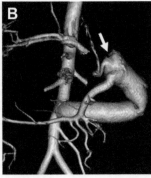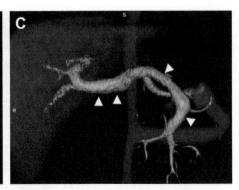

Fig. 9. Young woman in her early 30s status post modified multivisceral transplant (stomach, small bowel, and pancreas) for pseudo-obstruction. Coronal oblique reconstruction (*A*) image from CT angiogram demonstrates subocclusive thrombus (*black arrows*) in the distal portion of the aortic graft without extension to celiac axis and SMA (*black arrow heads*). Volume-rendered images from arterial (*B*) and venous (*C*) phases from the same examination demonstrate contour deformity of the distal portion of aortic graft from the subocclusive thrombus but the allograft SMV and native portal system (*white arrow heads*) are patent.

contraindicated, non-contrast MR angiogram can help in certain select scenarios.[32] Color Doppler ultrasound and contrast ultrasound are excellent options for the assessment of allograft hepatic vasculature and depending on body habitus and overlying structures may also be helpful in evaluation of allograft mesenteric vasculature.

Catastrophic bleeding can occur with rupture of a pseudoaneurysm, dehiscence of vascular anastomosis, or from an aortoenteric fistula and requires emergent management by catheter angiogram or surgery (**Fig. 8**). Arterial thrombosis more commonly involves the aortic conduit or the Carrel patch. When subocclusive and without extension to SMA, it can be managed conservatively with medications (**Fig. 9**). When occlusive or near occlusive thrombus is detected as a filing

defect involving SMA, the bowel should be scrutinized for signs of bowel ischemia such as mural hypoenhancement, mural thickening or thinning, pneumatosis, and pneumoperitoneum (**Fig. 10**). Immediate catheter-directed thrombolysis or surgical management should be considered to avoid loss of allograft or mortality.[11]

Allograft arterial pseudoaneurysms can occur secondary to infection, ischemia from disruption of vasa vasorum, or from high doses of immunosuppression (**Fig. 11**). Such pseudoaneurysms need prompt conventional angiographic management to avoid any untoward consequences.[33] Imaging features of allograft mesenteric venous thrombosis include filling defect involving mesenteric veins with or without extension to portal system and extensive mesenteric fat stranding and

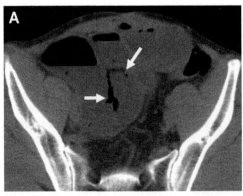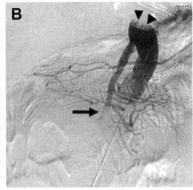

Fig. 10. Young man in his mid-30s status post modified multivisceral transplantation secondary to short gut syndrome resulting from a remote motor vehicle collision. Axial CT image (*A*) performed for abdominal pain demonstrated dilation and pneumatosis (*white arrows*) of allograft small bowel concerning for ischemia. Subsequent angiogram (*B*) with catheter tip in the aortic graft demonstrated complete thromboembolic occlusion of allograft SMA (*black arrow*) likely from a subocclusive thrombus (*black arrow* heads) in the distal portion of the aortic graft.

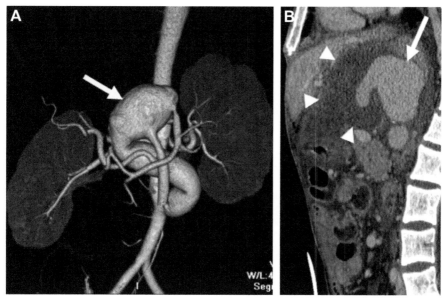

Fig. 11. Volume-rendered (*A*) and sagittal reconstruction (*B*) images from CT angiogram in a young man with a history of multivisceral transplantation demonstrate a pseudoaneurysm (*arrows*) involving distal portion of the aortic graft with large nonocclusive mural thrombus (*arrow heads*).

edema (**Fig. 12**). Bowel wall thickening, mural hyperdensity, pneumatosis, and portomesenteric venous gas are variably present. Risk factors associated with an increased risk of transmural intestinal necrosis include bowel dilation, elevated serum lactate, and organ failure.[34] Depending on the stability of the patient and potential risk of bowel infarction, mesenteric venous thrombosis is managed by anticoagulation therapy, transcatheter thrombolysis, or surgery. Portal vein thrombosis and stenosis can lead to hepatic perfusion anomalies or altered liver function tests. Hepatic venous outflow obstruction from thrombosis or stenosis of hepatic veins or inferior vena cava (IVC) can result in central hepatic hypertrophy and ascites. Such venous complications can be managed by percutaneous interventions such as transcatheter thrombolysis or balloon angioplasty but occasionally require surgical management.[35,36]

Gastrointestinal Complications

Gastrointestinal complications can occur in the early and late postoperative period. Intestinal

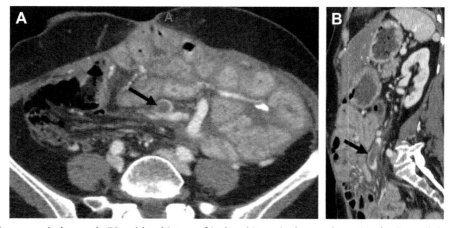

Fig. 12. A woman in her early 50s with a history of isolated intestinal transplantation for intra-abdominal desmoid tumor and short gut syndrome. Axial (*A*) and sagittal (*B*) images from venous phase of CT angiogram demonstrate a subocclsuive thrombus on the allograft SMV (*black arrows*). Patient was asymptomatic, a subsequent ileoscopy was normal and the thrombus resolved on a follow-up CT obtained a few weeks later.

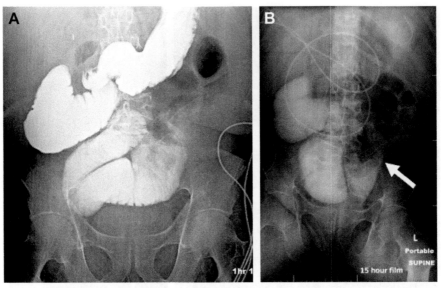

Fig. 13. One-hour (*A*) and 15-hour (*B*) delayed radiographs from small bowel follow through examination performed for vomiting and left lower quadrant pain in a middle-aged man who underwent isolated intestinal transplantation 1 year earlier demonstrate prolonged hold up of contrast in proximal small bowel with sharp angulated configuration at the transition point (*arrow*) consistent with high-grade mechanical obstruction from adhesions.

motility is often abnormal, especially in the early postoperative period. Delayed gastric emptying is seen in 76% of the fluoroscopic studies performed in the first 2 months after ITx, decreasing to 16% by 6 months. Allograft intestine can demonstrate hypomotility or hypermotility with small bowel transit times varying from 0.2 to 17.8 hours.[21] Anastomotic leaks and perforations are reported to occur in 2% to 8% of patients.[11,37] Anastomotic leaks are more common in the early postoperative period but can also occur several years after ITx. Anastomotic leaks can be diagnosed with fluoroscopic examination or CT scan with water soluble oral contrast.

Mechanical obstruction is an uncommon complication but can occur from usual postsurgical etiologies including adhesions (**Fig. 13**), stricture, internal or external hernia (**Fig. 14**), and volvulus. Enterocutaneous fistula is also an uncommon but important complication that can be associated with malnutrition, electrolyte abnormalities, and sepsis. Enterocutaneous fistula is best demonstrated by fistulogram performed under fluoroscopy (**Fig. 15**). Upper GI/small bowel follow-through examination can demonstrate larger fistulas but can be technically challenging for small fistulas. CT scan with water soluble oral contrast can also be used, though it is often inferior to

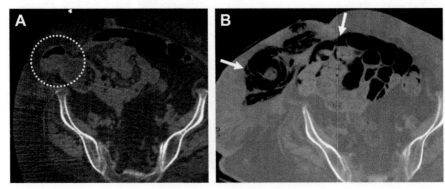

Fig. 14. Middle-aged man with a history of isolated intestinal transplantation and known right lower quadrant abdominal wall hernia containing cecum (*white circle*), seen on a CT 1 year earlier (*A*) presented with nausea and abdominal discomfort. Unenhanced CT scan (*B*) was performed which demonstrated perforated cecum with now incarcerated strangulated hernia with cecal wall pneumatosis and large pneumoperitoneum (*arrows*).

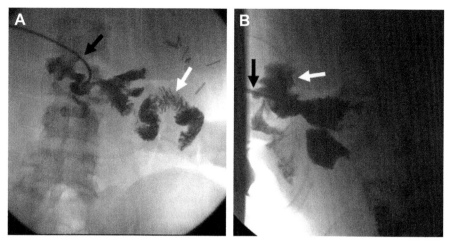

Fig. 15. Frontal (A) and lateral projection (B) images from fistulogram in a young man in his mid-30s with a history of modified multivisceral transplantation nearly 20 years earlier for hollow visceral myopathy and intestinal pseudo-obstruction, demonstrate enterocutaneous fistula with contrast injected through a red rubber catheter (black arrow) inserted through the cutaneous defect opacifying small bowel (white arrows).

fistulogram. Allograft stomach and small bowel can develop ulcers from ischemia or rejection. Larger ulcers in stomach and duodenum can be demonstrated on upper gastrointestinal examinations (Fig. 16).

Pancreaticobiliary Complications

Among the different types of ITx, pancreaticobiliary complications are most likely to occur in patients with L-ITx or MVTx with a prevalence of 17%. The risk of PB complications is higher in MVTx than in liver/small bowel (L/SB) transplants (25% vs 9%). Biliary complications include biliary leaks, biliary obstruction, choledocholithiasis, and cholangitis.[38,39]

Biliary leak

Biliary leak has an incidence of 2% and can occur at anastomotic sites such as choledocho-choledochal anastomosis or biliary-enteric anastomosis; at drain entry sites such as T-tube or percutaneous transheptic cholangiogram (PTC) insertion site; at resected components of biliary tree such as cystic duct stump or hepatic resection site; or at oversewn duodenal stump (Fig. 17). Where possible, biliary anastomoses are avoided during ITx to reduce the risk of biliary leak. For example, when L-Itx is performed, allograft duodenum is included in the transplant to ensure biliary continuity without requirement for choledocho-choledochostomy or choledochojejunostomy. Biliary leaks and resulting bilomas can

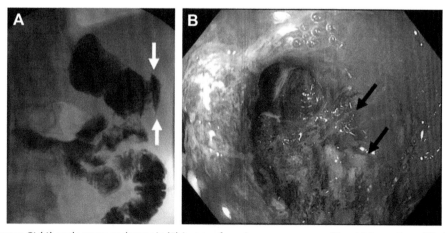

Fig. 16. Upper GI (A) and upper endoscopic (B) images from in a young man with a history of modified multivisceral transplantation nearly 15 years earlier, presenting with recurrent hematemesis, demonstrate a large outpouching of contrast from greater curvature (white arrows) and corresponding large, cratered ulcer (black arrows). Subsequent gastrectomy demonstrated multiple ischemic gastric ulcers.

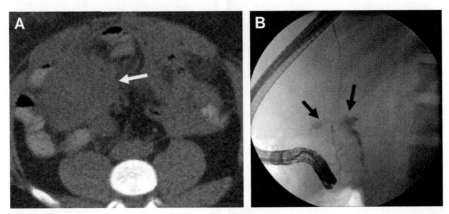

Fig. 17. Axial unenhanced CT (*A*) and ERCP (*B*) images demonstrating low-attenuation biloma (*white arrows*) in right mid-abdomen resulting from bile duct leak from T-tube insertion site (*black arrows*) in a young woman I month after modified multivisceral transplantation (stomach, duodenum, pancreas, and intestine) with choledocho-choledochal anastomosis.

be diagnosed by hepatobiliary scintigraphy or by MR imaging using a hepatobiliary agent such as gadoxetate disodium. Alternatively, they can be diagnosed by endoscopic retrograde cholangio-pancreatogram (ERCP) or PTC and simultaneously managed by placement of a biliary stent and percutaneous transhepatic biliary drainage catheter. Rarely, bile leaks may need surgical management.[7,38–40]

Biliary obstruction

Biliary obstruction can be caused by ampullary stenosis, anastomotic stenosis, bile duct stones, or casts. Patients with right upper quadrant pain or obstructive liver function tests are initially evaluated with ultrasound to assess for biliary dilation. MRCP is often used for better delineation of entire biliary tree to identify intraluminal filling defects and to detect presence as well as accurately localize site of obstruction. Although ERCP can provide diagnostic information, it is generally performed with a therapeutic intent. Depending on etiology, biliary obstruction is managed by sphincterotomy, balloon dilation, stenting, and/or removal of biliary calculi/casts.[39] Ampullary stenosis, one of the most common biliary complications of ITx, involves the allograft ampulla and is presumed to occur secondary to denervation of the common duct and the sphincter of Oddi, resulting in the loss of normal relaxation of the sphincter.[41]

Choledocholithiasis and bile duct casts can be seen incidentally on imaging but are often associated with ductal dilation and obstructive liver function tests (Fig. 18). They are more commonly encountered in the setting of ITx requiring biliary drainage procedures such as choledocho-

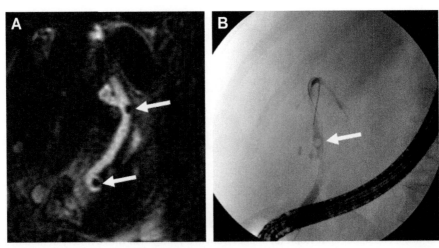

Fig. 18. Choledocholithiasis in a middle-aged man in his mid-50s with isolated intestinal transplantation for Crohn's disease. Oblique coronal 3D-MRCP (*A*) and ERCP (*B*) images demonstrate filling defects (*arrows*) in the common bile duct.

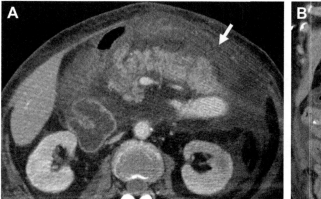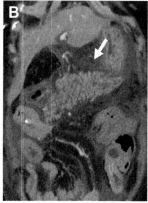

Fig. 19. Acute allograft pancreatitis in a woman in her mid-40s with a history of multivisceral transplantation more than 10 years earlier. Axial (*A*) and coronal (*B*) CT images demonstrate edematous enlargement of allograft pancreas with surrounding fat stranding (*arrows*) and fluid consistent acute interstitial pancreatitis.

choledochostomy or choledochojejunostomy. Bile duct casts are among the most common biliary complications. Factors contributing to formation of bile duct casts include sloughing of biliary epithelium from rejection or ischemia, biliary stasis, and infection. On ultrasound, stones and biliary casts are echogenic and often demonstrate acoustic shadowing. MRCP is more sensitive in detecting stones and casts, which are seen as intraluminal filling defects. Biliary casts and some biliary stones are T1-hyperintense and sometimes are much better appreciated on a T1-weighted sequence than even MRCP sequences. Most patients are successfully managed with ERCP.[38,39]

Cholangitis

Cholangitis occurs in association with choledo-cholithiasis, biliary intervention such as ERCP or PTC or due to reflux of enteric content through biliary-enteric anastomosis. Cholangitis is primarily a clinical diagnosis and suspected in patients presenting with right upper quadrant pain, fever and jaundice, or obstructive liver function tests

(Charcot's triad). Imaging may be negative or may show bile duct wall thickening and hyperenhancement, wedge-shaped T2 hyperintense or hyperenhancing areas of hepatic parenchyma and occasionally hepatic abscesses.[38,42]

Pancreatic complications

Pancreatic complications include acute pancreatitis, chronic pancreatitis, and pancreatic fistulas. With a prevalence of 5.5%, acute pancreatitis is the most common pancreatic complication after ITx and is usually seen with L-ITx and MVTx. Both allograft and native pancreata may be affected, although pancreas allograft is more commonly involved. Etiology is unclear but has been attributed to postsurgical altered perfusion and ischemia. Acute pancreatitis can sometimes be unrelated to transplantation. Pancreas divisum has been reported as the etiology for recurrent acute pancreatitis in a patient with MVTx.[38,39,43] Generic imaging findings of acute pancreatitis can be seen with both allograft and native pancreatitis. Edematous enlargement of pancreas,

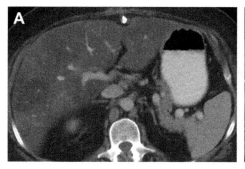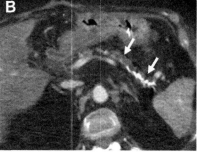

Fig. 20. Axial contrast-enhanced CT images before (*A*) and 6 years after (*B*) isolated intestinal transplantation for short gut syndrome from SMA thrombosis show new severe pancreatic parenchymal atrophy and calcifications (*arrows*) consistent with chronic calcific pancreatitis.

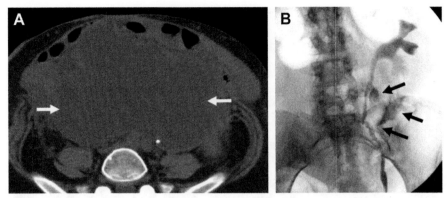

Fig. 21. Young woman in her mid-30s with a history of Gardner syndrome and modified multivisceral transplantation with chronic rejection now status post full multivisceral transplantation 1 month earlier. Unenhanced CT (*A*) showed a large deep-seated abdominal collection (*white arrows*) shown to be a urinoma on drainage. A subsequent retrograde pyelogram (*B*) showed ureteral leak (*black arrows*) presumed to be from intraoperative injury during transplantation.

decreased parenchymal T1 signal, increased signal on diffusion-weighted imaging, peripancreatic fat stranding, and peripancreatic fluid are typical findings of acute interstitial pancreatitis, whereas nonenhancing pancreatic parenchyma represents necrotizing pancreatitis (**Fig. 19**). Intrapancreatic or peripancreatic fluid collections may be present. Management is dictated by severity and associated complications and can include percutaneous drainage, endoscopic interventions, and rarely surgical debridement or drainage.[39] Severe acute pancreatitis can sometimes lead to allograft loss. In one study, severe acute pancreatitis was the second leading cause of intestinal allograft loss accounting for 11% of cases.[44]

Chronic pancreatitis is rare after ITx with prevalence of less than 1% but can affect both native and allograft pancreata.[38] CT scan findings of chronic pancreatitis include parenchymal atrophy, delayed parenchymal enhancement, intraductal and parenchymal calcifications, and irregular ductal dilation (**Fig. 20**). Similar findings are seen at MR imaging, although it is more sensitive and accurate than CT for depicting ductal changes especially when using secretin but is inferior to CT for detection of calcifications. Decreased parenchymal T1 signal is an additional MR imaging finding of chronic pancreatitis.[7,39]

Pancreatic fistula is a rare complication and may result from necrotizing pancreatitis or can occur postoperatively in cases of donor splenectomy. Transection of the donor pancreas was an etiology for pancreatic fistula in the past but has now been abandoned.[38,39]

Genitourinary Complications

Urologic complications may occur during or after transplantation. Urinary bladder and ureteral injuries have been reported during dissection of the native organs before allograft implantation in patients with preexisting adhesive disease. These

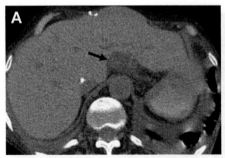
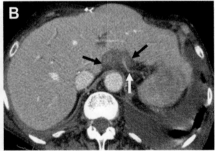

Fig. 22. Middle-aged woman with a history of multivisceral transplantation 5 years earlier for Gardner syndrome with recurrent desmoid tumor seen on routine follow-up imaging. Axial unenhanced (*A*) and post-contrast (*B*) CT images demonstrate a mildly enhancing soft tissue density mass (*black arrow*) in the gastrohepatic ligament encasing left gastric artery (*white arrow*). The mass was shown to be desmoid tumor on resection.

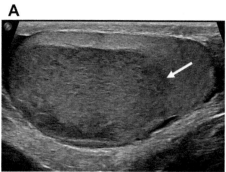 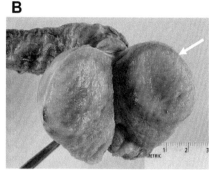

Fig. 23. Nearly 30-year-old man with a history of scrotal swelling 4 years after isolated intestinal transplantation. Scrotal ultrasound (*A*) showed a mildly heterogeneous hypoechoic testicular mass (*white arrow*). Orchiectomy specimen (*B*) on histopathology evaluation showed pure seminoma of the testis.

injuries can lead to urinary leak and urinoma formation. On imaging, urinomas are often noted to be loculated low-attenuation deep-seated or retroperitoneal collections. Diagnostic aspiration with estimation of fluid creatinine can help in confirming urinary leak. Alternatively, CT urogram or MR urogram with excretory phase imaging or retrograde pyelogram can establish the diagnosis (Fig. 21). In addition to cystitis, which is one of the common infectious complications after ITx, posttransplant genitourinary complications have been reported in approximately 13% of patients and include end-stage chronic renal failure, stress incontinence, ureteral stricture, renal hemorrhage, and testicular malignancy.[45]

Neoplastic Complications

In addition to PTLD, ITx recipients are prone to the increased incidence of other neoplasms. IITx, L-ITx, and MVTx have sometimes been performed in patients with unresectable tumoral involvement of mesentery such as from desmoids, neuroendocrine tumor, pancreatic adenocarcinoma, and lymphoma. These neoplasms demonstrate variable propensity for recurrence ranging from 100% recurrence of aggressive malignancy such as pancreatic adenocarcinoma to 35% recurrence for neuroendocrine tumor.[46,47] Recurrence of desmoid tumor is especially common in patients with Gardner syndrome (Fig. 22). After ITx, patients are also at risk of developing de novo primary nonlymphoid malignancies due to the long-term immunosuppression with the incidence of 3.2% and median time of nearly 5 years to cancer diagnosis after ITx. In a large study of 395 patients with ITx, Abu-Elmagd and colleagues reported occurrence of nonmelanocytic skin cancers (38% of all cancers) and other malignancies (62%). Previously reported de novo malignancies include primary lung, liver, gastrointestinal, and testicular malignancies as well as adenocarcinoma of unknown origin (Fig. 23). These malignancies can arise from recipient or donor tissue.[48] CT scan is the most frequently used imaging modality for assessment of the primary malignancy and for staging. PET/CT and MR imaging are alternative options.

SUMMARY

Thanks to several improvements in surgical technique, postoperative care, and immunosuppressive protocols in the last few decades, ITx patients are living longer. However, given the complex surgical technique, immunogenic nature of the allograft intestine and increased propensity for infections, ITx recipients are prone to a wide range of complications. Imaging plays a crucial role in detection of several critical complications. The awareness of the surgical technique, allograft components included in the transplantation, and timing of the surgery as well as familiarity with normal postoperative imaging appearances helps radiologists anticipate and accurately detect posttransplant complications.

CLINICS CARE POINTS

- Mild intestinal dilation, mesenteric fat stranding, mild mesenteric nodal enlargement, and small ascites are normal findings in the immediate postoperative setting due to the lack of normal intestinal innervation and lymphatic drainage.

- Chylous collections are common in the setting of intestinal transplantation due to disruption of the lymphatic drainage pathways in the mesentery. A characteristic imaging finding of chylous collections is the presence of nondependent layering fat attenuation.

- Overlapping imaging findings of acute cellular rejection, graft-versus-host disease, and infectious enteritis are nonspecific and include allograft bowel wall thickening, mucosal enhancement, and ascites.
- Vascular complications of intestinal transplantation including pseudoaneurysm, arterial and venous thrombosis, anastomotic stenoses, bleeding, and aortoenteric fistula can be imaged using CT angiogram, MR angiogram, color Doppler ultrasound, or catheter angiogram. Occlusive mesenteric arterial thrombus and catastrophic bleeding are among the most dreaded complications as they can result in loss of allograft or mortality.
- Bile leak is one of the most common biliary complications of intestinal transplantation and can be diagnosed by hepatobiliary scintigraphy, ERCP, percutaneous cholangiogram, or MR imaging with a hepatocyte specific contrast agent such as gadoxetate disodium.
- Recurrence of pretransplant neoplasms and development of de novo malignancies are late complications of intestinal transplantation.

DISCLOSURE

None of the authors have relevant commercial or financial conflicts of interest to disclose.

REFERENCES

1. Starzl TE, Rowe MI, Todo S, et al. Transplantation of multiple abdominal viscera. JAMA 1989;261(10):1449–57.
2. Garg M, Jones RM, Vaughan RB, et al. Intestinal transplantation: current status and future directions. J Gastroenterol Hepatol 2011;26(8):1221–8.
3. Available at: http://graphics.tts.org/ITR_2019_ReportSlides.pdf 2019. Accessed December 15, 2022.
4. Horslen S, Smith J, Weaver T, et al. OPTN/SRTR 2020 annual data report: intestine. Am J Transplant 2022;22:310–49.
5. Nickkholgh A, Contin P, Abu-Elmagd K, et al. Intestinal transplantation: review of operative techniques. Clin Transplant 2013;27:56–65.
6. Fishbein TM. Intestinal transplantation. N Engl J Med 2009;361(10):998–1008.
7. Rees MA, Amesur NB, Cruz RJ, et al. Imaging of intestinal and multivisceral transplantation. Radiographics 2018;38(2):413–32.
8. Pecchi A, De Santis M, Torricelli P, et al. Radiologic imaging of the transplanted bowel. Abdom Imag 2005;30(5):548–63.
9. Silva J, San-Juan R, Fernández-Caamaño B, et al. Infectious complications following small bowel transplantation. Am J Transplant 2016;16(3):951–9.
10. Loinaz C, Kato T, Nishida S, et al. Bacterial infections after intestine and multivisceral transplantation. In: Transplantation proceedings 35. Elsevier; 2003. p. 1929–30.
11. Abu-Elmagd KM, Costa G, Bond GJ, et al. Five hundred intestinal and multivisceral transplantations at a single center: major advances with new challenges. Ann Surg 2009;250(4):567–81.
12. Unsinn KM, Koenigsrainer A, Rieger M, et al. Spectrum of imaging findings after intestinal, liver-intestinal, or multivisceral transplantation: part 2, posttransplantation complications. Am J Roentgenol (1976) 2004;183(5):1285–91.
13. Smith J, Godfrey E, Bowden D, et al. Imaging of intestinal transplantation. Clin Radiol 2019;74(8):613–22.
14. Sigurdsson L, Reyes J, Kocoshis SA, et al. Bacteremia after intestinal transplantation in children correlates temporally with rejection or gastrointestinal lymphoproliferative disease. Transplantation 2000;70(2):302–5.
15. Merola J, Shamim A, Weiner J. Update on immunosuppressive strategies in intestinal transplantation. Curr Opin Organ Transplant 2022;27(2):119–25.
16. Ganoza A, Mazariegos GV, Khanna A. Current status of graft-versus-host disease after intestinal transplantation. Curr Opin Organ Transplant 2019;24(2):199–206.
17. Wozniak LJ, Mauer TL, Venick RS, et al. Clinical characteristics and outcomes of PTLD following intestinal transplantation. Clin Transplant 2018;32(8):e13313.
18. Lauro A, Marino IR, Matsumoto CS. Advances in allograft monitoring after intestinal transplantation. Curr Opin Organ Transplant 2016;21(2):165–70.
19. Crismale JF, Mahmoud D, Moon J, et al. The role of endoscopy in the small intestinal transplant recipient: a review. Am J Transplant 2021;21(5):1705–12.
20. Ramos E, Molina M, Sarría J, et al. Chronic rejection with sclerosing peritonitis following pediatric intestinal transplantation. Pediatr Transplant 2007;11(8):937–41.
21. Campbell W, Abu-Elmagd K, Federle M, et al. Contrast examination of the small bowel in patients with small-bowel transplants: findings in 16 patients. AJR Am J Roentgenol 1993;161(5):969–74.
22. McGuire MM, Demehri S, Kim HB, et al. Hypertrophic osteoarthropathy in intestinal transplant recipients. J Pediatr Surg 2010;45(11):e19–22.
23. Reber JD, McKenzie GA, Broski SM. Voriconazole-induced periostitis: beyond post-transplant patients. Skeletal Radiol 2016;45(6):839–42.
24. Kaufman SS, Hussan E, Kroemer A, et al. Graft versus host disease after intestinal transplantation:

a single-center experience. Transplant Direct, 2021; 7(8): e731.

25. Shimoni A, Rimon U, Hertz M, et al. CT in the clinical and prognostic evaluation of acute graft-vs-host disease of the gastrointestinal tract. Br J Radiol 2012; 85(1016):e416–23.

26. Courbage S, Canioni D, Talbotec C, et al. Beyond 10 years, with or without an intestinal graft: Present and future? Am J Transplant 2020;20(10):2802–12.

27. Borhani AA, Hosseinzadeh K, Almusa O, et al. Imaging of posttransplantation lymphoproliferative disorder after solid organ transplantation. Radiographics 2009;29(4):981–1000.

28. Camacho JC, Moreno CC, Harri PA, et al. Posttransplantation lymphoproliferative disease: proposed imaging classification. Radiographics 2014;34(7): 2025–38.

29. Kumar P, Singh A, Deshmukh A, et al. Imaging of bowel lymphoma: a pictorial review. Dig Dis Sci 2022;67(4):1187–99.

30. Fägerlind M, Gäbel M, Zachrisson-Jönsson K, et al. Vascular complications after intestinal transplantation-a single center experience. Transplantation 2017;101(6S2):S105.

31. Lacaille F, Irtan S, Dupic L, et al. Twenty-eight years of intestinal transplantation in Paris: experience of the oldest European center. Transpl Int 2017;30(2): 178–86.

32. Hakim B, Myers DT, Williams TR, et al. Intestinal transplants: review of normal imaging appearance and complications. Br J Radiol 2018;91(1090): 20180173.

33. Amesur NB, Zajko AB, Costa G, et al. Combined surgical and interventional radiologic management strategies in patients with arterial pseudo-aneurysms after multivisceral transplantation. Transplantation 2014;97(2):235–44.

34. Wang Y, Zhao R, Xia L, et al. Predictive risk factors of intestinal necrosis in patients with mesenteric venous thrombosis: retrospective study from a single center. Canadian Journal of Gastroenterology and Hepatology 2019;2019:8906803.

35. Rodríguez-Castro KI, Porte RJ, Nadal E, et al. Management of nonneoplastic portal vein thrombosis in the setting of liver transplantation: a systematic review. Transplantation 2012;94(11):1145–53.

36. Naidu SG, Alzubaidi SJ, Patel IJ, et al. Interventional radiology management of adult liver transplant complications. Radiographics 2022;42(6):1705–23.

37. Clouse JW, Kubal CA, Fridell JA, et al. Posttransplant complications in adult recipients of intestine grafts without bowel decontamination. J Surg Res 2018;225:125–30.

38. Papachristou GI, Abu-Elmagd KM, Bond G, et al. Pancreaticobiliary complications after composite visceral transplantation: incidence, risk, and management strategies. Gastrointest Endosc 2011; 73(6):1165–73.

39. Borhani AA, Dasyam AK, Papachristou G, et al. Radiologic features of pancreatic and biliary complications following composite visceral transplantation. Abdom Imag 2015;40(6):1961–70.

40. Kinner S, Dechêne A, Ladd SC, et al. Comparison of different MRCP techniques for the depiction of biliary complications after liver transplantation. Eur Radiol 2010;20(7):1749–56.

41. Pascher A, Neuhaus P. Biliary complications after deceased-donor orthotopic liver transplantation. J Hepato-Biliary-Pancreatic Surg 2006;13(6): 487–96.

42. Catalano OA, Sahani DV, Forcione DG, et al. Biliary infections: spectrum of imaging findings and management. Radiographics 2009;29(7):2059–80.

43. Nawaz H, Slivka A, Papachristou GI. Recurrent acute pancreatitis secondary to graft pancreas divisum in a patient with modified multi-visceral transplant. ACG Case Rep J 2014;1(2):103–5.

44. Ekser B, Kubal CA, Fridell JA, et al. Comparable outcomes in intestinal retransplantation: single-center cohort study. Clin Transplant 2018;32(7):e13290.

45. Akhavan A, Jackman SV, Costa G, et al. Urogenital disorders associated with gut failure and intestinal transplantation. J Urol 2007;178(5):2067–72.

46. Moon JI, Selvaggi G, Nishida S, et al. Intestinal transplantation for the treatment of neoplastic disease. J Surg Oncol 2005;92(4):284–91.

47. Duchateau NM, Canovai E, Vianna RM, et al. Combined liver-intestinal and multivisceral transplantation for neuroendocrine tumors extending beyond the liver: a systematic literature review. Transplant Rev 2022;36(1):100678.

48. Abu-Elmagd KM, Mazariegos G, Costa G, et al. Lymphoproliferative disorders and de novo malignancies in intestinal and multivisceral recipients: improved outcomes with new outlooks. Transplantation 2009;88(7):926–34.

Imaging of Uterine Transplantation

Sara A. Hunter, MD[a], Myra K. Feldman, MD[b],*

KEYWORDS

- Uterus transplantation • Absolute uterine factor infertility
- Mayer-Rokitansky-Küster-Hauser syndrome • Pelvic ultrasound • Pelvic MR imaging

KEY POINTS

- Uterine transplantation is an emergeing treatment for women with absolute uterine factor infertility (AUFI).
- The most common cause of early uterine transplant graft failure is thrombosis of uterine vessels.
- Imaging, particularly ultrasound imaging, is used to evaluate the uterine graft in the early post-operative period.

INTRODUCTION

Absolute uterine factor infertility (AUFI) impacts approximately 3% to 5% of women worldwide and is characterized by an absent or nonfunctional uterus. AUFI can be secondary to acquired causes, such as hysterectomy, or congenital causes, including Mayer-Rokitansky-Küster-Hauser syndrome (MRKH). Uterus transplantation (UTx), a novel procedure under study at several centers across the globe, is currently the only available treatment of AUFI.[1] UTx was first shown as a potential treatment of AUFI when a team from Sweden reported the first live birth of a woman following UTx in 2014.[2] At least 70 UTx procedures and 34 births have been reported as of November 2022, though this is likely an underestimation with additional cases not yet reported in the medical literature.[3]

UTx has been performed successfully with grafts from both living and deceased donors and each model is associated with unique advantages and drawbacks. In the living donor (LD) model, it is possible to obtain detailed information regarding the donor's medical history and control timing of the procedure. Drawbacks to this approach include the potential for physical and psychosocial harm to the donor. With the deceased donor (DD)

model, potential risks to the donor are completely eliminated. More tissue is available for the procurement surgery which, in theory, is advantageous. The main disadvantages of DD are the paucity of suitable donors, lack of information surrounding the donor's medical history, and inconvenience surrounding procedure timing.[4,5]

Unlike other solid organ transplantation procedures, success with UTx is defined by seven progressive stages: the technical success of the transplantation defined as graft viability at 3 months after surgery, menstruation, embryo implantation, pregnancy, delivery, and graft removal with long-term follow-up.[6] Imaging plays an important role throughout the life cycle of a uterus transplant. It is used for the evaluation of suitable donors and recipients, to monitor graft vasculature in the post-surgical setting, and to evaluate for suspected complications. Imaging also plays a role in the in vitro fertilization (IVF) process and monitoring of pregnancy. In this review, we will first describe the surgical technique of UTx. The article will then focus on the importance of imaging in the evaluation of potential recipients and donors and during the immediate post-surgical time course as graft viability is established. Imaging as part of IVF, pregnancy, and complications will also be discussed.

[a] Section of Abdominal Imaging, Imaging Institute, Cleveland Clinic, 9500 Euclid Avenue, L-10, Cleveland, OH 44195, USA; [b] Section of Abdominal Imaging, Imaging Institute, Cleveland Clinic, 9500 Euclid Avenue, A-21, Cleveland, OH 44195, USA
* Corresponding author.
E-mail address: feldmam2@ccf.org

Radiol Clin N Am 61 (2023) 889–899
https://doi.org/10.1016/j.rcl.2023.04.009
0033-8389/23/© 2023 Elsevier Inc. All rights reserved.

radiologic.theclinics.com

SURGICAL TECHNIQUE

UTx is performed in an orthotopic position with a composite graft that includes the uterus with surrounding parametria, a cuff of vaginal tissue, proximal segments of the paired (right and left) round ligaments, and paired uterine arterial and venous vascular pedicles. The length and specific vessels included with the vascular pedicles can vary significantly between institutions, and between LD and DD.[1,7]

The vascular anastomoses are the most critical component of the uterus transplantation procedure as the major cause of early graft failure is due to thrombosis of uterine vessels. The native human uterus is conventionally supplied by contributions from three pairs of vessels: the uterine, ovarian, and vaginal arteries. All uterine transplantation surgeries have been performed with two (paired right and left) uterine arteries, with some also including the internal iliac artery or anterior division of the internal iliac artery. With DD, longer lengths of the internal iliac artery can be included as part of the vascular pedicle. The arterial vascular pedicles are anastomosed in an end-to-side fashion to the external iliac arteries (**Fig. 1**).[8,9]

Establishing robust venous outflow is the most technically challenging component of UTx. There is confusion in the medical and UTx literature surrounding the naming and anatomy of the venous drainage of the uterus. The human uterus is drained by superior and inferior pairs of uterine

veins that extend from a periuterine venous plexus. There is variability in the number of tributaries and in the location and number of insertions to the internal iliac vein.[6,8] The most difficult portion of the graft retrieval is dissection of the uterine veins, given their thin walls, diminutive size, and proximity to the ureter.[10] Several different combinations of uterine vein (UV) anastomoses have been used including using the inferior UV, superior UV as well as ovarian veins, uteroovarian veins, and internal iliac vein for vascular pedicles from DD. The uterine graft venous anastomoses are performed in an end-to-side fashion to the external iliac veins.[1,9]

After the vascular anastomosis has been performed, the vaginal anastomosis can be completed between the graft vaginal cuff and the recipient vagina or neovagina. The recipient must have a patent vaginal canal to accommodate this anastomosis, to provide an outlet for menses, and for access to the cervix for routine biopsies necessary for rejection evaluation. The composite graft is further secured into place by attaching the graft ligaments to the recipient round ligaments, sacrouterine ligaments, or paravaginal connective tissue. Fixation to the rudimentary uterine tissue in a woman with MRKH has also been reported.[11,12]

IMAGING EVALUATION OF POTENTIAL RECIPIENTS

At present, UTx is offered to individuals assigned as female at birth, of child-bearing age with AUFI. In the future, the procedure may be expanded to include transgender women and those with other causes of uterine factor infertility that are not absolute, such as adenomyosis, endometriosis or other uterine anomalies.[13] Although specific inclusion and exclusion criteria vary by site, potential candidates typically undergo intense medical and psychosocial screening. Candidates must agree to undergo multiple surgical procedures including IVF, cesarean section, and hysterectomy. They must also agree to adhere to necessary medical therapies including antirejection regiments and vaccinations.[1]

Initially, imaging may be necessary to establish or confirm a diagnosis of AUFI. Transvaginal ultrasound (TVUS) is typically the first-line imaging modality used to evaluate women for infertility. MR imaging of the pelvis may also be necessary to confirm or better delineate anatomy, especially when congenital anomalies are the underlying cause of AUFI (**Fig. 2**).[14]

Imaging studies are also used to evaluate potential recipients for anatomic findings that could impact surgical planning or limit transplantation

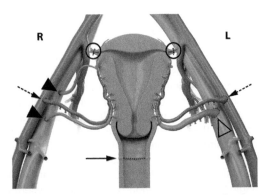

Fig. 1. Illustration of common anastomoses for UTx. The paired UA are anastomosed to the external iliac arteries in an end-to-side fashion (*dashed arrows*). Two different variations of UV anastomosis are shown, one with a single end-to-side anastomosis with the left external iliac vein (*open arrowhead*) and one with a superior and inferior UV end-to-side anastomoses (*right*) (*closed arrowhead*). The vaginal anastomosis is shown (*solid arrow*). The composite graft round ligaments (*black circles*) are typically secured to native round ligaments or sacrouterine ligaments. (Reprinted with permission, Cleveland Clinic Foundation ©2022. All Rights Reserved.)

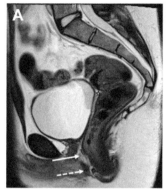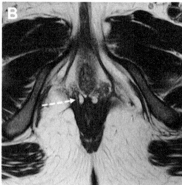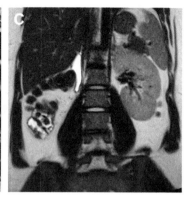

Fig. 2. Sagittal T2-weighted (T2W) MR imaging of the pelvis (*A*) in a woman with MRKH syndrome. The uterus and upper vagina are absent with a fat plane present in the expected location of the uterus (*star*) and upper two-thirds of the vagina (*white arrow*). Fibrous tissue corresponding with the atretic distal third of the vagina (*dashed arrow*) is noted on both the sagittal plane (*A*) and on an axial T2W image through the perineum (*B*). Large field of view Half-Fourier Acquisition Single-Shot Turbo spin Echo image through the upper abdomen (*C*) shows an associated renal anomaly with a single left kidney.

success. Most women who have undergone UTx have AUFI secondary to MRKH, a syndrome associated with renal, vascular, and skeletal anomalies.[15] Centers use abdominal US or computed tomography (CT) of the abdomen and pelvis to evaluate for associated anomalies, such as the presence of a pelvic kidney.[13] CT without contrast is used to evaluate for atherosclerotic calcifications, which could complicate the vascular anastomosis.[16] Some programs have described obtaining MR angiography (MRA) and CT angiography (CTA) studies to evaluate for potential congenital vasculature malformations and for vessel caliber (**Fig. 3**).[8,12,17] Chest x-rays are often obtained as part of the standard preoperative evaluation.

IMAGING EVALUATION OF POTENTIAL DONORS

Potential uterine graft donors must be screened for structural uterine anomalies that could interfere

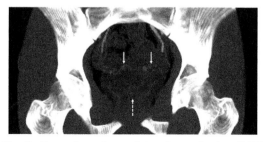

Fig. 3. Coronal maximum intensity projection (MIP) image from CTA of the abdomen and pelvis in a woman with MRKH. The uterine arteries are well seen bilaterally (*white arrows*) and measure 2 to 3 mm in diameter. The uterus is absent (*dashed arrow*), consistent with MRKH.

with implantation or support of a term pregnancy and also for vascular abnormalities that could be unfavorable for establishing a robust vascular supply to the allograft. Specific criteria and imaging evaluation of potential donors vary by institution and by type of donor, living or deceased.

UTx programs report screening for structural uterine abnormalities that could impact fertility such as leiomyomas, endometrial polyps, adenomyosis, Cesarian scar defects, vascular anomalies, and congenital uterine anomalies.[13] Programs using an LD model have reported using TVUS and MR of the pelvis for this assessment.[7] Programs that use a DD model may need to rely on prior imaging studies, if available, medical history from family members, or evaluation during procurement to assess for uterine pathology. It is sometimes possible to obtain a TVUS or CT from a potential DD before organ procurement (**Fig. 4**).

Evaluation of potential donor uterine vasculature is important as the major cause of early graft failure is thrombosis of uterine vessels, which is attributed to poor-quality vessels, hypoperfusion, and infection. Factors associated with poor outcomes include small caliber vessels and atherosclerotic disease. Detailed preoperative evaluation of vasculature is particularly important when LDs are used as these donors tend to be older or post-menopausal and, thus, at increased risk for atherosclerotic disease and smaller caliber vessels.[18] The vascular structures available to include as part of the allograft are limited for LD allografts which cannot include the larger caliber internal iliac arteries and veins.

Evaluation for uterine artery (UA) patency, vessel caliber, and the presence of atherosclerotic disease has thus been a focus of preoperative donor

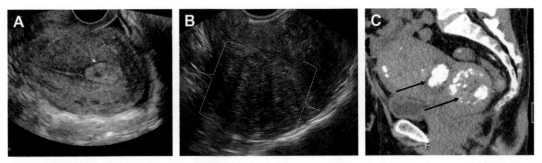

Fig. 4. Imaging findings that could exclude a potential uterine donor. The sagittal TVUS image of the uterus (*A*) shows an oval, hyperechoic endometrial polyp (*white arrow*). A sagittal TVUS image of the uterus from a different person (*B*) shows a globular shape of the uterus with asymmetric anterior wall thickening, diffuse myometrial heterogeneity, and shadowing (*brackets*), characteristic of adenomyosis. Sagittal unenhanced CT (*C*) from a different person shows several partially calcified uterine leiomyomas, some of which are either centered in or exert mass effect on the endometrium and lower uterine segment (*black arrows*).

evaluation for LD. In their initial cohort of 12 patients, Leonhardt and colleagues performed computed tomography angiogram (CTA), conventional digital subtracted angiography (DSA), and magnetic resonance angiography (MRA) on potential donors. The UA was measured in three locations along its course. In this cohort, most of the UAs were sufficiently evaluated by MRA. This group concluded that MRA could be used as a first-line imaging modality with CTA and possible DSA reserved for cases in which the UA was not well seen by MRA. This cohort showed US diameters ranging from 0.5 to 3.4 mm with an average of 2.1 mm, similar to other published data (**Fig. 5**).[18,19]

Kristek and colleagues reported a far more detailed imaging-based preoperative assessment of potential donor vasculature, evaluating both the donor arteries and veins using a novel vascular grading system. In this study, they concluded that MRA with venous phase imaging could be used to reliably access uterine venous characteristics as

well as arterial with CTA used as a problem-solving modality.[8]

Detailed assessment of vasculature is not possible with the DD model, however, information regarding the presence or absence of vascular calcifications can be determined if pre-procurement unenhanced CT is performed. Evaluation of vasculature can also be performed during the procurement surgery.[13]

POST-TRANSPLANTATION VASCULAR EVALUATION

In the early post-operative setting, technical success is defined by the establishment of vascular inflow and outflow to and from the allograft. Graft failure is most often associated with vascular complications, primarily attributed to the difficulties associated with graft supply by diminutive vessels. One-third of recipients undergo complications severe enough to require surgical or radiologic intervention, with 24% of grafts requiring removal,

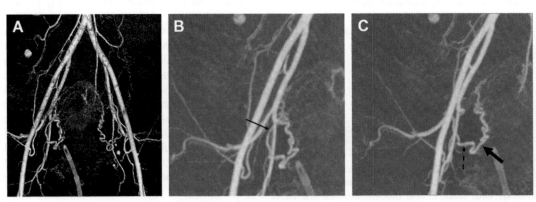

Fig. 5. Coronal three dimensional (3D) MIP CTA image (*A*) at the level of the uterine vasculature. Two MIP CTA images at slightly different obliquities through the right UA (*B, C*) show the location to obtain proximal (*thin black arrow*), mid (*dashed black arrow*), and distal (*thick black arrow*) UA caliber measurements.

predominantly related to vascular thrombosis or graft hypoperfusion from arterial disease or arteriosclerosis.[3] Most major complications occur during the first 2 weeks following transplantation.[20]

Complications will demonstrate abnormality on pelvic US, typically an increase in graft size and alteration of arterial flow. Some centers describe using Doppler implantable probes placed directly on the uterine arteries to monitor arterial flow in the early post-operative setting[16,17] while others use intraoperative US evaluation to ensure vascular patency before closing (**Fig. 6**).[12,16] Almost all centers describe using transabdominal US (TAUS) or TVUS with Doppler in the post-operative period to assess graft vasculature, however, very little information regarding specific imaging protocols and the timing and frequency of imaging has been published.[12,17,21–25]

In our experience, an imaging protocol similar to that used for renal transplant vasculature assessment can be applied (**Table 1**). Transabdominal technique with lower frequency curved linear or phased array transducers is preferred to allow time for the vaginal anastomosis to heal and also because many with MRKH cannot accommodate transvaginal technique. Color and spectral Doppler of the external iliac arteries and veins above, at, and below the vascular anastomoses is performed. Color and spectral Doppler imaging of the uterine arteries and veins bilaterally at the anastomosis and in the parametrial area is then documented if possible, followed by assessment of the intraparenchymal uterine arteries and veins of the upper, middle, and lower graft bilaterally.

Although standard criteria for normal uterine vascular waveforms and velocities are yet to be established, we expect arterial and venous vascular flow to be detectable within the graft by US. Venous flow may be slow and thus challenging to detect by Doppler imaging. Uterine arterial waveforms should show a brisk upstroke with antegrade flow throughout diastole (**Fig. 7**). The UAantegrade flow resistive index (RI) is higher in the non-gravid uterus (0.65–0.85) than in the gravid uterus.[26]

When US findings are indeterminate or concerning for a vascular complication, MR imaging, CT, MRA, or CTA may be performed for further evaluation (**Fig. 8**). Extrapolating on what is known from other solid organ transplants, decreased RIs (less than 0.55) can indicate upstream stenosis or inflow abnormality. Elevated arterial RIs are nonspecific and may be secondary to arteriosclerosis, venous thrombosis, or intrinsic graft dysfunction, such as from infection.[27] Reversal of diastolic flow is abnormal and should prompt further investigation into potential causes, if not readily apparent in US. CT or MR imaging can be used to identify abnormalities of the transplant arteries and veins. Vascular problems may also manifest as decreased, delayed, or absent parenchymal enhancement (**Fig. 9**).

POST-TRANSPLANTATION IMAGING TO EVALUATE GRAFT FUNCTION

Graft function is assessed by the onset of menstruation which typically occurs within the first 90 days. During this period, TAUS or TVUS initial grayscale imaging of the uterus may be used to evaluate for signs of cyclical endometrial change including measurement of endometrial thickness. As transplants are orthotopic, imaging appearance should mimic that of a native uterus, without significant change in appearance, size, or heterogeneity over time (14). Immediately post-transplant, the endometrium is not usually well seen but starts to react to hormonal changes over time, similar to that of a native uterus, and then follows the expected cyclical changes in appearance (**Fig. 10**).[28]

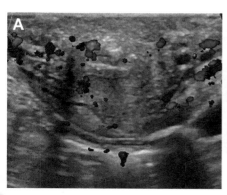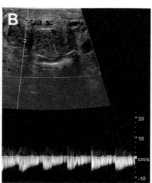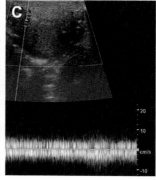

Fig. 6. Intraoperative US with color Doppler (*A*) shows uniform vascular flow throughout the uterus. The linear intraoperative probe is placed directly on the uterus in this open surgical procedure. Intraoperative US with color and spectral Doppler shows normal arterial (*B*) and venous (*C*) waveforms.

Table 1
Essential components of uterus transplant ultrasound evaluation

Technique	• Transabdominal with low frequency curved linear transducer and full bladder • Supplemental transvaginal may be used after the anastomosis has healed if tolerated
Doppler	• Color and spectral Doppler images of the external Iliac artery and vein (or other vessel if atypical anastomosis) bilaterally proximal to, at, and distal to the anastomosis • Color and spectral Doppler images of the transplant uterine arteries bilaterally at the anastomosis and parametrium • Color and spectral Doppler assessment of the transplant renal veins bilaterally at the anastomosis and parametrium • Color or power Doppler assessment of the entire uterus for global assessment of perfusion • Color and spectral Doppler assessment of the intrauterine arteries at superior, mid, and inferior poles • Color and/or spectral Doppler evaluation of the intrauterine veins
Greyscale	• Overall size measurement in longitudinal and transverse planes • Endometrial echo complex thickness • Peritransplant soft tissue evaluation for fluid collections.

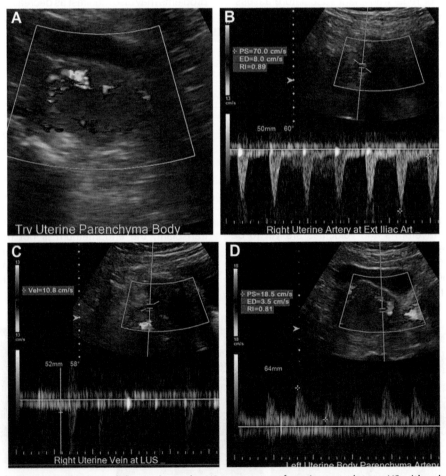

Fig. 7. Early post-operative transabdominal vascular US assessment of uterine vasculature. US with color Doppler (A) shows uniform, robust vascular flow throughout the graft. US with color and spectral Doppler at the level of the arterial anastomosis on the right (B) shows the transplant UA at the anastomosis is patent with normal waveform. US with color and spectral Doppler at the level of the right parametrium (C) shows patency of the UV with normal waveforms. US with color and spectral Doppler at the level of the transplanted uterus (D) shows robust vascular flow within the intraparenchymal UA on the left with a normal arterial waveform.

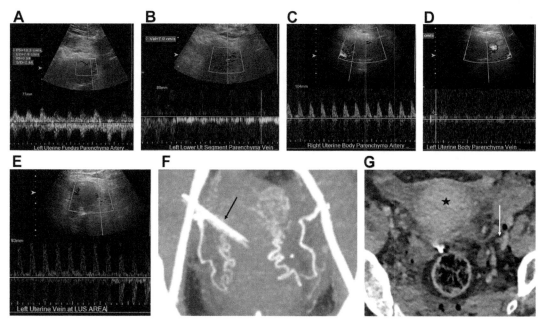

Fig. 8. Images from the first post-operative TAUS with color and spectral Doppler through an intra-parenchymal artery (*A*) and vein (*B*) show vessels are patent with normal waveforms. The transabdominal US with color and spectral Doppler through an intra-parenchymal artery the following day (*C*) shows a change in the waveform, now high resistance with areas of absent diastolic flow (RI = 1). Uterine venous waveforms were not identified within the uterus (*D*) or in the parametrial area (*E*) on the left. Given the change in findings, CTA with venous phase imaging at 90 and 180 seconds was performed. 3D MIP image from the arterial phase (*F*) shows the uterine arteries are patent bilaterally without stenosis. Surgical drain is present in the image (*black arrow*). Axial image at 90 seconds post-contrast (*G*) shows the left UV is patent at the anastomosis (*white arrow*). Although the vein was difficult to trace due to its small caliber and similar attenuation to parametrial soft tissues, the uterus showed symmetric enhancement (*black star*) during all phases of contrast enhancement. Patent vasculature was later confirmed during an exploratory laparotomy.

IMAGING DURING IN VITRO FERTILIZATION AND PREGNANCY

Most centers require recipients to undergo oocyte harvest with in vitro fertilization and have frozen high-quality blastocysts before consideration for ÚTx. Imaging associated with this process is thus completed before enrollment in a UTx program.

The graft is meant for up to two pregnancies and 5 to 7 years to limit the length of immunosuppression.[29] Embryo transfer can be considered once immunosuppression is stable, with centers reporting initiation of the process anywhere from 3 to

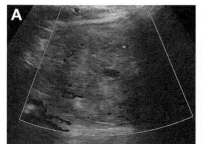
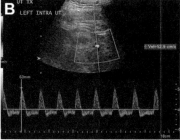
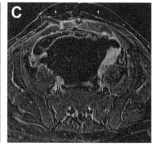

Fig. 9. Transabdominal US image of a uterus transplant with power Doppler (*A*) shows very little detectable flow throughout the myometrium. Color and spectral Doppler image through an intraparenchymal artery (*B*) shows an abnormal spectral waveform with reversal of diastolic flow. Axial T1 contrast-enhanced MR imaging from the venous phase of contrast enhancement with subtractions (*C*) shows absent enhancement throughout the graft. At explantation, the graft was found to be necrotic which was attributed to an underlying *Candida* infection.

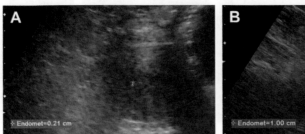
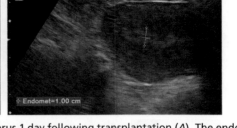

Fig. 10. Transabdominal US image of a transplanted uterus 1 day following transplantation (*A*). The endometrial echo complex (between calipers) is difficult to make out and measures 0.2 cm transabdominal US image of the same transplant uterus 6 months following transplantation (*B*). The endometrial echo complex (measurement *line*) is thicker, now measuring up to 1 cm and well seen with a trilaminar appearance characteristically seen during the proliferative phase of the menstrual cycle. This is a sign of graft function.

12 months post-transplantation. The process of embryo transfer is similar to that in a native uterus with imaging used according to the reproductive endocrinology protocol.[30] Once a pregnancy is established, the patient is followed closely by maternal–fetal-medicine, with regular sonographic interrogation of the graft and monitoring of the fetus following standard protocol. Fetal growth is monitored starting in the second trimester due to increased risk for fetal growth restriction, a known risk among women who have undergone other forms of solid organ transplantation.[14] Delivery is by low C-section to avoid disruption of the vaginal anastomosis. On average, children born from uterine transplants are delivered at 35 weeks, with an average weight for age.[31]

Multiple pregnancy complications have been reported in patients with a uterine transplant, including gestational hypertension and pre-eclampsia, which is at least in part related to the high rate of renal agenesis in this population.[32] Additional reported complications include cholestasis of pregnancy, premature rupture of membranes, pyelonephritis, oligohydramnios, polyhydramnios, placenta accreta (**Fig. 11**), and subchorionic hematoma.[3,10,12,33–35]

Due to immunosuppression, these patients are also at increased risk of infection and are monitored particularly closely for cytomegalovirus and toxoplasmosis due to the potential for teratogenic effects from these diseases.[3,36] Fortunately, no uterine transplant fetus has developed cytomegalovirus or toxoplasmosis infection to our knowledge. Of the 34 live births noted in the literature, there has only been one with congenital disease, which was an anteriorly and caudally displaced urethra.[37]

Following one to two successful deliveries (**Fig. 12**), the graft is removed and immunosuppression may be stopped.

NON-VASCULAR COMPLICATIONS AND THE ROLE OF IMAGING

Immunosuppression is started immediately following the transplant, with regimens paralleling that used for renal transplants. As there are no established, reliable imaging findings of rejection, routine cervical biopsies are performed to evaluate for rejection.[3]

Infection is a known complication of UTx. Most infections can be prevented through prophylactic therapy including vaccination and antimicrobial therapy. Infection may cause abnormal appearance of the graft on imaging studies (see **Fig. 9**).

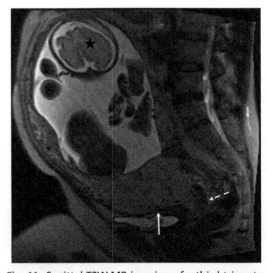

Fig. 11. Sagittal T2W MR imaging of a third-trimester fetus. The placenta is located inferiorly and covers the internal cervical os (*white arrow*), indicating placenta previa. There are placental vessels also extending outside the expected boundaries of the uterus (*dashed arrow*), consistent with placenta accrete. The fetus is also in breech position (*black star*).

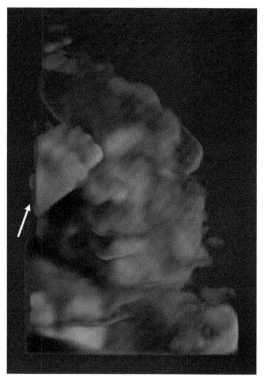

Fig. 12. 3D US image of a 34-week fetus in a uterine transplant patient. A foot (*white arrow*) is partially covering the fetus' face.

Severe infection may result in explantation.[1,30] Stenosis of the uterine-vaginal anastomosis has been described with one case developing a subsequent vesicovaginal fistula. This can be prevented with the use of vaginal dilators and vaginal estrogen.[28]

Cervical dysplasia has also occurred in patients following transplantation, despite being human papillomavirsu-negative before transplantation. Fortunately, as cervical biopsies are performed on a regular basis to evaluate for rejection, these cases of dysplasia are noted and managed early and there have not been any reports of subsequent development of cervical cancer in these cases.[3] There has been one case of an Epstein Barr Virus (EBV)-negative recipient received an EBV-positive graft, resulting in gastrointestinal post-transplant lymphoproliferative disorder (PTLD). The patient was treated with hysterectomy, which resolved the disease.[3]

The rate of post-surgical complications to living uterine donors, requiring surgical or radiologic intervention is 17%. Reported injuries include ureteric injury, uretovaginal fistula, and vaginal cuff dehiscence.[10,21,28,38] A single case of donor post-operative buttock/leg pain has been reported

presumably related to claudication from the removal of portions of the internal iliac artery to include in the graft.[10] If ureteral injuries are suspected, a CT urogram may be performed for identification of possible injury. A CT or fluoroscopic cystogram may be performed in conjunction with the urogram if there is suspicion of bladder injury or leakage.

SUMMARY

All members of the multidisciplinary care team are key to success in a UTx program. Radiologists play an instrumental role throughout the life cycle of a uterus transplant; from recipient work-up to donor selection, post-operative vascular assessment and investigation of complications. As the number of centers performing this procedure continues to expand, radiologists will need to focus on establishing diagnostic standards for donor evaluation and post-operative vascular assessment.

CLINICS CARE POINTS

- AUFI impacts approximately 3% to 5% of women worldwide and is characterized by an absent or non-functional uterus.

- Uterine transplantation (UTx) has been performed successfully with grafts from both living and DDs and each model is associated with unique advantages and drawbacks.

- Unlike other solid organ transplantation procedures, success with UTx is defined by seven progressive stages: the technical success of the transplantation defined as graft viability at 3 months after surgery, menstruation, embryo implantation, pregnancy, delivery, graft removal, and long-term follow-up.

- Potential uterine graft donors must be screened for structural uterine anomalies that could interfere with implantation or support of a term pregnancy and also for vascular abnormalities that could be unfavorable for establishing a robust vascular supply to the allograft.

- Graft failure is most often associated with vascular complications, primarily attributed to the difficulties associated with graft supply by diminutive vessels. One-third of recipients undergo complications severe enough to require surgical or radiologic intervention, with 24% of grafts requiring removal, predominantly related to vascular thrombosis or graft hypoperfusion from arterial disease or arteriosclerosis.

DISCLOSURE

The authors have nothing to disclose.

REFERENCES

1. Richards EG, Farrell RM, Ricci S, et al. Uterus transplantation: state of the art in 2021. J Assist Reprod and Gene 2021;38:2251–9.
2. Brännström M, Johannesson L, Bokström H, et al. Livebirth after uterus transplantation. Lancet 2015; 385(9968):607–16.
3. Ayoubi JM, Carbonnel M, Racowsky C, et al. Evolving clinical challenges in uterus transplantation. Reprod Biomed Online 2022;45(5):947–60.
4. Frisch EH, Falcone T, Flyct R, et al. Uterus transplantation: revisiting the question of deceased donors versus living donors for organ procurement. J Clin Med 2022;11(15):4516.
5. Bruno B, Arora KS. Uterus transplantation: the ethics of using deceased versus living donors. Am J Bioeth 2018;18:6–15.
6. Johannesson L, Testa G, Flyckt R, et al. Guidelines for standardized nomenclature and reporting in uterus transplantation: An opinion from the United States Uterus Transplant Consortium. Am J Transplant 2020;20:3319–25.
7. Favre-Inhofer A, Rafii A, Carbonnel M, et al. Uterine transplantation: review in human research. J Gynecol Obstet Hum Reprod 2018;47(6):213–21.
8. Kristek J, Johannesson L, Clemons MP, et al. Radiologic evaluation of uterine vasculature of uterus transplant living donor candidates: DUETS classification. J Clin Med 2022;11(4626):1–10.
9. Escandon JM, Bustos VP, Santamaría E, et al. Evolution and transformation of uterine transplantation: A systematic review of surgical techniques and outcomes. J Reconstr Microsurg 2021;28(6):429–40.
10. Testa G, Koon EC, Johannesson L, et al. Living Donor Uterus Transplantation: A Single Center's Observations and Lessons Learned From Early Setbacks to Technical Success. Am J Transplant 2017;17:2901–10.
11. Brannstrom M, Kahler PD, Greite R, et al. Uterus transplantation: a rapidly expanding field. Transplant J 2018;102(4):569–77.
12. Flyct R, Falcone T, Quintini C, et al. First birth from a deceased donor uterus in the United States: from severe graft rejection to successful cesarean delivery. Am J Obstet Gynecol 2020;143–51.
13. Johannesson L, Wall A. Uterus transplantation – donor and recipient work-up. Curr Opin Organ Transplant 2021;26(6):634–9.
14. Feldman MK, Hunter SA, Perni UC, et al. New Frontier: Role of the Radiologist in Uterine Transplantation. Radiographics 2019;40:291–302.
15. Wang Y, Lu J, Zhu L, et al. Evaluation of Mayer-Rokitansky-Küster-Hauser syndrome with magnetic resonance imaging: three patterns of uterine remnants and related anatomical features and clinical settings. Eur Radiol 2017;27(12):5215–24.
16. Brucker SY, Strowitzki T, Taran FA, et al. Living-donor uterus transplantation: pre intra- and postoperative parameters relevant to surgical success, pregnancy and obstetrics with live births. J Clin Med 2020;9: 2485.
17. Brannstrom M. First clinical uterus transplantation trial: a six-month report. Fertil Steril 2014;101(5): 1228–36.
18. Leonhardt H, Thilander-Klang A, Båth J, et al. Imaging evaluation of uterine arteries in potential living donors for uterus transplantation: a comparative study of MRA. CTA and DSA, Eur Radiol 2022;32:2360–71.
19. Mahmood S, Johannesson L, Testa G, et al. DUETS (Dallas UtErus Transplant Study): The role of imaging in uterus transplantation. SAGE open Medicine 2019;7.
20. Jones BP, Saso S, Bracewell-Milnes T, et al. Human uterine transplantation: a review of outcomes from the first 45 cases. BJOG 2019;126:1310–9.
21. Fageeh W, Raffa H, Jabbad H, et al. Transplantation of the human uterus. Int J Gynecol Obstet 2002;76: 245–51.
22. Ozkan O Akar ME, Ozkan O, et al. Preliminary results of the first human uterus transplantation from a multiorgan donor. Fertil Steril 2013;99:470–6.
23. Testa G, McKenna GJ, Gunby RT Jr, et al. First live birth after uterus transplantation in the United States. Am J Transplant 2018;18:1270–4.
24. Wei L, Xue T, Tao KS, et al. Modified human uterus transplantation using ovarian veins for venous drainage: the first report of surgically successful robotic-assisted uterus procurement and follow-up for 12 months. Fertil Steril 2017;108:346–56.
25. Fronek J, Kristek J, Chlupac J, et al. Human uterus transplantation from living and deceased donors: the interim results of the first 10 cases of the Czech trial. J Clin Med 2021;10:586.
26. Kurjak A, Kupesic-Urek S, Schulman H, et al. Transvaginal color flow Doppler in the assessment of ovarian and uterine blood flow in infertile women. Fertil Steril 1991;56(5):870–3.
27. McNaughton DA, Abu-Yousef MM. Doppler US of the liver made simple. Radiographics 2011;31:161–88.
28. Chmel R, Novackova M, Janousek L, et al. Revaluation and lessons learned from the first 9 cases of a Czech uterus transplantation trial: Four deceased donor and 5 living donor uterus transplantations. Am J Transplant 2019;19:855–64.
29. Johannesson L, Kvarnström N, Mölne J, et al. Uterus transplantation trial: 1-year outcome. Fertil Steril 2015;103:199–204.
30. Richards EG, Flyckt R, Tzakis A, et al. Uterus transplantation: organ procurement in a deceased donor model. Fertil Steril 2018;110(1):183.

31. Salomon LJ, Bernard JP, Ville Y. Estimation of fetal weight: reference range at 20–36 weeks' gestation and comparison with actual birth-weight reference range. Ultrasound Obstet Gynecol 2007;29:550–5.

32. Heinonen PK. Gestational hypertension and pre-eclampsia associated with unilateral renal agenesis in women with uterine malformations. Eur J Obstet Gynecol Reprod Biol 2004;114:39–43.

33. Jones BP, Williams NJ, Saso S, et al. Uterine transplantation in transgender women. Bjog. Wiley-Blackwell 2019;126:152.

34. Castellon LAR, Amador MIG, Gonzalez RED, et al. The history behind successful uterine transplantation in humans. JBRA assisted reproduction 2017; 21:126–34.

35. Ejzenberg D, Andraus W, Baratelli Carelli Mendes LR, et al. Livebirth after uterus transplantation from a deceased donor in a recipient with uterine infertility. Lancet 2019;392:2697–704.

36. Patel R, Paya CV. Infections in solid-organ transplant recipients. Clin Microbiol Rev 1997;10:86–124.

37. Johannesson A Wall, Putman JM, Zhang L, et al. Rethinking the time interval to embryo transfer after uterus transplantation – DUETS (Dallas UtErus Transplant Study). BJOG An Int J Obstet Gynaecol 2019;126(11):1305–9. https://doi.org/10.1111/1471-0528.15860.

38. Brannstrom MA, Belfort JM. Ayoubi Uterus transplantation worldwide: clinical activities and outcomes. Curr Opin Organ Transplant 2021;26(6): 616–26.

Unconventional Strategies for Solid Organ Transplantation and Special Transplantation Scenarios

Balasubramanya Rangaswamy, MD[a], Christopher B. Hughes, MD[b], Biatta Sholosh, MD[c], Anil K. Dasyam, MD[c],*

KEYWORDS

- Domino transplant • Paired organ donation • ABO incompatible Transplant • Split liver transplant
- Ex vivo liver resection and auto transplantation

KEY POINTS

- To supplement cadaveric and living liver transplantation, new methods have been developed to address transplant organ shortage.
- "Domino transplant" refers to transplanting relatively healthy liver from a patient with inborn error of metabolism, such as familial amyloid polyneuropathy, to a patient with liver failure.
- Ex vivo liver resection and auto transplantation is surgically challenging but is being done at tertiary transplant centers.

INTRODUCTION

Advances in surgical techniques and immunosuppressive treatments during the last few decades have improved long-term outcomes for patients receiving solid organ transplants.[1] Despite this progress, donor organ constraints limit the number of patients benefiting from organ transplantation. At the time of this writing, a total of 105,231 patients in the United States needed a lifesaving organ. The combined deceased and living donor pool for 2022 was 19,478 and the number of transplants performed using this pool was 39,241, per the latest data published by the United Network for Organ Sharing (UNOS) website.[2] Multiple unconventional strategies have been used to increase donor pool including sequential/domino transplant, Split liver transplant and paired organ transplant.[1,3] This article highlights some of these unconventional and special transplantation scenarios to increase

the donor pool. Although the overall number of these transplants is considerably lower compared with deceased or living donors, they nonetheless are an innovative approach to expand the donor pool.

DISCUSSION
Domino/Sequential Liver Transplantation

Principles

Many inborn errors of metabolism are usually cured with liver transplantation.[4] The metabolic enzymes that are lacking in these conditions are expressed in normal livers and therefore transplantation could cure these inborn errors of metabolism. A subset of these patients with such metabolic conditions retain structurally normal livers with preserved function that can still be used in other patients with liver failure (due to other causes) thus creating a domino effect.[1] The effects of these inborn errors of metabolism usually take

[a] Southwest Medical Imaging, 9700 North 91st Street, C-200, Scottzdale, AZ 85258, USA; [b] Department of Surgery, Liver Transplantation at the Thomas E. Starzl Transplantation Institute, 200 Lothrop Street, Pittsburgh, PA 15213, USA; [c] Department of Radiology, University of Pittsburgh School of Medicine, 200 Lothrop Street, Pittsburgh, PA 15213, USA
* Corresponding author.
E-mail address: dasyamak@upmc.edu

Radiol Clin N Am 61 (2023) 901–912
https://doi.org/10.1016/j.rcl.2023.04.012
0033-8389/23/© 2023 Elsevier Inc. All rights reserved.

years to become symptomatic and the premise is that downstream effects of the domino liver enzymatic defect would take years to become symptomatic in the recipient (**Fig. 1**).

Domino liver transplantation has been performed with multiple inborn errors of metabolism, most commonly with familial amyloid polyneuropathy (FAP).[5]

Familial Amyloid Polyneuropathy World Transplant registry (FAPWTR)/Domino Liver Transplant Registry is the online registry maintaining a list of domino liver transplants (DLTs) in centers around the world.[6] As per the registry, a total of 67 institutions across 21 countries are listed as of December 31, 2019. A total of 1289 domino transplants on 1268 patients have been registered so far. A total of 591 of these transplants are registered from Portugal alone comprising the country with the highest number of domino transplantation procedures.

Domino Liver Donor Candidates

DLT was first described by Furtado *and colleagues* in Portugal in 1996 using a liver from a donor with FAP.[7] It has since been adopted across several countries, and the list of inborn errors of metabolism has been expanded. Patients with FAP are by far the most common domino liver donors. Patients with inborn errors of metabolism who have been used as domino liver donors are listed in **Box 1**. A few of these common conditions are discussed below.

FAP is an autosomal dominant multisystem disorder with variable penetrance characterized by neuropathy secondary to amyloid deposits. Several mutations have been identified with the most common caused by the transthyretin (TTR) mutation. A point mutation causes valine to be replaced by methionine at position 30 of the TTR gene.[5,7] This mutation destabilizes the TTR protein and results in aggregation into amyloid fibrils that accumulate in different organs causing dysfunction. Besides FAP, amyloidosis can be seen in other medical conditions. The imaging manifestations are nonspecific and diverse with single or multiple organ involvement. It can present as a focal lesion, tumor-like observation, or infiltrative process[8] (**Fig. 2**).

Maple syrup urine disease (MSUD) is an autosomal recessive metabolic condition due to deficiency of branched-chain 2-ketoacid dehydrogenase resulting in toxic accumulation of branch chain amino acids—leucine, isoleucine, and valine and their metabolites.[1,9] The condition results in ketoacidosis and toxic encephalopathy.

Primary hyperoxaluria (PH) is a hereditary disease caused by the deficiency of liver-specific alanine glyoxylate aminotransferase resulting in overproduction of oxalate with precipitation in the kidneys and hence renal failure.[1,10] Liver alone or combined liver and kidney transplantation has been considered curative in these patients. Beside many skeletal imaging findings, the condition results in severe cortical nephrocalcinosis and nephrolithiasis associated with scarred small kidneys in infancy through young adulthood[11] (**Fig. 3**). The striking appearance of these kidneys occasionally allows the interpreting Radiologist to first raise the possibility of PH.

Familial hypercholesterolemia (FH) is caused by a deficiency in the low-density lipoprotein receptor on the cell membrane resulting in dysregulated

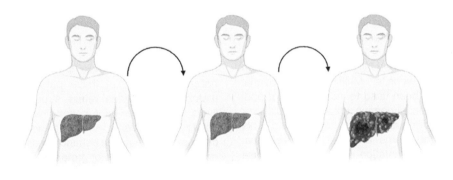

| Deceased or Living Donor | Structurally and functionally normal liver from a patient with inborn error of metabolism | Domino Recipient with Cirrhosis and multifocal HCC |

Fig. 1. Domino liver transplantation: Domino transplant involves transplanting relatively healthy liver from a patient with inborn error of metabolism (necessitating liver transplantation) to a patient with liver failure. (Created with BioRender.com.)

<table>
<tr><td>

Box 1
Domino liver donor candidates

Familial amyloid polyneuropathy

Fibrinogen A alpha chain amyloidosis

MSUD

Primary hyperoxalosis

FH

Hemochromatosis

Wilson disease

Methylmalonic acidemia

Hyperhomocysteinemia

Ornithine transcarbamylase deficiency

Citrullinemia

Crigler Najjar disease

Methioninemia

Propionic acidemia
</td></tr>
</table>

cholesterol production/metabolism, severe hyper-cholesterolemia, and premature atherosclerosis.[1,12]

Domino Liver Recipient Candidates

Domino livers offer distinct advantages. Usually, these livers are from younger patients and hence the liver harvests are from hemodynamically stable patients without portal hypertension. The planned nature of the harvest and subsequent transplant results in minimal cold ischemic times.[13] Such a transplant, however, can only be justified in a select group of recipients. These are usually elderly patients with shorter life expectancy and in whom palliative care rather than long-term cure remains the only option. In one study DLT recipients tended

to have lower MELD scores compared with deceased donor recipients (15 ± 5 vs 21 ± 10) and longer transplant wait times (584 ± 830 vs 272 ± 490 days).[14] The life expectancy of these recipients is estimated to be less than the duration to de novo development of the metabolic condition. As per FAPWTR, the median age of DLT recipients is 57.1 years. The sex distribution was 74% male and 26% female. Patients with already diagnosed hepatocellular carcinomas, hepatic metastases or patients with allograft failure being considered for retransplantation are usual candidates for DLT. Bridge treatment in pediatric age group to allow for growth until definitive transplantation is considered another indication for DLT.[1,6]

Surgical Considerations with Domino Liver Transplantation

Unique venous outflow reconstruction challenges are encountered at domino liver transplantation. Harvesting the domino liver with retrohepatic inferior vena cava (IVC) as is done with cadaveric transplant results in 2 major problems. First, harvesting the domino retrohepatic IVC would require cross clamping of the donor IVC with an external veno-venous bypass. Patients with FAP tend to have autonomic dysregulation and cardiac dysfunction due to amyloid deposits and cross clamping IVC results in dangerous intraoperative fluctuations in blood pressure.[15] Second, harvesting the retrohepatic IVC would result in a short suprahepatic IVC in the domino donor, which would then complicate their subsequent liver transplant venous anastomosis.[16] Several modifications of these conventional venous outflow reconstructions have been implemented. An end-to-side venous anastomosis after oversewing the suprahepatic IVC is one method to avoid

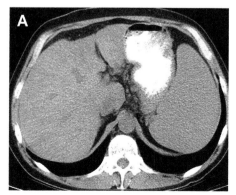 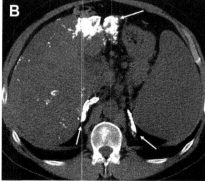

Fig. 2. A 48-year-old man with systemic amyloidosis. Axial noncontrast CT image through the abdomen (*A*) demonstrates dysmorphic liver with biopsy demonstrating extensive hepatic parenchymal involvement with hereditary apolipoprotein AI-associated amyloidosis. Follow-up unenhanced CT (*B*) several years later demonstrates dense calcifications (*arrows*) involving the liver and bilateral adrenal glands due to advanced amyloidosis.

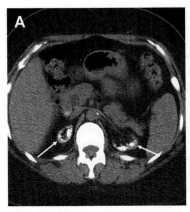 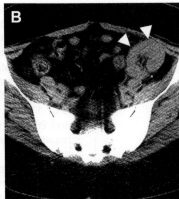 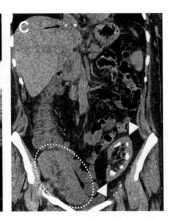

Fig. 3. A 30-year-old woman with delayed diagnosis of PH. Baseline axial unenhanced CT scan (*A*) in this patient with end-stage renal failure demonstrates atrophic kidneys with dense medullary calcifications (*white arrows*). Patient initially underwent isolated left lower quadrant renal transplantation (*arrowheads in B*). She then developed recurrent renal failure and allograft biopsy revealed PH following which a simultaneous liver and kidney transplantation was performed. Coronal image from an unenhanced CT (*C*) obtained 7 months later demonstrates new dense medullary calcifications involving failed old left lower quadrant allograft kidney (*arrowheads*) and new right lower quadrant renal allograft (*dashed oval*). Note the surgical clips near allograft hepatic venous anastomosis (*black arrow*).

complications from a foreshortened suprahepatic IVC.[16] A venous graft from tissue bank to increase the length of the suprahepatic IVC is another approach. "Caval sparing" techniques involve harvesting the domino liver without the retrohepatic IVC. One method is to harvest the domino liver and form a conjoined middle and left hepatic veins. A cadaveric IVC including the common iliac veins is then used to facilitate anastomoses of domino liver to the recipient. The 2 iliac veins are used to anastomose the common trunk of the left/middle hepatic veins and the right hepatic vein thus creating an inverted venous Y graft. Subsequently, the contiguous cadaveric IVC and domino recipient (DR) IVC are anastomosed in a standard piggyback fashion.[17] Another caval sparing technique is to conjoin the 3 hepatic veins to a venous patch. Such a patch is usually created from the cadaver IVC, cryopreserved portal vein, or the recanalized umbilical vein.[18–20] This recreated patch would then be standard piggyback anastomosed into the DR.

Long-Term Consequences and Outcomes after Domino Liver Transplantation

Data evaluating long-term outcomes of DRs are limited, which is not unexpected given the overall low frequency of this type of transplantation versus cadaver/living related donor transplantation. Much of the data are from Europe and Asia where DLTs are more common given the greater incidence of FAP. Portugal, Sweden, and Japan constitute the most endemic countries with FAP. Data from the

United States are not surprisingly very limited because only 0.1% of all transplants between 1996 and 2020 were domino transplants.[21]

The biggest concern for the DR is the risk of transmission of the monogenic metabolic condition into the recipient.[22] Most of the studies available to review such a risk of transmission are available for FAP liver recipients. In a study of 23 DRs, 17% (4 out of 23) of the patients developed biopsy proven de novo amyloidosis during an observation period of 10 years. Only 8% of these patients died due to complications from de novo amyloidosis such as arrhythmias secondary to cardiac amyloidosis. Recurrence of primary disease, sepsis, and multiorgan failure contributed to the majority of deaths in this group.[23] The study also reports an incubation period of 8 to 11-year for manifestations of de novo amyloidosis in DRs, comparatively symptoms develop after 20 years in patients with inherited FAP. The 1-year, 3-year, and 5-year survival rates of DRs in this study were 82%, 72%, and 70%, respectively.

Another study from Germany evaluated 61 DRs[24] 1-year, 3-year, 5-year survival rates were 82%, 71%, and 69%, respectively. About 3.3% (2 out of 61) DRs developed de novo amyloidosis. The largest outcomes study from Portugal with 114 DRs reports a 5-year survival of 59%. 11.4% (13 out of 114) DRs developed amyloidosis. The reported median time for developing clinical features of amyloidosis was 75 months (range 60–121 months).[25] Besides this small but tangible risk of transmission of disease, a study from Japan reported the mean time to de novo amyloidosis occurred earlier in older DRs than younger DRs. The time distribution was 5.8 versus 8.6 years in patients aged older than and younger than 50 years, respectively.[26] Hence, candidates for DLT need to be carefully selected and an appropriate surveillance protocol for the development of the metabolic condition is mandatory after transplantation. The diagnostic criteria are however not standardized. At Karolinska Institute in Sweden, postoperative monitoring of peripheral nerve function is performed with a standard Electroneurography index. Nerve conduction parameters are recorded at 1 month, 6 months, and then yearly after DLT.[27] Echocardiography and Cardiac MR imaging for cardiac amyloidosis, as well as abdominal fat, skin, gastric mucosa, labial salivary gland, and sural nerve biopsies are all variably reported in literature for the diagnosis of de novo amyloidosis.[1,23]

A US national transplant analysis reviewed the UNOS database between 1996 and 2020. A total of 181,976 liver transplants were performed during this period. Of these, there were only 185 DLTs (0.1%). FAP and MSUD accounted for 83% of the DLTs. The 3-year, 5-year, and 10-year patient survivals after DLT were 83%, 76%, and 57%, respectively.[21]

Based on available outcomes data, MSUD DRs tend to have a good prognosis. A study from the Children Hospital of Pittsburgh evaluated 17 MSUD DRs with 100% patient survival at median follow-up of 6.4 years (range 1.2–12.9 years).[9] Metabolic function assessed with serum branched chain amino acids and their metabolites were normal on an unrestricted protein diet. Another European study evaluated 14 MSUD DRs for a median follow-up of 23 months (range 2–31 months). Thirteen out of 14 patients were alive during the follow-up period.[28] One explanation for the good outcomes in MSUD DRs is that the liver is only responsible for about 9% to 13% of the branched-chain 2-ketoacid dehydrogenase activity and enzyme activity in the skeletal muscle, kidney, and brain adequately compensates in the DR.

Very limited data in the form of case reports are available for FH DRs. The liver contains approximately 50% to 75% of the total body's low-density lipoprotein receptors and hence liver transplantation is considered in patients with FH. However, the domino graft from a patient with FH may be compensated by extrahepatic low-density lipoprotein receptors in the DR. One of the case reports discusses a domino liver from a 25-year-old patient with FH was transplanted into a 46-year-old patient with hepatocellular carcinoma. Elevated levels of cholesterol were noted at follow-up, and these were partially controlled by diet and medications. This DR however did undergo coronary artery stenting for accelerated atherosclerosis.[12]

Several case reports and case series have been published detailing experiences with PH DLT. All reports seem to indicate recurrent oxalosis and renal failure needing dialysis in these DRs. One study discussed outcomes in 5 DRs from PH. All 5 patients developed dialysis-dependent renal failure within 14 days of transplantation and 4 out of 5 patients died with the only survivor undergoing retransplantation.[10] The dismal performance of the PH DLT is likely because of the presence of the alanine glyoxylate aminotransferase enzyme exclusively in the liver with no extrahepatic sources to back up in the DR. Given these reports, currently PH DLT is not recommended (**Fig. 4**).

Paired Organ Donation

Paired organ donation (POD) is commonly performed with renal transplantation and is simply known as "kidney swap." This type of transplantation is performed when the living donor and recipient in a pair are deemed ABO or human leukocyte antigen (HLA) incompatible. A "swap" between the donor of one pair with the recipient of the other pair and vice versa is performed to allow for more compatible matching.[3]

In its simplest form, a 2-way exchange is performed where 2 incompatible pairs come together to exchange their kidneys (**Fig. 5**). Three or more pairs can be used to perform multiple exchanges thereby leading to a chain of transplants. As can be imagined, the real success of paired organ exchange would be in expanding the living donor pool. This would increase the chances of finding an ABO/HLA compatible and appropriately sized organ from a living donor.

To this end, multicenter, national, and international kidney exchange programs are active to make PODs a success. The National Kidney Registry and UNOS launched programs for Kidney Paired Donation in 2007 and 2010, respectively. Local and regional programs such as the Johns Hopkins University Paired Kidney Exchange and New England Program for Paired Kidney Exchange have facilitated several renal transplants.

Nondirected altruistic donors can also enter such programs and initiate PODs. Such a kidney from an altruistic donor is matched to a recipient with an incompatible donor. The original donor would then donate to a compatible recipient on the list and so on. Ultimately, one of the POD donors would donate the organ to a patient on the deceased organ waiting list thereby closing the loop. Another variation to this cycle would be that the final donor instead of donating to

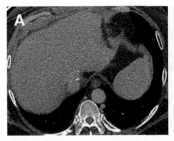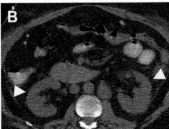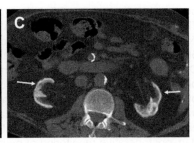

Fig. 4. A 51-year-old man with hepatitis C virus and alcohol-related cirrhosis who received DLT from a patient with PH. Baseline axial-unenhanced CT images (*A* and *B*) after liver transplantation demonstrate normal hepatic allograft and kidneys (*arrowheads*). Several months later, a random renal biopsy performed for "new unexplained renal failure" showed numerous intratubular calcium oxalate crystals and severe tubulointerstitial scarring confirming the "inheritance" of hyperoxaluria. Unenhanced CT a few years later (*C*) showed atrophic kidneys with dense cortical calcifications (*arrows*).

waitlisted recipient would become a bridge donor to start a new chain[3] (**Fig. 6**).

The POD program success can be further enhanced by hybrid techniques. This can be done by creating a list of ABO and HLA compatible participants within a single POD chain. Such a program is called Compatible Pair Participation.[3] Combining the POD with ABO desensitization protocols would also allow recipients to get more suitable donors against whom they have lower level of sensitization. Complex computational algorithms/artificial intelligence programs are also used to enhance the success of the POD programs to allow for the best matching depending on blood group, organ size, and sensitization status of recipients. This is usually done with multicenter or national level exchange programs. Alvin Roth and Lloyd Shapely received the 2012 Nobel Prize in economics for developing an algorithm to match large number of donors and recipients in Paired Kidney Exchange programs.[3]

Outcomes of paired kidney donation
Due to the living nature of these transplants, outcomes tend to be better and such exchange programs are gaining popularity. In fact, kidney paired exchange is now routinely performed in the United States and currently accounts for 12% of all living donor kidney transplants.[29] A study from the National Kidney Registry evaluated the outcomes of paired kidney transplants (n = 2363) versus living donor transplants (n = 54,497). When adjusted for donor, recipient, and transplant factors, there was no difference in graft failure or mortality between the groups. The 5-year and 7-year graft failure and mortality rates for the paired transplants were 6.4 years/8.7% and 6.8 years/10.9%, respectively. Statistics for the living donor group were 7.2 years/10.5% and 7.0 years/11.2%, respectively.[29]

Paired liver donation The liver counterpart of the POD is less commonly performed. This is because of the overall lower number of living donor liver transplants (LDLTs) and inherently more complex surgery. The first case of paired liver exchange was only performed as recently as 2020. As with paired kidney exchange, liver paired exchange can be used to overcome ABO incompatibility (ABOi) issues and organ size discrepancies. The

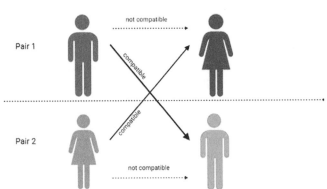

Paired Kidney Donation

Fig. 5. Paired kidney donation in a single pair. (Created with BioRender.com.)

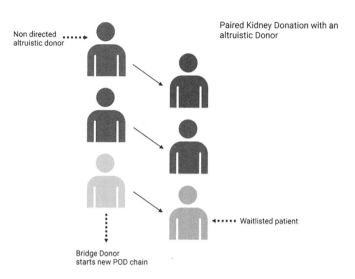

Non directed
altruistic donor

Paired Kidney Donation with an
altruistic Donor

Fig. 6. Paired kidney donation initiated by an altruistic donor.

Waitlisted patient

Bridge Donor
starts new POD chain

largest experience outside of Asia was described at the University of Pittsburgh with 10 paired liver exchanges (20 LDLTs). All 20 donors were alive and with no major complications at 12.7 months. Seventeen out of 20 recipients were alive and had good allograft function with a duration of follow-up of 12.5 months. One death was due to hepatic artery thrombosis while the other 2 deaths were unrelated to the transplant process.[30]

Limitations to POD Several impediments exist to the successful implementation of POD: (1) Organs have to be transported across cities/state lines as patients generally prefer to undergo transplantation close to home.[3] Such transportation raises concerns for an increase in cold ischemia time. However, a study reported good performance status of the kidney if the cold ischemia time is kept less than 14 hours[31]; (2) There is a risk of donors backing out of the program and revoking consent after the recipient has received the organ from another pair. This is especially true with bridge donors. To surmount this problem, all transplant surgeries must be performed simultaneously despite any logistic difficulties. Appropriate counseling and psychological assessments of all donors before transplantation is a must; (3) Within a POD program, there is a chance of inability to match all participants with their transplants. This is especially true in single-center programs with fewer pairs. The odds of matching more participants increase with higher numbers of registered pairs. Bingaman and colleagues showed a strong correlation between the number of successful paired kidney transplantations and addition of new pairs to the pool and suggested that a sharp increase occurs once pool size increases to 100 recipients[32]; and (4) O blood group is universal donor

and AB blood group is universal recipient. Hence, O group recipients and AB group donors accumulate in any POD chain. Registering more O donors and AB recipients or using both blood group and HLA compatible pairs can be used to balance any POD chain.

ABO Incompatible Organ Transplant

Another strategy to increase living donor pool is transplantation of organs despite ABOi. ABOi has long been considered a contraindication to organ transplant due to the risk of hyperacute rejection from preformed isoagglutinins and early graft loss.[33] Pretransplant desensitization techniques to prevent such rejection have been devised to allow for successful ABOi transplant.[34] Several desensitization protocols exist across various institutions. One such protocol at the University of Pittsburgh, ABOi Liver transplant program, is illustrated in **Fig. 7**. Uncertainty about the safety and efficacy of ABOi organ transplant exists and overall has not been universally accepted across various transplant centers. A study using the Scientific Registry of Transplant Recipients evaluated the outcome of 738 ABOi renal transplants to matched control group comprising of 77,455 ABO compatible (ABOc) transplants.[35] The median follow-up was 5 years (range 0–15 years). The graft loss was found to be significantly higher in the first 14 days after transplant while there was lesser difference after day 14. The patient survival with ABOi renal transplants at 1, 3, 5, and 10 years was 96.8%, 93.7%, 88.3%, and 74.5%, respectively, whereas the respective numbers for ABOc group were 97.8%, 94.9%, 90.7%, and 75.1%, respectively. A systematic review and meta-analysis evaluated 49 patient groups with renal

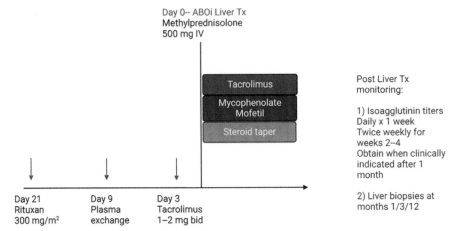

Fig. 7. ABO desensitization protocol at University of Pittsburgh Liver transplantation Center.

transplants comprising 65,063 participants.[36] This included 7098 patients with ABOi transplants. Compared with ABOc group, the ABOi group was associated with higher 1-year, 3-year, and 5-year mortality with odds ratio of 2.17, 1.89, and 1.47, respectively. Death-censored graft survival was lower in the ABOi than ABOc group at 1 and 3 years with odds ratio of 2.52 and 1.59, respectively. The graft loss and patient survival were similar after 5 and 8 years.

Another systematic review and meta-analysis evaluated 29 patient groups with liver transplants comprising 10,783 participants.[37] This included 2137 ABOi liver transplants. There was no statistically significant difference in all-cause mortality between ABOi and ABOc LDLTs at 1, 3, and 5 years with odds ratio, respectively, of 1.0, 0.78, and 0.96. The death-censored graft survival and complication rates were similar between the groups. There was however an increased all-cause mortality at 1 year between ABOi and

ABOc deceased liver donors with an odds ratio of 1.89. There was no significant difference in mortality between these groups at 3 and 5 years. The death-censored graft survival and complication rates tended to be worse than the ABOc group.

Despite uncertainties about ABOi solid organ transplantation, there is a continued upswing in the number of such transplants being performed especially in countries where paired organ transplantation is deemed unethical. Further advances and refinements in desensitization protocols will contribute to the success of ABOi transplantation.

Split Liver Transplantation

Split liver transplantation (SLT) is another method of increasing the donor liver pool by splitting the deceased donor liver into 2 parts based on one of the following techniques. In the classical split, the left hepatic lobe lateral segment (segments II and III) is used for a pediatric or a small adult

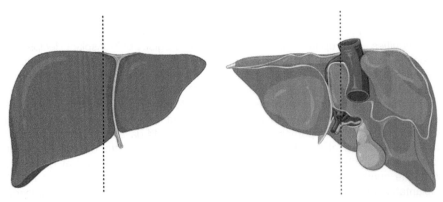

Fig. 8. Classic SLT: The plane of hepatic dissection is to the right of the falciform ligament. Split liver containing segments II and III is transplanted into a pediatric recipient while the split liver containing segments IV to VIII is transplanted into an adult recipient. (Created with BioRender.com.)

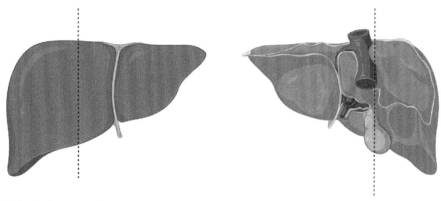

Fig. 9. Full SLT: The liver is split into segments I-IV and V-VIII. Each split liver is then transplanted into 2 adults. (Created with BioRender.com.)

recipient and the extended right hepatic lobe (segments I + IV-VIII) is used for an adult recipient (Fig. 8). In the full split technique, the liver is split into segments I-IV and V-VIII. Each of these portions is then transplanted into an adult recipient (Fig. 9). SLT is considered technically challenging with higher perioperative complications.[38] In general, SLT has been reserved for

the best donors (young and without comorbidities) and low-risk recipients (low-MELD score and low urgency).

Multiple studies have reviewed the outcomes of SLT in adult and pediatric recipients. A recent single-center study from Australia analyzed 1090 deceased adult liver donors including 155 SLTs.[39] Graft survival rates at 1, 3, and 5 years

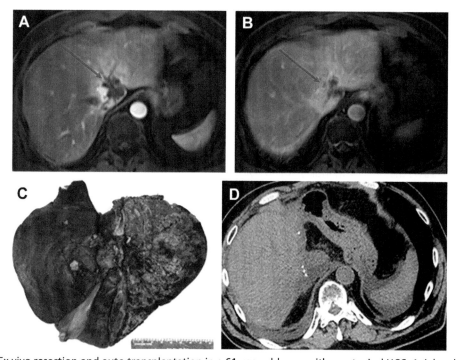

Fig. 10. Ex vivo resection and auto transplantation in a 61-year-old man with an atypical HCC. Axial early (A) and late phase (B) postcontrast MR images demonstrate a heterogeneous mass with progressive centripetal enhancement (arrows) centered on the confluence of the 3 hepatic veins invading IVC. The liver was completely mobilized outside the patient's body (C) and the patient was placed on portal bypass. Complex surgical dissection including back table dissection was performed with the removal of segments 1 to 4, 8 and portion of 7, resection of intrahepatic IVC and contiguous right hepatic vein with reconstruction using femoral vein and Dacron graft, and the liver was then auto transplanted (D). Final pathology revealed hepatocellular carcinoma.

were comparable between split and whole liver grafts. These were 82%, 79%, and 74% versus 86%, 81%, and 77%, respectively. The long-term patient survival was also comparable at 1, 3, and 5 years. However, the biliary complications and hepatic artery thrombosis were higher in the SLT group. A study from the European Liver Transplant Registry analyzed the left split graft outcomes in 1500 pediatric patients.[40] The graft and patient survival at 3 months and 5 years were 83.3% and 73.9% and 89.1% and 82.9%, respectively. At multivariate analysis, greater donor age (>50 years), increased cold ischemia time (>6 hours), urgent SLT, and lesser recipient body weight (<8 kg) were considered adverse factors.

Ex Vivo Liver Resection and Auto Transplantation

This technique is used in patients with conventionally unresectable liver tumors and involves complete hepatectomy and extracorporeal liver/tumor resection followed by autologous transplantation of the remaining liver parenchyma. It is generally chosen as last resort therapy to achieve Radical (R0) resection and reserved for a small group of patients with preserved hepatic function and sufficient predicted liver volumes. Ex vivo liver resection and auto transplantation (ERAT) has been used for various primary, metastatic liver malignancies and infectious conditions such as hepatic alveolar echinococcosis (**Fig. 10**). A systematic review and meta-analysis reviewed 53 studies with 244 patients.[41] The overall R0 resection rate was 93.4%, major complication rate was 24.5%, a 30-day mortality was 9.5% with a 1-year survival of 78.4%. The subset of patients with hepatic echinococcosis seemed to do better with ERAT, the 30-day mortality was 6.5% while the 1-year survival was 89.5%. Similar to liver, renal auto transplantation has also been described for patients with loin pain hematuria syndrome, ureteral stricture, and vascular anomalies.[42]

Summary

This article highlights the unconventional transplantation strategies most often described along with available evidence to argue for or against such techniques. These strategies, although not as common as conventional living or deceased organ donors, still offer a substantial addition to the pool of available organs. Such strategies should be explored, when possible, to overcome the persistent organ shortage. Indeed, these strategies are gaining traction in recent years with improvements in technology and awareness.

CLINICS CARE POINTS

- Donor organ constraints limit the success of solid organ transplantation across the world.
- Innovative techniques are essential to expand the organ pool and benefit more patients with end-stage organ damage.
- Domino transplant, POD, ABO incompatible transplantation, split liver transplant and ERAT are a few uncommon but innovative techniques to expand donor pool.
- Awareness of such techniques, application of appropriate advanced matching algorithms and effective immunosuppression will further increase the available organ pool and benefit patients in need of transplantation.

DISCLOSURE

None of the authors has relevant commercial or financial conflicts of interest to disclose.

REFERENCES

1. Kitchens WH. Domino liver transplantation: indications, techniques, and outcomes. Transplant Rev 2011 Oct;25(4):167–77.
2. Available at: https://www.unos.org. Accessed December 7, 2022.
3. Kher V, Jha PK. Paired Kidney exchange transplantation- pushing the boundaries. Transpl Int 2020;33:975–84.
4. Moini M, Mistry P, Schilsky ML. Liver transplantation for inherited metabolic disorders of the liver. Curr Opin Organ Transplant 2010;15:269–76.
5. Azoulay D, Samuel D, Castaing D, et al. Domino liver transplants for metabolic disorders: experience with familial amyloidotic polyneuropathy. JAMA 1999;189:584–93.
6. Available at: https://www.fapwtr.org. Accessed December 7, 2022.
7. Furtado A, Tomé L, Oliveira FJ, et al. Sequential liver transplantation. Transplant Proc 1997;29:467–8.
8. Georgiades CS, Neyman EG, Barish MA, et al. Amyloidosis: review and CT manifestations. Radiographics 2004;24(2):405–16.
9. Celik N, Kelly B, Soltys K, et al. Technique and outcome of domino liver transplantation from patients with maple syrup urine disease: Expanding the donor pool for live donor liver transplantation. Clin Transplant 2019;33(11):e13721.
10. Saner FH, Treckmann J, Pratschke J, et al. Early renal failure after domino liver transplantation using

organs from donors with primary hyperoxaluria type 1. Transplantation 2010 15;90(7):782–5.

11. Day DL, Scheinman JI, Mahan J. Radiological aspects of primary hyperoxaluria. AJR Am J Roentgenol 1986;146(2):395–401.

12. Popescu I, Habib N, Dima S, et al. Domino liver transplantation using a graft from a donor with familial hypercholesterolemia: seven-yr follow-up. Clin Transplant 2009;23(4):565–70.

13. Hemming AW, Cattral MS, Greig PD, et al. Domino liver transplantation for familial amyloid polyneuropathy: optimal use of a scarce resource. Transplant Proc 1999;31:515.

14. Geyer E, Burrier C, Tumin D, et al. Outcomes of domino liver transplantation compared to deceased donor liver transplantation: a propensity-matching approach. Transpl Int 2018;31:1200–6.

15. Escobar B, Taura P, Barreneche N, et al. The influence of the explant technique on the hemodynamic profile during sequential domino liver transplantation in familial amyloid polyneuropathy patients. LiverTranspl 2009;15:869–75.

16. Nishida S, Pinna A, Verzaro R. Domino liver transplantationwith end-to-side infrahepatic venacavocavostomy. J Am Coll Surg 2001;192:237–40.

17. Pacheco-Moreira LF, de Oliveira ME, Balbi E, et al. A new technical option for domino liver transplantation. Liver Transpl 2003;9:632–3.

18. Suarez-Munoz MA, Fernandez-Aguilar JL, Santoyo J, et al. An alternative method of reconstruction of hepatic venous outflow in domino liver transplantation. Transplant Proc 2010;41:994–5.

19. Soin A, Kumaran V, Mohanka R, et al. Bridge venoplasty: a new technique to simplify venous outflow reconstruction in living donor domino liver transplantation. Surgery 2010;148:155–7.

20. Mergental H, Gouw ASH, Slooff MJH, et al. Venous outflow reconstruction with surgically reopened obliterated umbilical vein in domino liver transplantation. Liver Transpl 2007;13:769–72.

21. Ahmed O, Vachharajani N, Chang SH, et al. Domino liver transplants: where do we stand after a quarter-century? A US national analysis. HPB 2022;24:1026–34.

22. Llado L, Baliellas C, Casasnovas C, et al. Risk of transmission of systemic transthyretin amyloidosis after domino liver transplantation. Liver Transpl 2010;16:1386.

23. Vollmar J, Schmid JC, Hoppe-Lotichius M, et al. Progression of transthyretin (TTR) amyloidosis in donors and recipients after domino liver transplantation—a prospective single-center cohort study. Transplant Int 2018;31:1207–15.

24. Bolte FJ, Schmidt HH, Becker T, et al. Evaluation of domino liver transplantations in Germany. Transpl Int 2013;26(7):715–23.

25. Marques HP, Ribeiro V, Almeida T, et al. Long-term Results of Domino Liver Transplantation for Hepatocellular Carcinoma Using the "Double Piggy-back" Technique: A 13-Year Experience. Ann Surg 2015;262(5):749–56.

26. Misumi Y, Narita Y, Oshima T, et al. Recipient aging accelerates acquired transthyretin amyloidosis after domino liver transplantation. Liver Transpl 2016;22(5):656–64.

27. Yamamoto S, Wilczek HE, Iwata T, et al. Long-term consequences of domino liver transplantation using familial amyloidotic polyneuropathy grafts. Transpl Int 2007;20(11):926–33.

28. Herden U, Grabhorn E, Santer R, et al. Surgical Aspects of Liver Transplantation and Domino Liver Transplantation in Maple Syrup Urine Disease: Analysis of 15 Donor-Recipient Pairs. Liver Transpl 2019;25(6):889–900.

29. Leeser DB, Thomas AG, Shaffer AA, et al. Patient and Kidney Allograft Survival with National Kidney Paired Donation. Clin J Am Soc Nephrol 2020;15(2):228–37.

30. Gunabushanam V, Ganesh S, Soltys K, et al. Increasing Living Donor Liver Transplantation Using Liver Paired Exchange. J Am Coll Surg 2022;234(2):115–20.

31. Segev DL, Veale JL, Berger JC, et al. Transporting live donor kidneys for kidney paired donation: initial national results. Am J Transplant 2011;11(2):356–60.

32. Bingaman AW, Wright FH Jr, Kapturczak M, et al. Single-Center Kidney paired donation: the Methodist San Antonio experience. Am J Transplant 2012;12(8):2125–32.

33. Hume DM, Merrill JP, Miller BF, et al. Experiences with renal homotransplantation in the human: report of nine cases. J Clin Invest 1955;34(2):327–82.

34. Tydén G, Kumlien G, Genberg H, et al. ABO incompatible kidney transplantations without splenectomy, using antigen-specific immunoadsorption and rituximab. Am J Transplant 2005;5(1):145–8.

35. Montgomery JR, Berger JC, Warren DS, et al. Outcomes of ABO-incompatible kidney transplantation in the United States. Transplantation 2012;93(6):603–9.

36. Scurt FG, Ewert L, Mertens P, et al. Clinical outcomes after ABO-incompatible renal transplantation: a systematic review and meta-analysis. Lancet 2019;393(10185):2059–72.

37. Gan K, Li Z, Bao S, et al. Clinical outcomes after ABO-incompatible liver transplantation: A systematic review and meta-analysis. Transpl Immunol 2021;69:101476.

38. Hackl C, Schmidt KM, Susal C, et al. Split liver transplantation: current developments. World J Gastroenterol 2018;24(47):5312–21.

39. Lau NS, Ly M, Liu K, et al. Is it safe to expand the indications for split liver transplantation in adults?

A single-center analysis of 155 in-situ splits. Clin Transplant 2022;36(7):e14673.

40. Angelico R, Nardi A, Adam R, et al. European Liver and Intestine Transplant Association (ELITA). Outcomes of left split graft transplantation in Europe: report from the European Liver Transplant Registry. Transpl Int 2018;31(7):739–50.

41. Zawistowski M, Nowaczyk J, Jakubczyk M, et al. Outcomes of ex vivo liver resection and auto transplantation: A systematic review and meta-analysis. Surgery 2020;168:631e642.

42. Cowan NG, Banerji JS, Johnston RB, et al. Renal autotransplantation: 27-year experience at 2 institutions. J Urology 2015;194(5):1357–61.

Immunosuppressive Therapy in Solid Organ Transplantation
Primer for Radiologists and Potential Complications

Varaha Sai Tammisetti, MD[a], Srinivasa R. Prasad, MD[b], Navya Dasyam, MD[c], Christine O. Menias, MD[d], Venkata Katabathina, MD[e],*

KEYWORDS

• Immunosuppression • Solid organ transplantation • Complications • Infections • Malignancies

KEY POINTS

• Transplant immunosuppression is divided into three phases: induction, maintenance, and anti-rejection. Drugs used in the first few days/weeks after transplantation are referred to as 'induction' agents, drugs that are useful in later life are called 'maintenance' agents, and drugs that aggressively treat rejection episodes are called 'anti-rejection' agents.

• Infections are the main cause of mortality, morbidity, and graft dysfunction during the first year after solid organ transplantation and both conventional and opportunistic infections may develop. "Net state of immunosuppression" resulting from the complex interaction of various factors, with significant determinants being dose, duration, intensity, type, and sequence of immunosuppressive regimens. This results in three overlapping periods of infectious risk after transplant based on the level of immunosuppression: (1) Early perioperative period (Phase 1–1 month) during which immunosuppression is not yet fully effective; (2) Intermediate period (Phase 2)–one to 6 months post-transplant when immunosuppression is at its peak; (3) The late period (Phase 3) is beyond 6 months post-transplant, by which immunosuppression is tapered.

• Solid organ transplant recipients have a two-to-three-fold increased risk of malignancies compared to the general population, which increases with time secondary to direct oncogenic effects of life-long immunosuppressive therapy, impaired immunosurveillance of tumor cells, and increased incidence of pro-oncogenic viral-driven malignancies. This also impacts allograft function and survival, causing morbidity and mortality.

INTRODUCTION

Solid organ transplantation is the treatment of choice for patients with end-stage organ failure that improves survival and quality of life. The kidney is the most commonly transplanted organ, followed by the liver, heart, and lung.[1,2] Sophisticated immunosuppressive (IS) regimens with potent drugs prevent allograft rejection, thus improving graft survival rates (up to 90% at 1 year and 75% at 5 years).[3,4] Complications due to chronic immunosuppression cause significant

[a] Department of Radiology, University of Texas Health, Houston, TX, USA; [b] Department of Radiology, University of Texas M. D. Anderson Cancer Center; [c] Department of Radiology, University of Pittsburgh Medical Center; [d] Department of Radiology, Mayo Clinic at Scottsdale; [e] Department of Radiology, University of Texas Health, San Antonio, TX, USA
* Corresponding author. 7703 Floyd Curl Drive, Mail code 7800, San Antonio, TX 78229.
E-mail address: katabathina@uthscsa.edu

Radiol Clin N Am 61 (2023) 913–932
https://doi.org/10.1016/j.rcl.2023.04.010
0033-8389/23/© 2023 Elsevier Inc. All rights reserved.

morbidity and mortality.[1] Therefore, IS drugs are used in combination regimens at relatively lower doses to prevent or reduce these complications.[5] These complications can be of two types: (1) drug-related adverse effects. (2) Sequela of immunosuppression: infections and malignancies.[3] Although clinical features and laboratory findings suffice in diagnosing drug-related side effects, cross-sectional imaging techniques, including ultrasound (US), computed tomography (CT), R imaging, and 18-flouro-deoxy glucose-PET (FDG-PET) play an essential role in the initial diagnosis, treatment follow-up, and long-term surveillance of infections and malignancies in solid organ transplant recipients (SOTRs).[1]

First, we will review the immunobiology of transplant rejection and the mechanism of action of commonly used IS drugs in solid organ transplantation. Then, we will discuss the pathogenesis and cross-sectional imaging findings of common infections and malignancies developing in the SOTRs and the role of imaging in screening, diagnosis, and surveillance.

IMMUNOBIOLOGY AND IMMUNOSUPPRESSIVE DRUGS IN SOLID ORGAN TRANSPLANTATION

The human immune response constitutes innate immunity (native response to microbes) and adaptive immunity (an acquired cellular or humoral antigenic response).[6] There are four phases of alloimmune response, (1) Recognition, (2) Activation with clonal expansion, (3) Recruitment of other effector mechanisms, and (4) Resolution.[5,6] T lymphocytes play a central role in the alloimmune response and transplant rejection; antigen-presenting cells (APCs) such as B lymphocytes, macrophages, and dendritic cells support this process.[7] T-cell activation and proliferation can be explained by a three-signal model that can help understand the specific targets of IS medications.[6,8] Signal 1—Alloantigen recognition: APCs bind to T-cell receptors and trigger T-cell recognition of foreign antigens, which activates three important signal transduction pathways in the T cells: the calcium-calcineurin, the nuclear factor-kB, and the RAS-mitogen-activated protein kinase.[3,6,7] Signal 2—Lymphocyte activation and co-stimulation: Co-stimulator molecules and ligands bind to each other resulting in increased production of interleukin (IL)-2, an effective stimulator of T-cell proliferation.[5,8] Signal 3—Clonal expansion: Binding of IL-2 to CD 25 (IL-2 receptor) on the surface of activated T cells leads to proliferation and differentiation of effector T cells resulting in rejection (Fig. 1).[7,8] In addition, activated B cells also start

producing alloantibodies against donor antigens.[7,9] Given the significant role of T cells in the rejection process, most of the IS drugs target the level of T-cell activation or proliferation or production; however, drugs targeting B lymphocytes with effect on alloantibodies production and components of the innate immune system (complement and macrophages) are also being investigated (see Fig. 1).[10] Current multidrug regimens that work at different signals of the immune system allow dose reduction of each drug with reduced drug toxicity but with increased efficacy.[1,3,8,10]

Transplant immunosuppression may be divided into three phases: induction, maintenance, and anti-rejection. Drugs used in the first few days/weeks after transplantation are referred to as 'induction' agents, drugs that are useful in later life are called 'maintenance' agents, and drugs that aggressively treat rejection episodes are called 'anti-rejection' agents.[10,11] The most used IS medications, as well as their mechanisms of action, are discussed below.

ANTIBODIES

Antibodies are commonly used as induction agents in most kidney and pancreas transplant recipients and less frequently in liver transplant recipients. They are also helpful in severe or steroid-resistant rejections. Polyclonal anti-thymocyte globulin (ATG), monoclonal antibodies, including alemtuzumab (anti-CD52 receptors) and muromonab (OKT3; anti-CD3 receptors), are depleting types of antibodies that act by reducing the number of circulating T cells and B cells (see Fig. 1).[9] Non-depleting antibodies, including basiliximab and daclizumab, block lymphocyte function by binding to IL-2 receptors on T cells and blocking the proliferative response of T cells to circulating IL-2.[3,7]

CORTICOSTEROIDS

Corticosteroids have been the mainstay of immunosuppression since the beginning of transplantation.[10] They exert immunomodulatory effects by down-regulating cytokine gene expression in lymphocytes, thus decreasing serum IL-2 levels and inhibiting macrophage differentiation and neutrophil functions (see Fig. 1).[3,12] Given the multiple effects at different sites of the immune system, corticosteroids are very effective in preventing and treating acute allograft rejection. Indeed, most acute rejection episodes are treated with pulse steroids.[10] Osteoporosis and avascular bone necrosis associated with chronic corticosteroid use can be detected on imaging studies.[13,14]

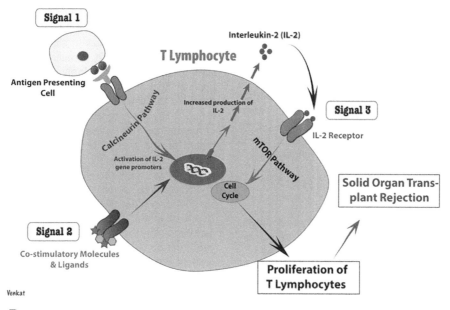

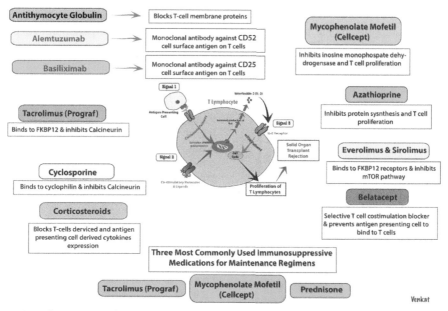

Fig. 1. Illustrations demonstrate the basic immunology of solid organ transplant rejection (*A*) and mechanisms of action of the commonly used immunosuppressive medications in solid organ transplant recipients (*B*). T lymphocyte activation and proliferation play a central role in alloimmune response and transplant rejection, which can be explained by a three-signal model. Antibodies such as ATG, alemtuzumab, and basiliximab are commonly used for induction. Prednisone, tacrolimus, and Mycophenolate mofetil are the three most commonly used immunosuppressive medications for maintenance therapy. (Courtesy of V Katabathina, MD, San Antonio, TX.)

CALCINEURIN INHIBITORS

Calcineurin inhibitors are the cornerstone of immunosuppression, especially long-term maintenance therapy in virtually all transplant programs.[8] Cyclosporine and tacrolimus (Prograf) are the two most commonly used agents in clinical practice.[1] The mechanism of action is by inhibiting calcineurin, thereby preventing the transcription of IL-2 and other nuclear growth factors impeding the T-cell activation cascade (see **Fig. 1**).[5] Tacrolimus is more potent than cyclosporine, with fewer side effects, and is frequently used in many transplant regimens.[7]

ANTIMETABOLITES (ANTIPROLIFERATIVE AGENTS)

Azathioprine and Mycophenolate mofetil (MMF) are two available antimetabolites used in maintenance therapy; MMF (Cellcept) is also used in anti-rejection therapy. Their mechanism of action is to inhibit purine base synthesis (deoxyribonucleic acid [DNA] and ribonucleic acid [RNA]) required for T-cell and B-cell proliferation.[8]

MAMMALIAN TARGET OF RAPAMYCIN (mTOR) INHIBITORS

In maintenance therapy regimens, sirolimus and everolimus are commonly used mTOR inhibitors.[8] Inhibition of the synthesis of mTOR protein that mediates the cytokine signal from the IL-2 receptor blocks the proliferation and differentiation of T cells and B cells.[5]

Other Novel Immunosuppressive Agents

Several novel immunosuppressive agents targeting T-cell and B-cell receptors are under various stages of validation; their goal is to improve potency and decrease adverse effects. Belatacept is a fusion protein that selectively blocks co-stimulation molecules of T-cell activation and can be used as an alternative to calcineurin inhibitors in induction and maintenance therapies.[6] Belimumab, Bortezomib, Janus Kinase inhibitors, Tofacitinib, Ruxolitinib, Eculizumab, Lulizumab, CFZ533, Tocilizumab, Voclosporin, anti-CD20 monoclonal antibodies such as Rituximab, and Sotrastaurin are newer agents in various stages of validation.[6]

COMPLICATIONS OF IMMUNOSUPPRESSIVE THERAPY IN SOLID ORGAN TRANSPLANT RECIPIENTS
Infections in Solid Organ Transplant Recipients

Infections are the main cause of mortality, morbidity, and graft dysfunction during the first year after SOT.[15] Approximately 30% to 60% of SOTRs develop an infection at some point of time post-transplant.[15] Owing to immunosuppression, physical signs of the immune response, such as fever, localizing signs, and elevated leukocyte counts, are usually lacking.[16] Therefore, diagnosis increasingly relies on imaging and invasive procedures that help obtain samples for histopathology, cell counts, and cultures.[16] SOTRs are at increased risk for both conventional and opportunistic infections,[15] based on the "net state of immunosuppression" (NSI). The NSI depends on a complex interaction of multiple factors, including pre-transplant characteristics (prior immune and non-immune conditions), type of transplanted organ, intraoperative events, and post-transplant factors, including IS therapy and immune-modulating viral infections.[15,16] Of these, the major determinant of the NSI is dose, duration, intensity, and sequence of IS agents. With the standardization of the IS regimens and changing risk factors over time, most post-transplant infections occur in a predictable pattern based on the timeline since the transplant.[1,16]

There are three overlapping periods of risk of infection post-transplant: (1) Early period–first month, which is the perioperative period, and immunosuppression is not yet fully effective; (2) Intermediate period–one to 6 months post-transplant when immunosuppression is at its peak and patients are also on antibiotic prophylaxis; (3) Late period—beyond 6 months post-transplant, by which time immunosuppression is tapered in patients with satisfactorily functioning grafts.[16] This timeline helps in the differential diagnosis of infections and helps design antimicrobial prophylaxis strategies (**Box 1**).[16]

Early period
During the first month post-transplant, common infections are from surgical complications, donor-derived infections, pre-existing infections, and hospital-acquired infections, including aspiration pneumonia, *Clostridium difficile* colitis, line infections, and wound infections.[15,16] Surgical complications that increase the risk of infection include bleeding, strictures, leaks, and graft injury. Infections specific to transplanted organs include urinary tract infection (renal recipients), biliary infections and bacteremia of *Enterobacteriaceae* (liver recipients, more so with choledochojejunostomy compared to bile duct–bile duct anastomosis), mediastinitis (heart recipients who had pre-transplant ventricular assist devices), and severe pneumonia (lung recipients due to impaired cough reflex).[15]

Box 1
Timeline of infections and infectious complications developing in solid organ transplant recipients

Timeline of infections and infectious risk following solid organ transplantation (SOT)

Early period (Phase 1–First month after SOT)

- Surgical complications

Bleeding, strictures, leaks, graft injury

- Hospital-acquired infections

Aspiration pneumonia, *C. difficile* colitis, line infections and wound infections

- Donor-derived infections

HSV, Rabies, West Nile virus, HIV, Parasites, non-albicans Candida species,

- Recipient pre-existing infections

MRSA, Pseudomonas, Acinetobacter, Aspergillus

- Infections specific to the transplanted organ

Renal Tx-urinary tract infection; liver Tx-biliary infections and bacteremia of *Enterobacteriaceae* ; heart Tx-mediastinitis; lung Tx-severe pneumonias

Intermediate period (Phase 2–1 to 6 months)

  Without prophylaxis:

    Immunomodulatory viral infections that predispose to other infections (CMV, EBV)

    Opportunistic infections (Aspergillus, *P jirovecii*, Toxoplasma, Legionella, Listeria, Nocardia, endemic fungal infections: *Histoplasma, Coccidioides, Cryptococcus)*

    Reactivation of latent infections (Cytomegalovirus, HSV, VZV, Hepatitis-B and C, Mycobacteria)

  With prophylaxis:

    Lingering early period infections (*C. difficile* colitis, surgical leaks)

    Polyomavirus BK infection, Nephropathy, HCV infection, Adenovirus, Influenza, *Cryptococcus neoformans* , Mycobacteria

Late period (Phase 3—beyond 6 months)

  Recipients with satisfactory allograft function:

- Community acquired infections
- Infections from underlying conditions such as diabetes mellitus
- Malignancies from chronic viral infections

  "High-risk" recipients with poor allograft function on immunosuppressive therapy:

- Hospitalizations from recurrent infections, infections with drug-resistant organisms
- Severe infections from common and uncommon opportunistic pathogens

---

Intermediate period

SOTRs are in a state of maximal immunosuppression and diminished cell-mediated immunity due to T-cell dysfunction from IS therapy that predisposes them to infections from intracellular pathogens and human herpes viruses (HHV).[1,16] Infections during this time are predominantly immunomodulatory viral infections (cytomegalovirus [CMV], Epstein-Barr virus [EBV]), opportunistic infections (*Aspergillus, Pneumocystis, Toxoplasma, Legionella, Listeria, Nocardia*, endemic fungal infections : *Histoplasma, Coccidioides, Cryptococcus)* or reactivation of latent infections (CMV, Herpes Simplex virus [HSV], Varicella-Zoster Virus (VZV), hepatitis-B and C, Mycobacteria).[1,15]

Late period

SOTRs with satisfactory allograft function that tolerate lowered levels of immunosuppression have lowered the risk of infections.[16] This group of healthy recipients can develop community acquired infections like the general population or infections from their underlying conditions.[16] Chronic or progressive viral infections without antiviral therapies can also cause direct organ damage or contribute to malignant transformation.[5,16] Recipients with poor allograft function require high levels of immunosuppression and are at "high risk" for infections from common and unusual opportunistic pathogens.[16] **Box 2** summarizes the common viral, fungal, bacterial, mycobacterial, and parasitic infections that arise from persistent immunosuppression in SOTRs.

Viral Infections

Cytomegalovirus

The incidence of CMV infection ranges from 25% to 50% of patients after SOT.[17,18] High-risk factors include CMV donor/recipient-seropositivity, lung

---

> **Box 2**
> **Common malignancies in solid organ transplant recipients**
>
> Malignancies in Solid Organ Transplant Recipients
>
>   De novo Malignancies
>
>   NMSCs
>
>   PTLD
>
>   Anogenital cancers
>
>   KS
>
>   Head and neck cancers
>
>   Lung cancer
>
> Donor-related (pre-existing or de novo within donor tissue)
>
>   DTCs
>
>   RCC
>
>   Pancreatic adenocarcinoma
>
>   Malignant melanoma
>
>   Choriocarcinoma
>
>   DDCs
>
>   Kaposi's sarcoma (from donor-derived HHV-8 infected cells)
>
>   Hepatocellular carcinoma (from donor-derived Hepatitis-B infection)
>
>   Donor-origin adenocarcinoma or small-cell carcinoma, or leukemia
>
> Recurrence after transplantation (pre-existing malignancy in the recipient)
>
>   Hepatocellular carcinoma
>
>   Cholangiocarcinoma
>
>   Neuroendocrine liver metastases
>
>   Malignant melanoma

---

and intestinal transplants, use of T-cell depleting IS agents, allograft rejection, and defects in innate immune responses.[17,18]

Manifestations of CMV disease are from direct tissue-invasive disease or indirect immunomodulatory effect causing secondary bacterial and invasive fungal infections, recurrent hepatitis C, and organ-specific injuries causing allograft rejection and failure.[18] Direct tissue-invasive CMV disease is associated with specific organ involvement, such as enteritis, pneumonitis, hepatitis, nephritis, myocarditis, and retinitis, with gastrointestinal (GI) involvement being the most common.[18] Imaging manifestations of CMV infection of the GI tract include mucosal ulcers, plaques, and diffuse irregular bowel wall thickening with fat stranding; bowel wall pneumatosis and pneumoperitoneum may be seen in severe cases (**Fig. 2**).[19,20] The esophagus and colon are common target sites of involvement. CMV pneumonitis, the second most common site of direct tissue-invasive disease, manifests on CT imaging as bilateral, multifocal areas of ground-glass opacities, poorly defined centrilobular nodules, and consolidations (see **Fig. 2**).[21] Transplant-specific CMV disease by direct allograft involvement manifests as hepatitis/hepatic artery thrombosis, nephritis/allograft nephropathy, pneumonitis/bronchiolitis obliterans, myocarditis/coronary vasculopathy, and pancreatitis in the liver, kidney, lung, heart, and pancreas transplants, respectively.[18] Ganciclovir is commonly used for treating and prophylaxis CMV infections; novel prophylaxis, preemptive therapy, and treatment options for ganciclovir-resistant CMV infections are currently being used.[17]

Other Herpes virus infections

Other Herpes serotypes, such as HSV, VZV, EBV, and human herpesvirus (HHV) 6, 7, and 8, might emerge in SOTRs as a result of the reactivation of a dormant infection.[22] Although oral or genital mucocutaneous ulcers are the usual clinical manifestations of HSV, severe disease can cause pneumonitis, esophagitis, hepatitis, encephalitis, and disseminated visceral disease.[23,24] Infections with VZV and HHV-6 can result in encephalitis, pneumonitis, and a hemorrhagic rash. VZV, in addition, can cause cerebellitis, cerebritis, vasculopathy, and meningitis.[24]

Fungal Infections

Invasive fungal infections can be seen in up to 40% of SOTRs; risk factors include large doses of immunosuppression (especially steroids), hyperglycemia, immunomodulatory viral infections, multiple rejection episodes, poor allograft function, and old age.[25–27] Candida and Aspergillus are the most

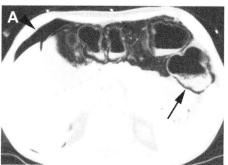
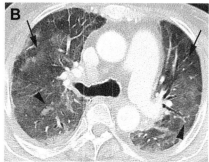

Fig. 2. Imaging findings of CMV in two different solid organ transplant recipients. (A) CMV colitis with perforation in a 32-year-old man, a kidney transplant recipient presenting with diarrhea and severe abdominal pain. Axial CT image of the abdomen shows pneumatosis (*arrow*) of the transverse colon and pneumoperitoneum (*arrowhead*). The diagnosis of CMV colitis was proved on pathology. (B) CMV pneumonitis in a 65-year-old woman, post bilateral lung transplant. Axial CT image of the chest shows multifocal, bilateral patchy pulmonary ground-glass opacities (*arrows*) and multiple centrilobular nodules (*arrowheads*).

common fungal infections; infections with *Pneumocystis*, *Cryptococcus*, Mucormycosis, *Actinomyces*, and endemic fungi (*Histoplasma*, *Coccidioides*, and *Blastomyces*) are also seen. Amphotericin B and voriconazole are commonly used antifungal agents in treatment and prophylaxis.[26]

Candidiasis

Invasive candidiasis is the most common fungal infection accounting for 80% of fungal infections, with *Candida albicans* accounting for half of those. Liver transplant recipients with choledochojejunostomy are at the greatest risk, followed by pancreas and lung transplant recipients due to colonization.[26] Oral thrush is the most common clinical presentation. Candida esophagitis can be seen as multiple, longitudinal, plaque-like filling defect that carpet the entire esophagus along the longitudinal folds and small round ulcers on double contrast barium esophagogram.[20] Disseminated candidiasis presents with both thoracic and abdominal involvement. Pulmonary candidiasis can present as patchy consolidations, diffuse reticulonodular opacities, and pleural effusions on imaging (**Fig. 3**).[26,27] Abdominal manifestations include multiple abscesses, diffuse peritonitis, hepatosplenic microabscesses, cystitis, and renal lesions.[28]

Aspergillosis

Invasive aspergillosis (IA) accounts for 15% to 20% of fungal infections in SOTRs, and is associated with high rates of graft loss and mortality ranging from 80% to 90% in liver transplants and 15% to 25% in non-liver transplants.[25,26,29] *Aspergillus fumigatus* is the most common organism. Pulmonary disease, tracheobronchitis, sinusitis, and central nervous system (CNS) abscesses are

common manifestations of IA.[30,31] Although pulmonary parenchymal and airway disease is frequently seen in lung transplants, CNS involvement may be seen in up to 50% of patients with disseminated IA.[23]

Imaging findings of pulmonary aspergillosis include multiple nodules with or without a peripheral ground-glass halo (bleeding due to angioinvasiveness), ill-defined consolidations, and multiple masses (**Fig. 4**).[25,30] Irregular wall thickening and enhancement involving the trachea and main bronchi resulting in luminal narrowing suggest tracheobronchitis and commonly occurs near the anastomotic site in lung transplants (see **Fig. 4**).[25,30] CNS disease can appear as multiple, non-enhancing hemorrhagic foci involving the cerebral parenchyma or as enhancing soft tissue thickening at the orbital apex, extending into the

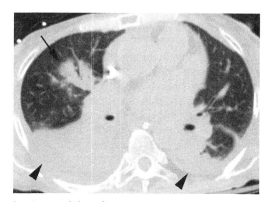

Fig. 3. *Candida* infection in a 65-year-old woman, liver transplant recipient. Axial CT image of the chest depicts patchy consolidation in the right lung parenchyma (*arrow*) and bilateral pleural effusions (*arrowheads*). *Candida albicans* was isolated from bronchial washings.

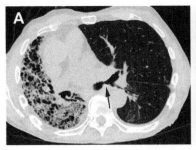
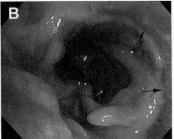
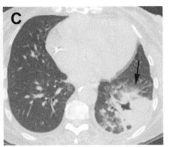

Fig. 4. Imaging findings of aspergillosis in two different solid organ transplant recipients. (*A* and *B*) Aspergillus bronchitis along the wall of the left lung bronchial anastomosis causing bronchial stenosis in a 72-year-old man, 2 years following left single lung transplantation. (*A*) Axial noncontrast CT image of the chest shows stenosis and focal wall thickening along the posterior wall of the left major bronchus at the anastomosis (*arrow*). (*B*) An optical bronchoscopy image of the left major bronchus at the anastomosis shows yellowish-appearing pseudomembranes (*blue arrows*). (*C*) IA of the left lung parenchyma in a 72-year-old man, 2 years following orthotopic heart transplantation. Axial CT image of the chest shows left lower lobe consolidation with cavitation and surrounding ground-glass haziness (*arrow*).

cranial cavity, resulting in cavernous sinus thrombosis.[1,31]

Pneumocystis jirovecii

Up to 15% of SOTRs develop *Pneumocystis jirovecii* pneumonia (PJP), most commonly during the first 6 months, and it has a rapid progression and high fatality rate without trimethoprim-sulfamethoxazole (TMP-SMX) prophylaxis.[23] Patients with PJP typically present with fever, dyspnea, nonproductive cough, and hypoxemia out of proportion to the radiographic and physical findings. PJP manifests as interstitial infiltrates on radiographs.[24,32] On chest high-resolution computed tomography (HRCT), widespread ground-glass opacities with upper lobe predominance are typical features; other findings include patchy consolidations, nodules, cysts, and spontaneous pneumothorax (**Fig. 5**).[33]

Cryptococcus neoformans

Cryptococcus neoformans infection has been reported in up to 5% of SOTRs; inhalation of the organisms is the primary mode of transmission with the development of pulmonary disease.[25–27,32] Hematogenous dissemination, most frequently to the CNS, bones, and skin, may occur, mainly secondary to intense immunosuppression. Common chest CT abnormalities include multiple, ill-defined, small nodules, large masses, diffuse interstitial infiltrates, and cavitary nodules (**Fig. 6**).[1] Common CNS manifestations include hydrocephalus, dilated Virchow-Robin spaces, widespread meningeal enhancement, cyst-like structures, and choroid plexus granulomas.[1]

Mucormycosis

Mucormycosis accounts for 2% of invasive fungal infections in SOTRs; *Rhizopus* species and *Mucor*

species are the most frequently isolated organisms.[26,34] Infection usually arises due to inhalation, ingestion, or direct traumatic inoculation of fungal spores.[24,26] Risk factors include diabetic ketoacidosis, use of steroids, and bicarbonate leakage in pancreas transplants. Rhinocerebral, pulmonary, renal, gastrointestinal, and disseminated diseases are common. Paranasal sinuses and orbital disease, followed by rapid and progressive involvement of the cavernous sinus, vascular structures, and intracranial contents, are characteristic MR imaging findings of rhinocerebral mucormycosis.[35] Single or multiple lung masses surrounded by ground-glass opacities are commonly seen on chest CT. Necrotic areas involving multiple intra-abdominal organs, including the kidneys and GI tract, can be seen on imaging; irregular bowel wall thickening with associated pneumatosis and pneumoperitoneum can be seen (**Fig. 7**).[36,37]

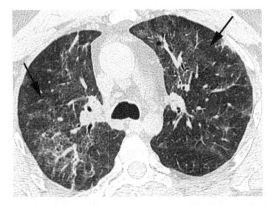

Fig. 5. *PJP* in a 42-year-old man, a renal transplant recipient. Axial CT image of the chest demonstrates widespread ground-glass opacities involving bilateral lung parenchyma (*arrows*).

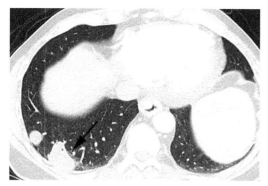

Fig. 6. *Cryptococcus neoformans* infection in a 56-year-old man, renal transplant recipient for autosomal dominant polycystic kidney disease. Axial CT image of the chest shows two well-defined nodules in the right lower lobe lung parenchyma (*arrow*).

Bacterial Infections

Most bacterial infections in SOTRs occur during the first month after transplant involving the surgical site and graft.[38] Opportunistic infections during the intermediate period after transplant are from *Nocardia species, Listeria monocytogenes, and Legionella pneumophila.*[38] Community acquired bacterial infections such as pneumococci are seen in the late period.[38] Additionally, latent mycobacterial infections can be reactivated due to suppressed immune system.

Nocardiosis

Nocardial infections are rare in SOTRs, with *Nocardia asteroides* being the most common species. Pulmonary involvement is the most common presentation, although meningitis and brain abscesses may also be seen.[24] Imaging manifestations of pulmonary involvement are nonspecific, with multiple nodules, masses, consolidation, pleural effusions, and chest wall involvement, and they need to be differentiated from other infections and tumors (**Fig. 8**).[39,40]

Mycobacterial infections

Mycobacterial infection results from the reactivation of latent infection during the intermediate period.[16] SOTRs are at an increased risk of developing tubercular and atypical mycobacterial infections. *Mycobacterium tuberculosis* (TB) is 20 to 75 times higher than in the general population and may occur in up to 15% of these patients.[24,41] TB most commonly presents with lung involvement in 50% of patients, disseminated disease in 33%, and extra-pulmonary involvement in 16%.[42] Significant morbidity is also caused by anti-TB chemotherapy-induced changes in the metabolism of immunosuppressive IS medications, resulting in increased infection and rejection.[41] On imaging, lung parenchymal infiltrates and cavitary nodules/masses with predominant upper lobe involvement are common findings. Irregular bowel wall thickening with associated lymphadenopathy is the common imaging feature of GI TB; multiple, ill-defined, hypoattenuating nodules and masses characterize hepato-splenic TB (**Fig. 9**).[43]

Other bacterial infections

Listeria monocytogens commonly involve CNS and cause meningitis and encephalitis. Pneumonia with or without abscess formation and cavitation represent common manifestations of *Legionella pneumophilia.*[24,32] Legionella pneumonitis can be seen in heart/lung and lung allograft recipients occurring any time after transplant.[38] Disseminated infections involving multiple organs may occur during the state of severe immunosuppression.

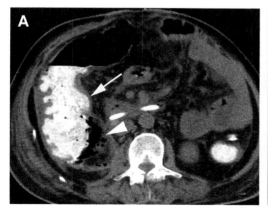
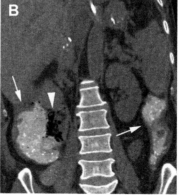

Fig. 7. Mucormycosis infection of the colon with perforation 6 weeks following OLT in a 56-year-old man. (*A* and *B*) Axial (*A*) and coronal (*B*) unenhanced CT images of the abdomen show irregular wall thickening of the ascending and descending colon (*arrows*) and focal perforation with pneumatosis and extraluminal gas along the medial wall of ascending colon (*arrowheads*).

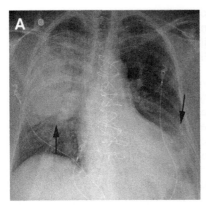
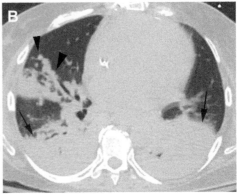

Fig. 8. Pulmonary Nocardiosis in a 57-year-old woman, 4 months following orthotopic heart transplantation. (*A*) A frontal chest radiograph shows right upper lobe and left lower lobe consolidations (*arrows*) (*B*) Axial unenhanced CT image of the chest depicts bilateral lower lobe consolidations (*arrows*) and right middle lobe confluent and discrete nodules (*arrowheads*). *Nocardia veterana* was identified on bronchioalveolar lavage.

Parasitic Infections

As *Toxoplasma gondii* cysts prefer muscle tissue, heart transplant recipients are at a high risk of infection.[44] Reactivation of latent infection in the myocardium is a common etiology of toxoplasmosis and carries a mortality rate of up to 100%.[32] Meningo-encephalitis, brain abscess, myocarditis, and pneumonia are common imaging findings.[24] *Strongyloides stercoralis* infection presents either with GI tract (small bowel obstruction and ileus) or pulmonary disease (alveolar or interstitial infiltrates).[24,44]

Malignancies in Solid Organ Transplant Recipients

Post-transplant malignancies are the third most common cause of death in SOTRs after cardiovascular disease and infections.[45] Compared to the general population, SOTRs have a two- to three-fold higher risk of developing malignancies.[45,46] This risk rises over time due to lifelong IS therapy's direct oncogenic effects, impaired immune surveillance of tumor cells, and an increased incidence of pro-oncogenic viral-driven malignancies. Mortality from post-transplant malignancies ranges from 10% to 20% and increases with longer allograft survival and time since transplant.[47] The risk of death from malignancy in SOTRs compared to the general population is higher.[48] These poor outcomes could be explained by biologically more aggressive cancers and the need to balance cancer-directed therapies and impact on allograft function from the decreased intensity of pharmacological immunosuppression.[46,48,49]

IS medications have both direct and indirect effects on developing post-transplant malignancies in SOTRs.[50] The type, intensity, and duration of

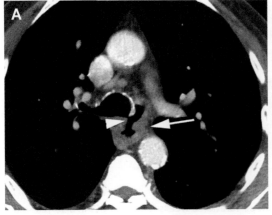
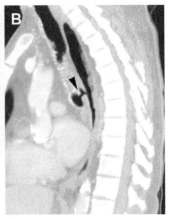

Fig. 9. Esophageal tuberculosis in a 72-year-old man, 2 years following renal transplantation. (*A* and *B*) Contrast-enhanced axial (*A*) and sagittal (*B*) images of the chest show irregular wall thickening of the mid-thoracic esophagus (*arrows*) with associated tracheoesophageal fistula (*arrowheads*).

Table 1
Clinical and imaging pearls in common malignancies developing in solid organ transplant recipients

Type of Malignancy in SOTRs	Clinical Pearls	Imaging Pearls
Post-Transplant Lymphoproliferative Disorder (PTLD)	Frequently EBV-associated. Bimodal (Early—first 2 y post-transplant and Late—5–10 y post-transplant). 50%–75% within the abdomen	Bulky retroperitoneal lymph nodes or extra-nodal masses in GI tract, liver, lung, bone marrow, and CNS Most common target site is in the GI tract Peritransplant PTLD as hepatic hilar or renal hilar mass
Non-melanoma skin cancers	Risk factors include fair skin, high sun exposure Squamous cell carcinoma is the most common type, followed by basal cell carcinoma	Diagnosis is by clinical examination Imaging with CT and FDG-PET to detect and map metastatic disease
Kaposi sarcoma	90%— mucocutaneous 20%—visceral disease	Mucocutaneous KS: Enhancing nodules Visceral KS: Nodular bowel wall thickening, hypervascular hepatic and splenic masses, hypervascular lymphadenopathy, and hypervascular mesenteric masses
Anogenital cancers	More common in women Risk factors: HPV infection, high levels of immunosuppression, smoking Treatment based on depth of invasion	Large, aggressive, and multicentric masses in anal canal or genital tract MR imaging to detect depth of invasion FDG-PET to detect metastatic disease
Lung cancer	Highest risk in lung transplant recipients and pre-transplant smokers Most common— adenocarcinoma	Locally aggressive lung mass(es) in the native lung or lung allograft
Renal cell carcinoma	Seen in renal allografts and native kidneys also with longer duration of dialysis	Incidentally detected small (<4 cm) renal masses. Most commonly either hypervascular clear cell (46%) or hypovascular papillary (42%) RCC subtypes. Annual ultrasound surveillance
Recurrent hepatocellular carcinoma	Pre-transplant predictors of recurrence: large size, vascular invasion, high AFP levels, histologic differentiation. Recurrence rate is 6%–16%; 90% recur in the first 6 mo post-transplant	Recurrent HCC within the orthotopic liver transplant or as diffuse metastatic disease Regular surveillance with CT/MR imaging for 2–3 y, serial AFP levels
Recurrent cholangiocarcinoma	Recurrence rate is 20%. Increased risk in patients with primary sclerosing cholangitis	Imaging patterns of recurrence include multifocal hepatic masses, malignant biliary stricture with biliary wall thickening at the anastomotic site and perihilar masses

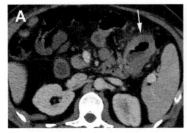
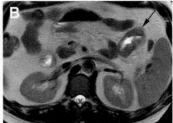
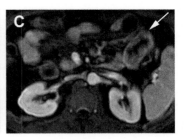

Fig. 10. Small bowel PTLD in a 45-year-old man following OLT (*A*) Axial contrast-enhanced CT image of the abdomen demonstrates irregular, circumferential wall thickening and aneurysmal dilation of a jejunal loop (*arrows*) in the left upper quadrant. (*B* and *C*) Axial T2-weighted (*B*) and axial contrast-enhanced T1-weighted (*C*) images of the abdomen show irregular, circumferential wall thickening and aneurysmal dilation of the jejunal loop (*arrows*). The diagnosis of PTLD was made on the pathology.

immunosuppression influence carcinogenesis.[51] Among biological agents, intensive immunosuppression with T-cell-depleting antibody induction using anti-thymocyte globulins and belatacept is associated with an increased risk of EBV-driven post-transplant lymphoproliferative disorder (PTLD). Corticosteroids have a direct pro-oncogenic effect on lymphoid cells and also impair immunosurveillance. Among antimetabolites, azathioprine directly affects the post-replicative DNA mismatch repair exacerbating the ultraviolet light-induced DNA damage and increasing the risk of non-melanoma skin cancers (NMSCs). Among calcineurin inhibitors, both cyclosporine and tacrolimus promote carcinogenesis by directly affecting the cells causing inhibition of DNA repair and apoptosis, increased production of transforming growth factor-beta (TGF-β) (enables invasive and metastatic potential), and vascular endothelial growth factor (angiogenesis) and decreased production of IL-2 from helper T cells.[50] This is associated with an increased risk of EBV-driven PTLD with increasing doses. mTOR inhibitors are associated with decreased cancer risk due to their antiproliferative effects.

Oncogenic virus-induced malignancies in SOTRs include PTLD with EBV, NMSCs, and anogenital cancers with HPV, Kaposi sarcoma with human herpes virus-8 (HHV-8), hepatitis-B and hepatitis C with HCC, and Merkel cell carcinoma with Merkel cell polyomavirus.[49] The combined effect of oncogenic viruses and impaired immunosurveillance with chronic immunosuppression promote carcinogenesis by various pathways, including activation of oncogenes, suppression of tumor suppressor genes, and activation of cellular proliferation. Cancer immunosurveillance is a function of the innate and adaptive immune system crucial to eliminating cancer cells and defends against metastatic processes such as vascular emboli, lymphatic invasion, and perineural invasion.[52]

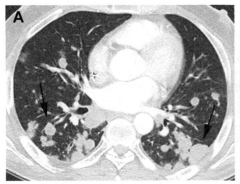
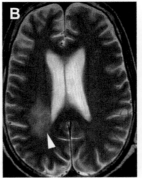
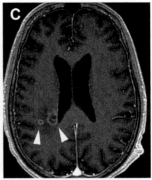

Fig. 11. Intrathoracic and intracranial PTLD in a 49-year-old man following liver transplantation. (*A*) Axial CT image of the chest demonstrates multiple nodules involving bilateral lung parenchyma (*arrows*). (*B* and *C*) Axial T2-weighted (*B*) and axial contrast-enhanced (*C*) MR images of the brain demonstrate heterogeneously T2 hyperintense, ring-enhancing lesions in the right posterior periventricular region (*arrowheads*) with associated perilesional edema. The diagnosis of PTLD was made on the pathology.

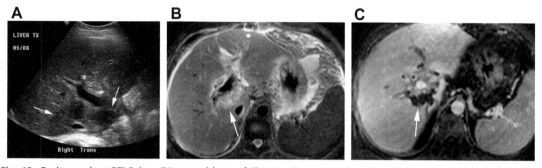

Fig. 12. Peritransplant PTLD in a 51-year-old man following liver transplantation. (*A*) Axial US image of the liver shows ill-defined iso-to hypoechoic lesions at the porta hepatis abutting the main portal vein (*arrows*). (*B* and *C*) Axial T2-weighted (*B*) and axial contrast-enhanced (*C*) MR images of the liver demonstrate heterogeneously T2 hyperintense enhancing masses at the porta hepatis abutting the portal vein (*arrows*). The diagnosis of PTLD was made on the pathology.

Classification of post-transplant malignancies

Malignancies in SOTRs are broadly categorized into three groups based on their origin and pathogenesis. De novo malignancies are new cancers originating separately from the transplanted organ; donor-related cancers are either donor-transmitted or donor-derived cancers; and recurrent malignancies are from recurrence of pre-existing malignancies in the recipient (see **Box 2**; **Table 1**).[49,53] Cancer-specific screening and early detection of malignancies remain integral approaches in SOTRs.[49]

De Novo Malignancies

Post-transplant lymphoproliferative disorder

PTLD is a spectrum of lymphoproliferative disorders seen in up to 20% of SOTRs that varies with the type of transplant and is frequently EBV-associated.[54] SOT-PTLDs are frequently bimodal,

with an early-onset form that is seen within the first 2 years after transplant and a late-onset form that is seen between 5 and 10 years after transplant.[54] Early-onset PTLD is EBV-positive with polymorphic B cell lesions, and late-onset PTLD is EBV-negative.[54]

Imaging is critical in the surveillance, diagnosis, staging, and assessment response to therapy in patients with PTLD.[54] On imaging, PTLD can manifest as either bulky retroperitoneal nodes or extranodal masses in diverse sites, including the GI tract, liver, lungs, bone marrow, and CNS.[49,55] Approximately 50% to 75% of PTLDs are seen in the abdomen. The most common site is the GI tract (small bowel loops), manifesting as irregular bowel wall thickening, eccentric mural masses, and aneurysmal dilation (**Fig. 10**). Multiple lung nodules/masses with associated mediastinal lymphadenopathy are the common manifestation

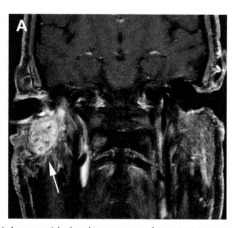
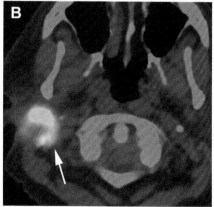

Fig. 13. Right parotid gland metastases from SCC in a 52-year-old man following heart transplantation. (*A*) Coronal contrast-enhanced MR image of the neck shows heterogeneously enhancing mass in the right parotid gland (*arrow*). (*B*) Axial fused [18]FDG-PET-CT image of the neck demonstrates increased FDG uptake within the parotid mass (*arrow*).

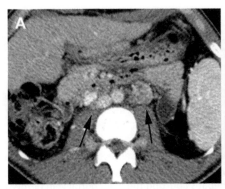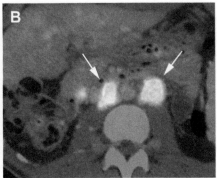

Fig. 14. HHV-8 positive KS in a 31-year-old man, 12 years following liver transplantation. (*A*) Axial contrast-enhanced CT image of the abdomen shows multiple avidly enhancing retroperitoneal lymph nodes (*arrows*). (*B*) Axial fused FDG-PET-CT image of the abdomen demonstrates FDG-avid retroperitoneal lymph nodes (*arrows*).

of thoracic PTLD; rarely, PTLD can develop in the brain parenchyma and present as heterogeneously enhancing masses with perilesional edema (**Fig. 11**). Peritransplant PTLD may present as a focal mass near the hepatic hilum of the liver transplant or parapelvic mass in renal transplant recipients (**Fig. 12**).[49,51,55] PTLD has a high incidence of cancer-associated mortality ranging from 22% to 70%; early diagnosis with imaging is critical for improved survival. A marked reduction in immunosuppression with chemotherapy and anti-CD 20 therapy is well tolerated in terms of graft function in PTLD.[56]

Non-melanoma skin cancers
NMSCs are the most common malignancies seen in more than half of SOTRs, with up to a 250-fold increase in incidence and a 30-fold increase in mortality compared to the general population.[48,57,58] NMSCs are more aggressive, typically presenting with multiple lesions, local recurrences, and metastatic disease.[51] Risk factors include fair skin, high sun exposure, HPV infection, and prolonged immunosuppression. Squamous cell carcinoma (SCC) is the most common type, followed by basal cell carcinoma.[58] Although diagnosis is by clinical examination, imaging with CT and FDG-PET/CT is essential to map the extent of disease spread (**Fig. 13**). Cessation, reduction, or modification of IS therapy is essential to treatment along with ablative/surgical therapies and adjuvant chemotherapy/radiation based on the extent of the disease.[51]

Kaposi sarcoma
Kaposi sarcoma (KS) is a multifocal angio-proliferative endothelial malignancy driven by HHV-8 infection.[51] There is a 400-to-500-fold increased incidence of KS in SOTRs compared to the general population.[51] Mucocutaneous KS

is seen in 90% of SOTRs and visceral disease in 20%.[51] Mucocutaneous KS manifests as lower extremity angiomatous plaques and nodules. Visceral KS involves the GI tract, lymph nodes, and lungs; allograft involvement is rare.[51] On imaging, cutaneous KS manifests as enhancing nodules; visceral manifestations include nodular bowel wall thickening, hypervascular hepatic and splenic masses, hypervascular lymph nodes, and vascular mesenteric masses (**Fig. 14**).[51]

Anogenital cancers
Anogenital cancers account for 3% of all post-transplant malignancies involving the anal canal, perianal skin, vulva, perineum, penis, and scrotum.[51] There is a 30- to 100-fold increased incidence compared to the general population. Risk factors include HPV infection, high levels of immunosuppression, and smoking; tumors are seen

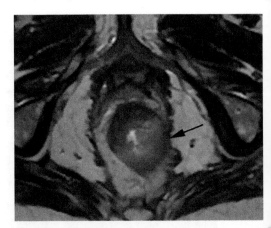

Fig. 15. Rectal adenocarcinoma in a 72-year-old woman, 6 years following renal transplantation. Axial T2-weighted MR image of the pelvis shows moderately T2 hyperintense rectal wall thickening along the left lateral and posterior walls (*arrow*).

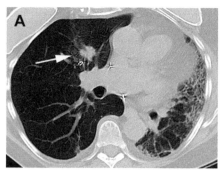
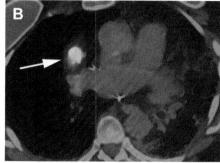

Fig. 16. Lung adenocarcinoma in a 76-year-old woman, 15 years following right lung transplantation. (A) Axial unenhanced CT image of the chest shows a spiculated mass in the lung parenchyma (arrow). Also note, end-stage fibrosis of the left lung parenchyma. (B) Axial fused FDG-PET-CT image of the chest demonstrates FDG-avid right lung mass (arrow).

more commonly in women.[1,45] Anogenital cancers in SOTRs are typically large, aggressive, multicentric, and refractory to treatment. The treatment is dependent on the depth of invasion. Therefore, MR imaging is the preferred imaging modality for local staging; FDG-PET/CT is used for mapping nodal and distant metastatic disease (Fig. 15).

Lung cancer

There is a six-fold increased risk of lung cancer in lung transplant recipients; this risk is higher during the first 6 months following lung transplantation. Other non-lung SOTRs also have a two - to three-fold higher risk of developing lung cancer and more in pre-transplant smokers. Clinically, post-transplant lung cancer can be seen either in the native lung, lung allograft (donor-related), or recurrent lung cancer (when the transplant indication is lung cancer).[59] The most common histologic subtypes include adenocarcinoma and SCC, and imaging findings are similar to lung cancers in the general population (Fig. 16).[51] Smoking cessation is mandated to prevent lung cancer,

and regular imaging surveillance with chest CT helps in early detection.[59]

Donor-Related Malignancies

Donor-related cancers account for up to 2% of malignancies in SOTRs. They are further classified into two subtypes: donor-transmitted cancers (DTCs) that originate from transmission of pre-existing cancer in the donor to the recipient and typically become evident during the first 2 years after transplant; donor-derived cancers (DDCs) that are new cancers that develop from neoplastic transformation of donor cells following solid organ transplantation from a donor without pre-existing malignancy and are extremely rare.[53,60] Renal cell carcinoma (RCC), melanoma, and choriocarcinoma are common donor-related cancers. The risk of donor transmission varies with the type of pre-existing cancer within a donor, and each cancer has specific cancer-free intervals before being considered for organ donation.[50]

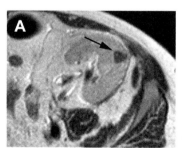
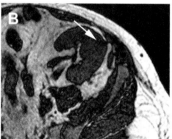
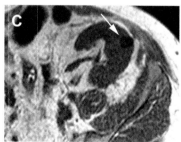

Fig. 17. Papillary RCC in the left lower quadrant transplant kidney. (A–C) Axial T2-weighted (A), T1-weighted opposed-phase (B), and in-phase (C) MR images of the pelvis demonstrate a small mass in the transplanted kidney, which is isointense on T1-weighted opposed-phase image and hypointense on T2-weighted image and shows signal loss on the in-phase image (arrows). These findings are suggestive of intralesional hemosiderin, diagnostic of papillary RCC.

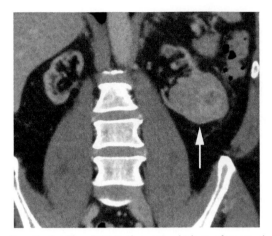

Fig. 18. Papillary RCC in the native kidney after renal transplantation. Coronal contrast-enhanced CT images of the abdomen show a homogenously hypoenhancing mass in the lower pole of the left kidney (*arrow*), which was proved to be papillary RCC on pathology. Also note, atrophic native kidneys.

Renal cell carcinoma

RCC accounts for 2% of post-transplant malignancies. Although donor-transmitted and donor-derived RCCs can be seen in renal allografts, the risk of de novo RCC in native kidneys is higher in patients with a history of longer duration of dialysis and acquired renal cystic disease.[61] Most post-transplant RCCs are small, incidentally detected on imaging surveillance, and are most commonly either clear cell (46%) or papillary (42%) histologic subtypes.[51] Annual ultrasound surveillance of

renal allograft and native kidneys helps in early diagnosis.[61] Imaging features of RCC depend on the histologic subtype; papillary RCC is typically hypovascular, and clear cell RCC is typically hypervascular.[51] On MR imaging, a drop in signal on the in-phase indicating presence of hemosiderin also aids in the diagnosis of papillary RCC (**Figs. 17 and 18**).

Malignant melanoma

Malignant melanoma is an immune-driven malignancy due to the reactivation of dormant tumor cells from immunosuppression.[51] Malignant melanoma can originate de novo, be donor-related, or present as a recurrent malignancy.[51] Donor-transmitted malignant melanoma more commonly presents with disseminated metastatic disease and can involve any organ presenting as soft tissue masses on imaging (**Fig. 19**).[51]

Recurrent Malignancies

Recurrent malignancies of recipient origin are further categorized into two subtypes: recurrence of malignancy that led to the transplant and recurrence of malignancy that is unrelated to the transplanted organ.[51] To avoid the recurrence of pre-existing malignancy in the recipients, there are recommendations specific to each cancer subtype in regard to cancer-free wait times before receiving the transplant.[51] The recurrence rate is higher (>25%) in patients with previously treated sarcoma, myeloma, urinary bladder carcinoma, RCC, and melanoma.

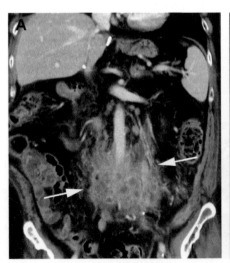
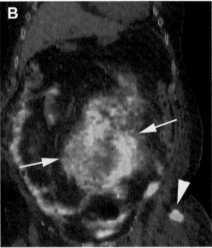

Fig. 19. Disseminated malignant melanoma with peritoneal carcinomatosis in a 58 year old man, following liver transplantation. (*A*) Coronal contrast-enhanced CT image of the abdomen and pelvis demonstrate heterogeneously enhancing retroperitoneal mass (*arrows*). (*B*) Axial fused FDG-PET-CT image of the abdomen and pelvis demonstrate demonstrates increased FDG uptake in the retroperitoneal mass and peritoneal carcinomatosis (*arrows*). Also note, a metastatic focus with increased uptake in the left thigh muscles (*arrowhead*).

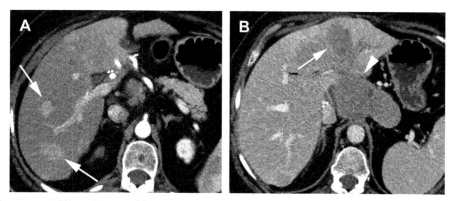

Fig. 20. Recurrent HCCin a 62-year-old man with orthotopic liver transplant. (*A, B*) Axial contrast-enhanced CT images of the liver in the arterial phase (*A*), and portal venous phase (*B*) shows multiple arterially enhancing focal hepatic lesions with portal venous washout (*arrows*) and an enlarged lymph node at porta hepatis (*arrowhead*).

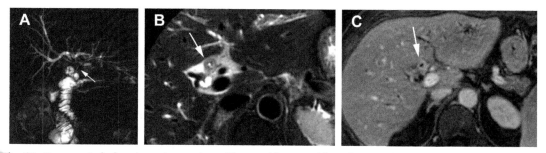

Fig. 21. Recurrent cholangiocarcinoma in a 47-year-old man with orthotopic liver transplant. (*A–C*) Axial 2D MRCP (*A*), T2-weighted (*B*), and axial contrast-enhanced T1-weighted (*C*) MR images of the liver demonstrate focal irregular wall thickening and stricture of the bile duct at the hepatico-jejunostomy site that demonstrates diffuse enhancement after contrast administration (*arrows*) concerning for recurrent cholangiocarcinoma.

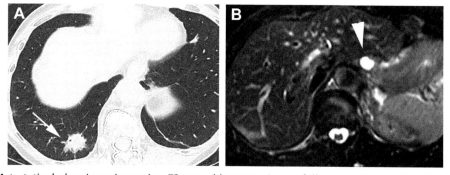

Fig. 22. Metastatic cholangiocarcinoma in a 73-year-old woman, 2 years following orthotopic liver transplant. (*A*) Axial CT image of the chest shows a spiculated mass in the right lung parenchyma (*arrow*) concerning for metastatic disease. (*B*) Axial T2-weighted MR image of the liver shows an enlarged lymph node abutting the left lobe of the liver (*arrowhead*). The diagnosis of metastatic, recurrent cholangiocarcinoma was proved on pathology.

Hepatocellular carcinoma

Pre-transplant predictors of recurrence of hepato-cellular carcinoma (HCC) include tumor size, vascular invasion, high alpha-fetoprotein (AFP) levels, and histologic differentiation.[51] The recurrence rate of HCC is 6% to 16%, and the majority (90%) manifest in the first 6 months after transplant.[62] Imaging and morphologic patterns of recurrent HCC include recurrent mass localized to the allograft and diffuse metastatic disease (**Fig. 20**). Regular surveillance with CT/MR imaging for 2 to 3 years, serial AFP levels, and control of HCV and HBV infection is a widely accepted practice that helps in the early detection and prevention of recurrent HCC.[62]

Cholangiocarcinoma

Orthotopic liver transplantation (OLT) is an established treatment option in select patients with localized unresectable, lymph node-negative cholangiocarcinoma following neoadjuvant chemo-radiotherapy; recurrence rate after OLT is 20%[63] Additionally, liver transplant recipients with a history of primary sclerosing cholangitis and ulcerative colitis are at increased risk for cholangiocarcinoma and colon cancer. Imaging manifestations of recurrent cholangiocarcinoma include multifocal hepatic masses, malignant biliary stricture, typically at the anastomotic site with focal biliary wall thickening, perihilar masses, lymphadenopathy, and distant metastatic disease (**Figs. 21** and **22**).

SUMMARY

Advances in IS regimens allowed the usage of potent immunosuppressants at lower doses, resulting in improved graft survival, but this has increased the number of chronically immunosuppressed patients. Immunosuppression is associated with either drug-related side effects or can be complicated by infections and malignancies. Imaging plays a crucial role in the surveillance, diagnosis, and management of these infectious and neoplastic complications of IS therapy.

CLINICS CARE POINTS

- Transplant-related immunosuppression is divided into three phases: induction, maintenance, and anti-rejection. Although ATG and alemtuzumab constitute commonly used induction agents, the usual maintenance agents are tacrolimus (Prograf), Mycophenolate mofetil (Cellcept), sirolimus, and prednisone. Corticosteroids comprise commonly used anti-rejection agents.

- Transplant-related immunosuppression predisposes to characteristic infections and malignancies that account for increased morbidity and mortality. The transplant recipients are at increased risk for a variety of both conventional and opportunistic infections in a predictable pattern based on the timeline of the NSI during early, intermediate, and late post-transplant periods.

- Early period infections during the first month after transplant are most commonly perioperative infections from surgical complications and hospital-acquired infections. Intermediate period infections between 1 and 6 months are dependent on viral prophylaxis and commonly include immunomodulatory viral infections (CMV, EBV), opportunistic infections (*Aspergillus, Pneumocystis*, endemic fungal infections), and reactivation of latent infections (CMV, HSV, VZV, hepatitis-B, and hepatitis-C, Mycobacteria). Late-period infections beyond 6 months after transplant include community acquired infections in patients with good allograft function. Imaging findings are specific to the type of infection.

- Post-transplant malignancies are categorized into de novo, donor-related and recurrent malignancies. Non-melanoma skin cancer is the most common post-transplant malignancy in SOTRs. PTLD, lung cancer, anogenital carcinoma, RCC, and recurrent HCC are other commonly seen malignancies.

- Imaging plays a pivotal role in the surveillance, diagnosis, and management of infectious and neoplastic complications of immunosuppressive therapy.

DISCLOSURE

No financial disclosures.

REFERENCES

1. Katabathina V, Menias CO, Pickhardt P, et al. Complications of Immunosuppressive Therapy in Solid Organ Transplantation. Radiol Clin North Am 2016; 54(2):303–19.
2. Organ Procurement and Transplantation Network (OPTN). Available at: https://insights.unos.org/OPTN-metrics/. Accessed November 28, 2022.
3. Girlanda R. Complications of Post-Transplant Immunosuppression. Regenerative Medicine and Tissue Engineering. Prof. Jose A. Andrades (Ed.), ISBN: 978-953-51-1108-5, InTech, DOI.
4. Nelson J, Alvey N, Bowman L, et al. Consensus recommendations for use of maintenance immunosuppression in solid organ transplantation: Endorsed by the American College of Clinical Pharmacy,

American Society of Transplantation, and the International Society for Heart and Lung Transplantation. Pharmacotherapy 2022;42(8):599–633.

5. Reske A, Reske A, Metze M. Complications of immunosuppressive agents therapy in transplant patients. Minerva Anestesiol 2015;81(11):1244–61.

6. Parlakpinar H, Gunata M. Transplantation and immunosuppression: a review of novel transplant-related immunosuppressant drugs. Immunopharmacol Immunotoxicol 2021;43(6):651–65.

7. Halloran PF. Immunosuppressive drugs for kidney transplantation. Review. N Engl J Med 2004; 351(26):2715–29.

8. Enderby C, Keller CA. An overview of immunosuppression in solid organ transplantation. Am J Manag Care 2015;21(1 Suppl):s12–23.

9. Raffaele Girlanda CSM, Keith J. Melancon and Thomas M. Fishbein Current Immunosuppression in Abdominal Organ Transplantation, Immunosuppression - Role in Health and Diseases, Dr. Suman Kapur (Ed.), ISBN: 978-953-51-0152-9, InTech, DOI: 10. 5772/26683. 2012.

10. Moini M, Schilsky ML, Tichy EM. Review on immunosuppression in liver transplantation. World J Hepatol 2015;7(10):1355–68.

11. Mahmud N, Klipa D, Ahsan N. Antibody immunosuppressive therapy in solid-organ transplant: Part I. mAbs 2010;2(2):148–56.

12. van Sandwijk MS, Bemelman FJ, Ten Berge IJ. Immunosuppressive drugs after solid organ transplantation. Neth J Med Jul-Aug 2013;71(6):281–9.

13. Hedri H, Cherif M, Zouaghi K, et al. Avascular osteonecrosis after renal transplantation. Transplant Proc 2007;39(4):1036–8.

14. Maalouf NM, Shane E. Osteoporosis after solid organ transplantation. J Clin Endocrinol Metab 2005; 90(4):2456–65.

15. Timsit JF, Sonneville R, Kalil AC, et al. Diagnostic and therapeutic approach to infectious diseases in solid organ transplant recipients. Intensive Care Med 2019;45(5):573–91.

16. Fishman JA. Infection in Organ Transplantation. Am J Transplant 2017;17(4):856–79.

17. Haidar G, Boeckh M, Singh N. Cytomegalovirus Infection in Solid Organ and Hematopoietic Cell Transplantation: State of the Evidence. J Infect Dis 2020;221(Suppl 1):S23–31.

18. Ramanan P, Razonable RR. Cytomegalovirus infections in solid organ transplantation: a review. Infect Chemother 2013;45(3):260–71.

19. Poghosyan T, Ackerman SJ, Ravenel JG. Infectious complications of solid organ transplantation. Semin Roentgenol 2007;42(1):11–22.

20. Itani M, Kaur N, Roychowdhury A, et al. Gastrointestinal Manifestations of Immunodeficiency: Imaging Spectrum. Radiographics May-Jun 2022;42(3): 759–77.

21. Moon JH, Kim EA, Lee KS, et al. Cytomegalovirus pneumonia: high-resolution CT findings in ten non-AIDS immunocompromised patients. Korean J Radiol Apr-Jun 2000;1(2):73–8.

22. Jenkins FJ, Rowe DT, Rinaldo CR Jr. Herpesvirus infections in organ transplant recipients. Clin Diagn Lab Immunol 2003;10(1):1–7.

23. Singh N. Infections in solid-organ transplant recipients. Am J Infect Control 1997;25(5):409–17.

24. Patel R, Paya CV. Infections in solid-organ transplant recipients. Clin Microbiol Rev 1997;10(1):86–124.

25. Silveira FP, Husain S. Fungal infections in solid organ transplantation. Med Mycol 2007;45(4):305–20.

26. Shoham S, Marr KA. Invasive fungal infections in solid organ transplant recipients. Future Microbiol 2012;7(5):639–55.

27. Samanta P, Clancy CJ, Nguyen MH. Fungal infections in lung transplantation. J Thorac Dis 2021; 13(11):6695–707.

28. Pastakia B, Shawker TH, Thaler M, et al. Hepatosplenic candidiasis: wheels within wheels. Radiology 1988;166(2):417–21.

29. Neofytos D, Garcia-Vidal C, Lamoth F, et al. Invasive aspergillosis in solid organ transplant patients: diagnosis, prophylaxis, treatment, and assessment of response. BMC Infect Dis 2021;21(1):296.

30. Singh N, Paterson DL. Aspergillus infections in transplant recipients. Clin Microbiol Rev 2005;18(1):44–69.

31. Ruhnke M, Kofla G, Otto K, et al. CNS aspergillosis: recognition, diagnosis and management. CNS Drugs 2007;21(8):659–76.

32. Fischer SA. Infections complicating solid organ transplantation. Surg Clin 2006;86(5):1127–45. v-vi.

33. Kanne JP, Yandow DR, Meyer CA. Pneumocystis jiroveci pneumonia: high-resolution CT findings in patients with and without HIV infection. AJR Am J Roentgenol 2012;198(6):W555–61.

34. Lanternier F, Sun HY, Ribaud P, et al. Mucormycosis in organ and stem cell transplant recipients. Clin Infect Dis 2012;54(11):1629–36.

35. Herrera DA, Dublin AB, Ormsby EL, et al. Imaging findings of rhinocerebral mucormycosis. Skull Base 2009;19(2):117–25.

36. Hamdi A, Mulanovich VE, Matin SF, et al. Isolated renal mucormycosis in a transplantation recipient. J Clin Oncol 2015;33(10):e50–1.

37. Spellberg B. Gastrointestinal mucormycosis: an evolving disease. Gastroenterol Hepatol 2012;8(2): 140–2.

38. Simon DM, Levin S. Infectious complications of solid organ transplantations. Infect Dis Clin North Am 2001;15(2):521–49.

39. Kanne JP, Yandow DR, Mohammed TL, et al. CT findings of pulmonary nocardiosis. AJR Am J Roentgenol 2011;197(2):W266–72.

40. Raby N, Forbes G, Williams R. Nocardia infection in patients with liver transplants or chronic liver disease:

radiologic findings. Radiology 1990;174(3 Pt 1): 713–6.

41. Munoz P, Rodriguez C, Bouza E. Mycobacterium tuberculosis infection in recipients of solid organ transplants. Clin Infect Dis 2005;40(4):581–7.

42. Singh N, Paterson DL. Mycobacterium tuberculosis infection in solid-organ transplant recipients: impact and implications for management. Clin Infect Dis 1998;27(5):1266–77.

43. Burrill J, Williams CJ, Bain G, et al. Tuberculosis: a radiologic review. Radiographics 2007;27(5):1255–73.

44. Barsoum RS. Parasitic infections in transplant recipients. Nature Clinical Practice Nephrology 2006;2(9): 490–503.

45. Engels EA, Pfeiffer RM, Fraumeni JF Jr, et al. Spectrum of cancer risk among US solid organ transplant recipients. JAMA 2011;306(17):1891–901.

46. Engels EA. Cancer in Solid Organ Transplant Recipients: There Is Still Much to Learn and Do. Am J Transplant 2017;17(8):1967–9.

47. Noone AM, Pfeiffer RM, Dorgan JF, et al. Cancer-attributable mortality among solid organ transplant recipients in the United States: 1987 through 2014. Cancer 2019;125(15):2647–55.

48. Asch WS, Perazella MA. Cancer and Mortality in Solid-Organ Transplantation: Preventable or Inevitable? Am J Kidney Dis 2016;68(6):839–42.

49. Gogna S, Ramakrishna K, John S. Post transplantation cancer. StatPearls. StatPearls Publishing LLC.; 2022.

50. Stallone G, Infante B, Grandaliano G. Management and prevention of post-transplant malignancies in kidney transplant recipients. Clin Kidney J 2015; 8(5):637–44.

51. Katabathina VS, Menias CO, Tammisetti VS, et al. Malignancy after Solid Organ Transplantation: Comprehensive Imaging Review. Radiographics 2016;36(5):1390–407.

52. Gutierrez-Dalmau A, Campistol JM. Immunosuppressive therapy and malignancy in organ transplant recipients: a systematic review. Drugs 2007;67(8): 1167–98.

53. Greenhall GHB, Ibrahim M, Dutta U, et al. Donor-Transmitted Cancer in Orthotopic Solid Organ Transplant Recipients: A Systematic Review. Transpl Int 2021;35:10092.

54. Dharnidharka VR, Webster AC, Martinez OM, et al. Post-transplant lymphoproliferative disorders. Nat Rev Dis Primers 2016;2:15088.

55. Borhani AA, Hosseinzadeh K, Almusa O, et al. Imaging of posttransplantation lymphoproliferative disorder after solid organ transplantation. Radiographics 2009;29(4):981–1000 [discussion: 1000-2].

56. Roberts MB, Fishman JA. Immunosuppressive Agents and Infectious Risk in Transplantation: Managing the "Net State of Immunosuppression". Clin Infect Dis 2021;73(7):e1302–17.

57. D'Arcy ME, Castenson D, Lynch CF, et al. Risk of Rare Cancers Among Solid Organ Transplant Recipients. J Natl Cancer Inst 2021;113(2):199–207.

58. Mittal A, Colegio OR. Skin Cancers in Organ Transplant Recipients. Am J Transplant 2017;17(10): 2509–30.

59. Shtraichman O, Ahya VN. Malignancy after lung transplantation. Ann Transl Med 2020;8(6):416.

60. Morath C, Schwenger V, Schmidt J, et al. Transmission of malignancy with solid organ transplants. Transplantation 2005;80(1 Suppl):S164–6.

61. Dahle DO, Skauby M, Langberg CW, et al. Renal Cell Carcinoma and Kidney Transplantation: A Narrative Review. Transplantation 2022;106(1):e52–63.

62. Agarwal PD, Lucey MR. Management of hepatocellular carcinoma recurrence after liver transplantation. Ann Hepatol 2022;27(1):100654.

63. Sapisochín G, Fernández de Sevilla E, Echeverri J, et al. Liver transplantation for cholangiocarcinoma: Current status and new insights. World J Hepatol 2015;7(22):2396–403.

Moving?

Make sure your subscription moves with you!

To notify us of your new address, find your **Clinics Account Number** (located on your mailing label above your name), and contact customer service at:

Email: journalscustomerservice-usa@elsevier.com

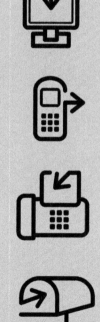

800-654-2452 (subscribers in the U.S. & Canada)
314-447-8871 (subscribers outside of the U.S. & Canada)

Fax number: 314-447-8029

Elsevier Health Sciences Division
Subscription Customer Service
3251 Riverport Lane
Maryland Heights, MO 63043

ELSEVIER